Update on Immunotherapy for Aeroallergens, Foods, and Venoms

Editors

LINDA S. COX
ANNA NOWAK-WEGRZYN

IMMUNOLOGY AND ALLERGY CLINICS OF NORTH AMERICA

www.immunology.theclinics.com

Consulting Editor
LINDA S. COX

February 2020 • Volume 40 • Number 1

ELSEVIER

1600 John F. Kennedy Boulevard • Suite 1800 • Philadelphia, Pennsylvania, 19103-2899

http://www.theclinics.com

IMMUNOLOGY AND ALLERGY CLINICS OF NORTH AMERICA Volume 40, Number 1

February 2020 ISSN 0889-8561, ISBN-13: 978-0-323-71854-7

Editor: Katerina Heidhausen

Developmental Editor: Kristen Helm

Immunology and Allergy Clinics of North America (ISSN 0889–8561) is published quarterly by Elsevier Inc., 360 Park Avenue South, New York, NY 10010-1710. Months of issue are February, May, August, and November. Periodicals postage paid at New York, NY and additional mailing offices. Subscription prices are $344.00 per year for US individuals, $623.00 per year for US institutions, $100.00 per year for US students and residents, $423.00 per year for Canadian individuals, $100.00 per year for Canadian students, $791.00 per year for Canadian institutions, $447.00 per year for international individuals, $791.00 per year for international institutions, $220.00 per year for international students. To receive student/resident rate, orders must be accompanied by name of affiliated institution, date of term, and the *signature* of program/residency coordinator on institution letterhead. Orders will be billed at individual rate until proof of status is received. Foreign air speed delivery is included in all *Clinics* subscription prices. All prices are subject to change without notice. **POSTMASTER:** Send address changes to *Immunology and Allergy Clinics of North America,* Elsevier Health Sciences Division, Subscription Customer Service, 3251 Riverport Lane, Maryland Heights, MO 63043. **Customer Service: 1-800-654-2452 (U.S. and Canada); 314-447-8871 (outside U.S. and Canada). Fax: 314-447-8029. E-mail: journalscustomerservice-usa@elsevier.com** (for print support); **journalsonlinesupport-usa@elsevier.com (for online support).**

Reprints. For copies of 100 or more, of articles in this publication, please contact the Commercial Reprints Department, Elsevier Inc., 360 Park Avenue South, New York, New York 10010-1710. Tel. 212-633-3874, Fax: 212-633-3820, E-mail: reprints@elsevier.com.

Immunology and Allergy Clinics of North America is covered in MEDLINE/PubMed (Index Medicus), Current Contents/Life Sciences, Science Citation Index, ISI/BIOMED, Chemical Abstracts, and EMBASE/Excerpta Medica.

Contributors

CONSULTING EDITOR

LINDA S. COX, MD, FACP, AAAAI
Adjunct Faculty at University of Miami Medical School, Department of Medicine and Dermatology, Associate Professor of Medicine and Dermatology, Nova Southeastern University, Casper, Wyoming, USA; Associate Professor of Medicine, Nova Southeastern University, Fort Lauderdale, Florida, USA

EDITORS

LINDA S. COX, MD, FACP, AAAAI
Adjunct Faculty at University of Miami Medical School, Department of Medicine and Dermatology, Associate Professor of Medicine and Dermatology, Nova Southeastern University, Casper, Wyoming, USA; Associate Professor of Medicine, Nova Southeastern University, Fort Lauderdale, Florida, USA

ANNA NOWAK-WEGRZYN, MD, PhD
Professor of Pediatrics, Allergy and Immunology, Department of Pediatrics, Hassenfeld Children's Hospital, NYU Langone Health, New York, NY, USA; Department of Pediatrics, Gastroenterology and Nutrition, Collegium Medicum, University of Warmia and Mazury, Olsztyn, Poland

AUTHORS

CEZMI A. AKDIS, MD
Swiss Institute of Allergy and Asthma Research (SIAF), Christine Kühne – Center for Allergy Research and Education, Davos Wolfgang, Switzerland

MÜBECCEL AKDIS, MD, PhD
Swiss Institute of Allergy and Asthma Research (SIAF), Christine Kühne – Center for Allergy Research and Education, Davos Wolfgang, Switzerland

SULTAN ALBUHAIRI, MD
Assistant Professor, Department of Pediatrics, College of Medicine, Majmaah University, Majmaah, Saudi Arabia

MONTSERRAT ALVARO-LOZANO, MD, PhD
Consultant in Pediatric Allergy and Clinical Immunology, Allergy and Clinical Immunology Department, Hospital Sant Joan de Deu, Secció d'Al-lergia i Immunologia Clínica, Barcelona, Spain

STEFANIA ARASI, MD, PhD
Consultant and Researcher in Pediatric Allergy, Pediatric Allergology Unit, Department of Pediatric Medicine, Bambino Gesù Children's Research Hospital (IRCCS), Rome, Italy

JOSEPH L. BAUMERT, PhD
Food Allergy Research and Resource Program, Department of Food Science and Technology, University of Nebraska, Food Innovation Center, Lincoln, Nebraska, USA

DAVID I. BERNSTEIN, MD
Division of Immunology, Allergy and Rheumatology, Department of Medicine, University of Cincinnati College of Medicine, Bernstein Clinical Research Center, Cincinnati, Ohio, USA

J. ANDREW BIRD, MD
Departments of Pediatrics and Internal Medicine, Division of Allergy and Immunology, The University of Texas Southwestern Medical Center, Dallas, Texas, USA

CHRIS CALABRIA, MD
Department of Allergy and Immunology, Wilford Hall Medical Center, Lackland Air Force Base, San Antonio, Texas, USA

LINDA S. COX, MD, FACP, AAAAI
Adjunct Faculty at University of Miami Medical School, Department of Medicine and Dermatology, Associate Professor of Medicine and Dermatology, Nova Southeastern University, Casper, Wyoming, USA; Associate Professor of Medicine, Nova Southeastern University, Fort Lauderdale, Florida, USA

MONTSERRAT FERNÁNDEZ-RIVAS, MD, PhD
Head, Allergy Department, Hospital Clinico San Carlos, Associate Professor, Medicine UCM, IdISSC, ARADyAL, Madrid, Spain

THEODORE M. FREEMAN, MD
San Antonio Asthma and Allergy Clinic, San Antonio, Texas, USA

DAVID B.K. GOLDEN, MD
Associate Professor, Department of Medicine, Division of Allergy-Immunology, Johns Hopkins University, Baltimore, Maryland, USA

CHERYL HANKIN, PhD
President and Chief Scientific Officer, BioMedEcon, Moss Beach, California, USA

PALOMA JAQUETI, MD
Consultant Allergist, Allergy Department, Hospital Clinico San Carlos, IdISSC, Madrid, Spain

EDWIN H. KIM, MD, MS
Assistant Professor of Medicine and Pediatrics, University of North Carolina at Chapel Hill School of Medicine, Chapel Hill, North Carolina, USA

ZSOLT ISTVÁN KOMLÓSI, MD, PhD
Department of Genetics, Cell and Immunobiology, Semmelweis University, Budapest, Hungary

NÓRA KOVÁCS, MD
Department of Genetics, Cell and Immunobiology, Semmelweis University, Budapest, Hungary; Lung Health Hospital, Törökbálint, Hungary

MICHAEL D. KULIS, PhD
UNC Department of Pediatrics, UNC Food Allergy Initiative, The University of North Carolina at Chapel Hill, Chapel Hill, North Carolina, USA

PAXTON LOKE, MBBS, PhD, FRACP
Department of Pediatrics, The University of Melbourne, Allergy Immunology, Murdoch Children's Research Institute, Melbourne, Australia

ADRIANA C. LOZINSKY, MSc, MD
Allergy Immunology, Murdoch Children's Research Institute, Melbourne, Australia

ADRIANNA MACHINENA, MD
Consultant in Pediatric Allergy and Clinical Immunology, Allergy and Clinical Immunology Department, Hospital Sant Joan de Deu, Secció d'Al-lergia i Immunologia Clínica, Barcelona, Spain

ANDREW MURPHEY, MD
Asthma Allergy and Sinus Center, West Chester, Pennsylvania, USA

RORY E. NICOLAIDES, MD
Departments of Pediatrics and Internal Medicine, Division of Allergy and Immunology, The University of Texas Southwestern Medical Center, Dallas, Texas, USA

CHRISTOPHER P. PARRISH, MD
Departments of Pediatrics and Internal Medicine, Division of Allergy and Immunology, The University of Texas Southwestern Medical Center, Dallas, Texas, USA

RIMA RACHID, MD
Division of Immunology, Associate Professor, Department of Pediatrics, Boston Children's Hospital, Harvard Medical School, Boston, Massachusetts, USA

BENJAMIN C. REMINGTON, PhD
Food Allergy Research and Resource Program, Department of Food Science and Technology, University of Nebraska, Food Innovation Center, Lincoln, Nebraska, USA; Remington Consulting Group B.V., Utrecht, The Netherlands

MARIO SÁNCHEZ-BORGES, MD
Allergy and Clinical Immunology Department, Centro Médico Docente La Trinidad and Clínica El Avila, Caracas, Venezuela

JOHANNA M. SMEEKENS, PhD
UNC Department of Pediatrics, UNC Food Allergy Initiative, The University of North Carolina at Chapel Hill, Chapel Hill, North Carolina, USA

DEREK M. SMITH, MD
Department of Allergy/Immunology, Wilford Hall Ambulatory Surgical Center, San Antonio, Texas, USA

MILENA SOKOLOWSKA, MD, PhD
Swiss Institute of Allergy and Asthma Research (SIAF), Christine Kühne – Center for Allergy Research and Education, Davos Wolfgang, Switzerland

MIMI L.K. TANG, MBBS, PhD, FRACP, FRCPA, FAAAAI
Allergy Immunology, Murdoch Children's Research Institute, Department of Pediatrics, The University of Melbourne, Department of Allergy and Immunology, The Royal Children's Hospital, Melbourne, Australia

SONIA VÁZQUEZ-CORTÉS, MD
Consultant Allergist, Allergy Department, Hospital Clinico San Carlos, IdISSC, ARADyAL, Madrid, Spain

WILLEM VAN DE VEEN, PhD
Swiss Institute of Allergy and Asthma Research (SIAF), Christine Kühne – Center for Allergy Research and Education, Davos Wolfgang, Switzerland

JAMIE WALDRON, MD
Fellow-in-Training, University of North Carolina at Chapel Hill School of Medicine, Chapel Hill, North Carolina, USA

Contents

Allergen immunotherapy (AIT) is considered to be the only treatment option with the promise of healing and induction of long-lasting allergen tolerance, persisting even after discontinuation of therapy. Despite a more than 100-year-long history, still only a minority of patients are being treated with AIT. Substantial developments took place in the last decade to overcome problems in standardization, efficacy, safety, high costs, long duration of treatment; and new guidelines have also been implemented. Major advancements in the understanding of AIT mechanisms with the focus on recent findings of subcutaneous and sublingual AIT have been summarized.

Increasing safety while maintaining or even augmenting efficiency are the main goals of research for novel vaccine development and improvement of treatment schemes in allergen immunotherapy (AIT). To increase the efficacy of AIT, allergens have been coupled to innate immunostimulatory substances and new adjuvants have been introduced. Allergens have been modified to increase their uptake and presentation. Hypoallergenic molecules have been developed to improve the safety profile of the vaccines. Administration of recombinant IgG4 antibodies is a new, quick, passive immunization strategy with remarkable efficiency. Results of some current investigations aiming at further improvement of AIT vaccines have been summarized.

Subcutaneous immunotherapy (SCIT) is effective for allergic rhinitis and conjunctivitis, asthma, and insect venom hypersensitivity. The risk of severe allergic reactions induced by SCIT remains low, and mild systemic reactions have recently shown a tendency to decline. However, near-fatal and fatal anaphylactic reactions may occur. Clinicians administering allergen-specific immunotherapy should receive specialized training and be aware of risk factors and preventive measures to avoid severe allergic reactions induced by SCIT.

Derek M. Smith and Theodore M. Freeman

There is some evidence to support the use of sublingual immunotherapy (SLIT) in food allergy, although its role is unclear. One randomized, double-blind, placebo-controlled trial supports the safe and efficacious use of dust mite SLIT in children with mild to moderate atopic dermatitis, but these data have not been confirmed. Although there are several randomized, double-blind, placebo-controlled trials to support the use of SLIT-LATEX, this product is not available in the United States and extrapolation of these effects to latex extracts is unsubstantiated. There is also insufficient evidence to support the use of SLIT for venom hypersensitivity at this time.

David B.K. Golden

Questions and controversies regarding venom immunotherapy (VIT) remain. It is important to recognize risk factors for severe sting anaphylaxis that guide the recommendation for testing, epinephrine injectors, and VIT. Premedication, rush VIT, and omalizumab are successful in overcoming recurrent systemic reactions to VIT. A maintenance dose is adequate in children, but higher doses are needed in high-risk patients. The consensus on risk of β-blockers and angiotensin-converting enzyme inhibitors in patients on VIT has shifted to the belief that risk is small. The decision to stop VIT after 5 years rests on known risk factors rather than any diagnostic tests.

Linda S. Cox, Andrew Murphey, and Cheryl Hankin

This article evaluates the cost-effectiveness of allergy immunotherapy (AIT) in the treatment of allergic rhinitis, asthma, and other allergic conditions. An extensive search of the PubMed and Medline databases (up to December 2018) was conducted. There is strong evidence in the collective literature, which included individual studies and systematic reviews, that AIT is cost-effective in the management of allergic rhinitis and asthma as compared with standard drug treatment alone. The magnitude of AIT's cost-effectiveness is likely underestimated because most of the studies considered during-treatment costs and not the long-term benefits or preventive or prophylactic effects of AIT.

Johanna M. Smeekens and Michael D. Kulis

Food allergies are a growing public health concern affecting approximately 8% of children and 10% of adults in the United States. Several immunotherapy approaches are under active investigation, including oral immunotherapy, epicutaneous immunotherapy, and sublingual immuno-therapy. Each of these approaches uses a similar strategy of administering small, increasing amounts of allergen to the allergic subject. Immunologic studies have described changes in the T-cell compartment, serum and salivary immunoglobulin profile, and mast cell and basophil degranulation status in response to allergens. This review highlights the immunologic changes induced by food allergen-specific immunotherapy and discusses future directions in this field.

Mimi L.K. Tang, Adriana C. Lozinsky, and Paxton Loke

Cumulative evidence shows that peanut oral immunotherapy (OIT) is effec-tive at inducing desensitization through downregulation of effector path-ways in the allergic reaction cascade; however, only a subset of patients achieve sustained unresponsiveness (remission), which requires redirec-tion of the underlying allergic response toward tolerance. A recent meta-analysis of peanut OIT randomized trials found that OIT is associated with a threefold greater risk of anaphylaxis and twofold greater risk of epinephrine use than allergen avoidance. Strategies to reduce adverse events associated with OIT and improve the ability for OIT to induce sustained unresponsiveness are required to improve the benefit-risk of peanut OIT.

Sonia Vázquez-Cortés, Paloma Jaqueti, Stefania Arasi, Adrianna Machinena, Montserrat Alvaro-Lozano, and Montserrat Fernández-Rivas

Oral immunotherapy (OIT) for food allergy entails a risk of adverse reac-tions, including anaphylaxis. This safety concern is the major barrier for OIT to become a therapeutic option in clinical practice. The high heteroge-neity in safety reporting of OIT studies prevents setting the safety profile accurately. An international consensus is needed to facilitate the analysis of large pooled clinical data with homogeneous safety reporting, that together with integrated omics, and patients/families' opinions, may help stratify the patients' risk and needs, and help developing safe(r) individual-ized care pathways. This will give OIT the right place in the food allergy therapy.

Jamie Waldron and Edwin H. Kim

This article reviews research advances for sublingual and patch immuno-therapy for food allergy with a focus on peanut allergy. Published studies on sublingual immunotherapy (SLIT) and epicutaneous immunotherapy (EPIT) were summarized in this review. Sublingual and epicutaneous methods have emerged as alternatives to oral immunotherapy. SLIT studies have shown modest desensitization with a robust safety profile. EPIT studies have high adherence rates, an excellent safety profile, and potential for desensitization in children. Advances in food immunotherapy

IMMUNOLOGY AND ALLERGY CLINICS OF NORTH AMERICA

SERIES OF RELATED INTEREST

Pediatric Clinics of North America
Available at: https://www.pediatric.theclinics.com/

THE CLINICS ARE AVAILABLE ONLINE!
Access your subscription at:
www.theclinics.com

Foreword

Allergy Immunotherapy: Are We Making Progress or Just Standing Still?

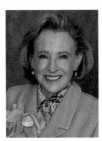

Linda S. Cox, MD, FACP, AAAAI
Consulting Editor

It has been over a century since Noon and Freeman began injecting allergic patients with allergens.[1-4] Their rationale was based on the work of Edward Jenners, who had demonstrated that injecting cow pox conveyed immunity to smallpox. Surprisingly, Noon and Freeman were right. Not only did they "cure" many of their patients, they did not kill any of them. However, they did have to administer epinephrine a few times during "rapid desensitization." Interesting, they realized early on that "leisurely inoculations" (ie, conventional buildup schedules) were inconvenient for the patients and began experimenting with more rapid buildup schedules, rush and cluster immunotherapy. Although their treatment was successful, it was not until 1969 that it was discovered that the immune response involved a totally different immunoglobulin than immunoglobulin G. This was when Kimishige Ishizaka and his wife Teruko Ishizaka discovered immunoglobulin E. In the 1950s, Frankland, Lowell, and Franklin proved allergen immunotherapy was dose dependent and allergen specific.[5,6] But it was not until the 1980s that we began to elucidate the complex mechanisms of allergen immunotherapy.

This is the third issue of *Immunology and Allergy Clinics of North America* of which I've had the honor of being an editor. In the first issue, the entire focus was aeroallergen immunotherapy.[7] In the second issue, it was apparent that food allergy immunotherapy was making progress, and so I asked Anna Nowak-Wegrzyn to guest edit that issue.[8] In this issue, we decided to include venom immunotherapy (VIT).

The issue begins with 2 excellent review articles by Mübeccel Akdis and Cezmi Akdis and colleagues on the mechanisms of subcutaneous and sublingual immunotherapy and highlights of novel vaccination strategies in allergen immunotherapy. They are followed by Mario Sánchez-Borges and colleagues' article reviewing subcutaneous

Immunol Allergy Clin N Am 40 (2020) xiii–xiv
https://doi.org/10.1016/j.iac.2019.10.002
0889-8561/20/© 2019 Published by Elsevier Inc.

immunotherapy safety and risk factors. Sublingual immunotherapy for other indications, such as venom large local reactions, latex and food allergy, and atopic dermatitis, is reviewed in Smith and Freeman's article. David Golden's article addresses some provocative and unanswered questions regarding Hymenoptera allergy and VIT, such as when to stop recommending an epinephrine autoinjector at all times and when is it safe to stop VIT. The cost-effectiveness of allergen immunotherapy is explored in an article I wrote alongside Andrew Murphey and Cheryl Hankin. Smeekens and Kulis review the evolution of the immune responses in food immunotherapy. Mimi Tang and colleagues present the "state-of-the-art" in peanut oral immunotherapy. Vázquez-Cortés and colleagues tell us "what we need to know" about the safety of food oral immunotherapy. Next, Waldron and Kim's article explores sublingual and epicutaneous immunotherapy for food allergy. The use of adjuvants with food immunotherapy is explored in Nicolaides, Parrish, and Bird's article. Albuhairi and Rachid explore novel therapies for the treatment of food allergy. The issue concludes with Remington and Baumert's article on risk reduction in peanut immunotherapy.

This issue is packed with cutting-edge review articles written by some of the world's experts in allergy and immunology. It may not be as engaging as an Agatha Christie murder mystery novel, but it should be a "must-read," and after all, you are physicians/scientists, not police detectives.

Linda S. Cox, MD, FACP, AAAAI
Department of Medicine and Dermatology
Nova Southeastern University
1108 South Wolcott Street
Casper, WY 82601, USA

E-mail address:
lindaswolfcox@msn.com

REFERENCES

1. Noon L. Prophylactic inoculation against hay fever. Lancet 1911;1:1572–3.
2. Freeman J. Further observations of the treatment of hay fever by hypodermic inoculations of pollen vaccine. Lancet 1911;2:814–7.
3. Freeman J. Vaccination against hay fever: report of results during the last three years. Lancet 1914;183:1178–80.
4. Freeman J. "Rush Inoculation", with special reference to hay fever treatment. Lancet 1930;1:744–7.
5. Frankland AW, Augustin R. Prophylaxis of summer hay-fever and asthma: a controlled trial comparing crude grass-pollen extract with isolated main protein component. Lancet 1954;266(6821):1055–7.
6. Lowell FC, Franklin W. A double-blind study of the effectiveness and specificity of injection therapy in ragweed hay fever. N Engl J Med 1965;273:675–9.
7. Cox L. Preface allergen immunotherapy: the first centenary and beyond. Immunol Allergy Clin North Am 2011;31:xvii–xix.
8. Nowak-Wegrzyn AH, Cox LS. Allergen-specific immunotherapy–turning the tables on the immune system. Immunol Allergy Clin North Am 2016;36:xv–xxi.

Preface

Leaps and Bounds in Allergen Immunotherapy

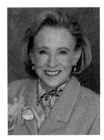 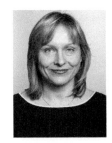

Linda S. Cox, MD, FACP, AAAAI   Anna Nowak-Wegrzyn, MD, PhD
Editors

It has been almost one hundred ten years since allergen immunotherapy (AIT) was first recognized as a treatment for allergic diseases by the English physicians, Noon and Freeman. However, it was applied thousands of years earlier. Snake handlers learned that if they swam in snake-infested waters, they would acquire immunity to the cobra's venom.[1] This was likely the first use of oral immunotherapy (OIT) because the snake-infested waters contained venom, and the snake handlers swallowed it as they swam.

This issue begins with an outstanding review by Komlósi and colleagues[2] of the mechanisms of subcutaneous and sublingual AIT. It was not until the last 3 decades that we began to understand the mechanisms of AIT. Although I, Linda S. Cox, have lectured on this subject and consider myself relatively up-to-date, every time I read a "review" of this subject, there have been 4 or 5 new regulatory cells, cytokine, or CD whatever. So, I encourage you to spend time reading and digesting this article. This article is followed by an article on novel vaccination strategies in AIT by Komlósi and colleagues[3] and Sánchez-Borges' article[4] on reducing risk with subcutaneous immunotherapy (SCIT). Not only does Sánchez-Borges' article provide guidance on clinical practice interventions that can reduce mortality and morbidity associated with SCIT but also it presents the newly revised World Allergy Organization System for classifying systemic allergic reactions due to any causative agent.[5] The article by Smith and Freeman[6] provides a truly "up-to-date" discussion of sublingual immunotherapy (SLIT), which covers venom large local reactions, atopic dermatitis, and food and latex allergy. Golden's article[7] addresses many of the "unanswered" questions regarding venom immunotherapy, such as when is it really safe to stop, when can I tell a patient to stop carrying an epinephrine autoinjector, as well as the guidelines in the newest Venom Allergic Practice Parameter.[8] The next article is

Immunol Allergy Clin N Am 40 (2020) xv–xvii
https://doi.org/10.1016/j.iac.2019.10.001
0889-8561/20/© 2019 Published by Elsevier Inc.

devoted to the cost-effectiveness of AIT compared with that of pharmacotherapy for the treatment of allergic rhinitis and asthma by Cox and colleagues.[9]

The field of food AIT is undergoing a dramatic development. The first published report of the allergen-specific immunotherapy dates back to 1908, when Schofield described successful oral desensitization to raw egg in a teenage boy with anaphylactic egg allergy.[10] The renewed interest in food immunotherapy emerged in the first decade of the twenty-first century in response to the growing global burden of food allergy. Following the ground-breaking investigator-initiated studies that were limited in size, we have entered a stage of international clinical trials and pharmaceutical product development. Our understanding of the mechanisms of immunomodulation is also improved by Smeekens and Kulis.[11] OIT remains at the forefront of this progress, with the first biologic drug (AR101, Palforzia™) being currently reviewed by the Food and Drug Administration. AR101 has shown promising efficacy in desensitizing peanut-allergic children to a minimum 300-mg peanut protein (equivalent to 1 peanut kernel) following 12 months of treatment by Tang and colleagues.[12] However, concerns remain regarding the treatment-emergent adverse events (AEs), uncertainty regarding permanent tolerance development, the need for long-term treatment, and the lack of long-term safety data by Vázquez-Cortés and colleagues.[13] SLIT has not been developed commercially, although recent long-term follow-up data from peanut SLIT demonstrate a favorable risk-to-benefit ratio and suggest that SLIT may lead to tolerance (sustained unresponsiveness [SU]) in a subset of treated patients by Waldron and Kim.[14] These allergen-specific strategies pose a significant burden of long-term daily maintenance dosing and raise concerns about real-world adherence. Epicutaneous patch immunotherapy (EPIT) with Viaskin Peanut™ 250 is another commercial product evaluated in a phase 3 clinical trial in children with peanut allergy. Peanut EPIT offers superior safety compared with OIT with AEs mostly limited to local skin reactions at the site of patch application, but lower efficacy. OIT with probiotic and other adjuvants is being investigated to address the safety and efficacy concerns by Nicolaides and colleagues.[15] Alternative strategies involving omalizumab and dupilumab as monotherapies or in combination with allergen-specific therapies are being investigated as means of enhancing achievement of SU as well as improving safety and adherence by Albuhairi and Rachid.[16] As the OIT for other and multiple foods remains the subject of investigator-initiated studies, there is an urgent need to harmonize the international efforts regarding protocol design, efficacy endpoints, and safety reporting. Finally, it is important to determine the risk reduction afforded by therapies that induce desensitization but not SU by Remington and Baumert.[17]

Linda S. Cox, MD, FACP, AAAAI
Department of Medicine and Dermatology
Nova Southeastern University
1108 South Wolcott Street
Casper, WY 82601, USA

Anna Nowak-Wegrzyn, MD, PhD
Professor of Pediatrics
Allergy and Immunology, Department of Pediatrics
Hassenfeld Children's Hospital
NYU Langone Health, New York, NY, USA

Department of Pediatrics
Gastroenterology and Nutrition
Collegium Medicum University of Warmia and Mazury
Olsztyn, Poland
403 East 34th Street
New York, NY 10016, USA

E-mail addresses:
lindaswolfcox@msn.com (L.S. Cox)
Anna.nowak-wegrzyn@nyulangone.org (A. Nowak-Wegrzyn)

REFERENCES

1. Fitzhugh DJ, Lockey RF. Allergen immunotherapy: a history of the first 100 years. Curr Opin Allergy Clin Immunol 2011;11(6):554–9.
2. Komlósi ZI, Kovács N, Sokolowska M, et al. Mechanisms of subcutaneous and sublingual aeroallergen immunotherapy: what is new? Immunol Allergy Clin N Am 2019;40(1):1–14.
3. Komlósi ZI, Kovács N, Sokolowska M, et al. Highlights of novel vaccination strategies in allergen immunotherapy immunol allergy. Clin N Am 2019;40(1):15–24.
4. Sánchez-Borges M, Bernstein DI, Calabria C. Subcutaneous immunotherapy safety: incidence per surveys and risk factors immunol allergy. Clin N Am 2019;40(1):25–39.
5. Cox LS, Sanchez-Borges M, Lockey RF. World Allergy Organization systemic allergic reaction grading system: is a modification needed? J Allergy Clin Immunol Pract 2017;5(1):58–62.e5.
6. Smith DM, Freeman TM. Sublingual immunotherapy for other indications: venom large local, latex, atopic dermatitis, and food immunol allergy. Clin N Am 2019; 40(1):41–57.
7. Golden DBK. Venom immunotherapy: questions and controversies immunol allergy. Clin N Am 2019;40(1):59–68.
8. Golden DB, Moffitt J, Nicklas RA, et al. Stinging insect hypersensitivity: a practice parameter update 2011. J Allergy Clin Immunol 2011;127(4):852–4.e23.
9. Cox LS, Murphey A, Hankin C. The cost-effectiveness of allergen immunotherapy compared with pharmacotherapy for treatment of allergic rhinitis and asthma. Immunol Allergy Clin N Am 2019;40(1):69–85.
10. Schofield AT. A case of egg poisoning. Lancet 1908;1:716.
11. Smeekens JM, Kulis MD. Evolution of immune responses in food immunotherapy immunol allergy. Clin N Am 2019;40(1):87–95.
12. Tang MLK, Lozinsky AC, Loke P. Peanut oral immunotherapy: state of the art immunol allergy. Clin N Am 2019;40(1):97–110.
13. Vázquez-Cortés S, Jaqueti P, Arasi S, et al. Safety of food oral immunotherapy: what we know, and what we need to learn immunol allergy. Clin N Am 2019; 40(1):111–33.
14. Waldron J, Kim E. Sublingual and patch immunotherapy for food allergy immunol allergy. Clin N Am 2019;40(1):135–48.
15. Nicolaides R, Parrish CP, Bird JA. Food allergy immunotherapy with adjuvants immunol allergy. Clin N Am 2019;40(1):149–73.
16. Albuhairi S, Rachid R. Novel therapies for treatment of food allergy immunol allergy. Clin N Am 2019;40(1):175–86.
17. Remington BC, Baumert JL. Risk reduction in peanut immunotherapy immunol allergy. Clin N Am 2019;40(1):187–200.

Mechanisms of Subcutaneous and Sublingual Aeroallergen Immunotherapy: What Is New?

Zsolt István Komlósi, MD, PhD[a,*], Nóra Kovács, MD[a,b],
Milena Sokolowska, MD, PhD[c,d], Willem van de Veen, PhD[c,d],
Mübeccel Akdis, MD, PhD[c,d], Cezmi A. Akdis, MD[c,d]

KEYWORDS

- Allergy • Aeroallergen • Allergen immunotherapy
- Subcutaneous allergen immunotherapy • Sublingual allergen immunotherapy
- Treg cells • Breg cells • Innate lymphoid cells

KEY POINTS

- The two most widely used forms of allergen immunotherapy (AIT) for treatment of aeroallergen-induced allergic diseases are the subcutaneous and the sublingual AIT. Substantial developments in AIT took place in the last decade to overcome problems in standardization, efficacy, safety, long duration of treatment, and costs.

- However, accurate descriptions of AIT-responsive disease endotypes with well-defined biomarkers continues to be an unmet need.

- AIT uses general mechanisms of immune tolerance to allergens with changes in allergen-specific memory T- and B-cell responses, regulation of allergen-specific IgE and IgG production, and modification of mast cell and basophil activation thresholds or dendritic cell phenotypes.

- The main highlights of recent years are advances in the understanding of innate lymphoid cells (ILC) including involvement of type 2 ILCs in development of allergic airway inflammation, and contribution of type 3 ILCs to B_{reg} cell–mediated immune tolerance.

- There is a need for further investigation of AIT mechanisms and biomarkers to identify the best candidates for AIT, the long-term responders.

[a] Department of Genetics, Cell- and Immunobiology, Semmelweis University, Nagyvárad Sqr. 4, Budapest 1089, Hungary; [b] Lung Health Hospital, Munkácsy Mihály Str. 70, Törökbálint 2045, Hungary; [c] Swiss Institute of Allergy and Asthma Research (SIAF), Hermann-Burchard Strasse 9, Davos Wolfgang CH7265, Switzerland; [d] Christine Kühne – Center for Allergy Research and Education, Hermann-Burchard Strasse 1, Davos Wolfgang CH7265, Switzerland
* Corresponding author.
E-mail addresses: komlosi.zsolt@med.semmelweis-univ.hu; drkomlo@yahoo.com

Immunol Allergy Clin N Am 40 (2020) 1–14
https://doi.org/10.1016/j.iac.2019.09.009   **immunology.theclinics.com**

INTRODUCTION

The two biggest success stories in allergy treatment are topical glucocorticosteroids and allergen immunotherapy (AIT). Glucocorticosteroids, the principal pharmaceuticals of allergy treatment, efficiently treat inflammation without curing the disease. AIT is the only therapeutic approach exerting profound effect on basic mechanisms of the disease, and is able to modify the disease course. Although glucocorticosteroid treatment also exerts some tolerance-inducing effects via its regulatory T (T_{reg}) cell–inducing capacity,[1,2] AIT is considered to be the only treatment option with the promise of healing and induction of long-lasting tolerance, persisting even after discontinuation of therapy. Glucocorticosteroid treatment is efficient, but not effective enough, whereas AIT is effective but not efficient enough.[3] Consequently, aiming for the ideal therapy to overcome the global burden of allergy, a disease-modifying treatment, such as AIT, is the best choice. Substantial progress has been made in the last decade to overcome problems in standardization, efficacy, safety, long treatment duration, patient adherence, and costs of AIT, and as a result, new guidelines have been implemented.[4–12] Here, we summarize some major advancements of the last years in the understanding of AIT mechanisms. This review is focused on recent findings and better understanding of the mechanisms of subcutaneous and sublingual aeroallergen immunotherapy (SCIT and SLIT, respectively).

Difficulties in the management of allergic disease originate from its heterogeneity in patient population. Phenotyping allergic diseases helps identify clinical and morphologic characteristics and unique responses to treatment. However, phenotypes do not seem to be directly linked to molecular mechanisms of the disease. Endotypes of allergy and asthma describe certain mechanisms of the subgroups of the diseases, such as metabolic, inflammatory, immunologic, and remodeling pathways involved in the pathogenesis.[13–15] The relationship of the endotypes to AIT responsiveness is unclear thus far. It is hoped that detailed description of allergy endotypes and identification of their biomarkers will enable more successful, endotype-driven AIT strategies in the future. In particular, AIT-responsive endotypes should be identified and biomarkers of these endotypes should be discovered and become available at the point of care. These biomarkers should define AIT-responsive patients as early as possible.

ROLE OF VARIOUS T CELLS IN ALLERGEN TOLERANCE AND IMMUNOTHERAPY
Regulatory T Cells

Immune tolerance to allergens implies changes in memory-type allergen-specific T- and B-cell responses, regulation of allergen-specific IgE and IgG production, and modification of mast cell and basophil activation thresholds or dendritic cell (DC) phenotypes (**Fig. 1**). Different levels of evidence from direct in vivo data and in vitro experiments demonstrate the role of allergen-specific T_{reg} cells in allergen tolerance in humans.

Strong in vivo evidence has been obtained by investigation of biopsies of affected tissue and skin late-phase responses. A decrease in T helper cell type 2 (T_H2) and eosinophils and a parallel increase in T_{reg} cells and their cytokines in the tissue is observed after AIT.[16] In the last two decades, the pivotal role of T_{reg} cells in induction and maintenance of immune tolerance has been demonstrated. This is further supported by the fact that adoptive transfer of T_{reg} cells, depending on the timing of administration, can play a role in the prevention or treatment of several T-cell-mediated diseases, including allergic airway inflammation and hyperresponsiveness,[17] a large spectrum of autoimmune diseases (eg, diabetes mellitus, experimental autoimmune encephalomyelitis, inflammatory bowel disease,

Mechanisms of allergen immunotherapy   Desensitization, suppression of
                                                effector cell functions

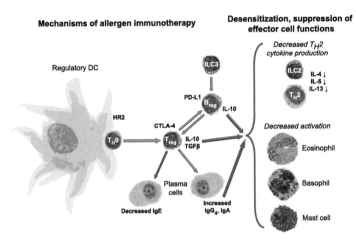

Fig. 1. Overview of the basic mechanisms of allergen immunotherapy. Regulatory T and B cells play a central role in the suppression of allergic inflammation, mainly by means of their interleukin-10 and transforming growth factor-β production. *Green arrows* indicate induction; *red arrows* indicate inhibition. B_{reg}, regulatory B cell; IL, interleukin; TGF, transforming growth factor.

systemic lupus erythematosus, rheumatoid arthritis), and graft-versus-host disease after allogeneic hematopoietic stem cell transplantation; and inhibit rejection of the graft after allogeneic solid organ transplantation in mouse models of these conditions. The human application of adoptive T_{reg} cell transfer therapy is currently being pursued in many studies.[18,19] In the clinical setting, SCIT and SLIT have been shown to induce allergen-specific T_{reg} cells in humans. Peripheral T-cell tolerance is characterized mainly by generation of allergen-specific T_{reg} cells and decrease of T_H2 cells.[20–24]

Direct ex vivo analysis of human peripheral blood cells without any in vitro culture also provided evidence to support the role of T_{reg} cells in maintenance of immune tolerance. Samples were collected from patients allergic to bee venom during AIT and from healthy beekeepers, who were not allergic to bee venom, on acquiring natural tolerance to high-dose allergen exposure during beekeeping season. Allergen-specific $CD4^+$ T cells, identified using major histocompatibility complex class II tetramers, and interleukin (IL)-4, interferon (IFN)- γ, and IL-10 cytokine-secreting cells have been analyzed in these studies. These data demonstrate that allergen-specific T_{reg} cells increase and allergen-specific and nonspecific T_H2 cells decrease in parallel with the induction of natural or clinical immune tolerance in beekeepers during beekeeping season and AIT-treated patients with allergy, respectively.[24,25] AIT also promotes allergen-specific IL-22 and IFN-γ producing T_H cells.[24,26] It is now well understood that allergen-specific T_{reg} cells and allergen-specific and nonspecific effector T cells contain several distinct phenotypic compartments.[27] AIT involves upregulation of the activated T_{reg} and downregulation of allergen-specific immunoglobulin-like transcript 3 (ILT3)-expressing, dysfunctional T_{reg} cells.[24] ILT3+ T_{reg} cells were identified as dysfunctional T_{reg} cells, because they have impaired suppressive potency and they are unable to control the maturation of T_H2-inducing DCs.[28]

Additional evidence has been obtained from cell cultures. IL-10 and transforming growth factor-β are produced by antigen-specific T_{reg} cells. T_{reg} cells from donors with atopy have a reduced capability to suppress T-cell proliferation. Immune tolerance induced by SLIT is associated with an increase in T_{reg} cell numbers; elevated IL-10 production in sublingual FOXP3-expressing T_{reg} cells; and elevated allergen-specific IgG_4, IgA levels and serum blocking activity for IgE-facilitated allergen binding (IgE-FAB) to B cells.[23,29,30] IL-10-producing T_{reg} cells suppress T_H2-type immune response and IL-17-producing T_H cells.[31,32]

It has been recently demonstrated that a significant increase in the numbers of allergen-specific $FOXP3^+Helios^+CD25^+CD127^-$ T_{reg} cells took place at the end of up-dosing phase (10 weeks), which only slightly decreased at the end of the maintenance phase (3 years) of house dust mite (HDM) SCIT.[24] In contrast, $ILT3^+$ dysfunctional T_{reg} cells[28] decreased substantially after 3 years of SCIT.[24] Additionally, $IL-10^+$ allergen-specific T_{reg} cells are still present at high frequency at the end of SCIT. Increased number of $FOXP3^+Helios^+$ and $IL-10^+$ T_{reg} cell and decreased $ILT3^+$ T_{reg} cell responses correlated with improved allergic symptoms. These data further confirm that the induction of allergen-specific functional T_{reg} cells is one of the key events of AIT.[24] In all of these mechanisms, the H_2 receptor plays an important role. It has been shown that it can suppress DCs, T cells, natural killer T cells, and basophils. This results in antagonizing the proallergic effects of histamine via the H_1 receptor.[33–35] Histamine signaling is a newly determined link between microbiome and immune tolerance. It has been recently shown that histamine-secreting commensal bacteria exist in human gut and are linked to severity of asthma[36] and have pleiotropic effects on tolerance in the lungs.[37,38]

Taken together, the critical role for allergen-specific T_{reg} cell–mediated immune tolerance in successful AIT is well established. However, this is not the only mechanism operational in the AIT-induced tolerance.

The equally important immunologic phenomenon that warrants the favorable clinical outcome of AIT is the eradication of allergen-specific T_H2 cells (**Fig. 2**). It has been recently demonstrated that there are subsets of allergen-specific T_H2 cells, such as $CD27^-CD45RB^-CRTH2^+CD49d^+CD161^+$ T_H2 memory cells, $CRTH2^+CCR4^+CD27^-CD4^+$ T_H2 cells,[32] or $ST2^+CD45RO^+CD4^+$ cells,[39] of special importance in the pathogenesis of allergic diseases. These so-called T_H2A cells or pathogenic T_H2 cells are specifically targeted during AIT, and their eradication is indicative of favorable clinical response.[3,39,40] These cells are characterized by high

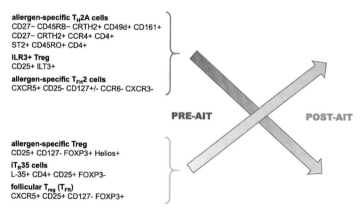

Fig. 2. Direction of change in some important T-cell subsets in response to AIT. Allergen-specific pathogenic T cells decrease and regulatory T cells increase during a successful AIT.

expression of *IL17RB* (gene encoding IL-25 receptor), *IL1RL1* (gene encoding ST2, a receptor for IL-33), and *CRLF2* (gene encoding TSLP receptor), and they highly express *IL13* and *IL5* genes.[40,41]

Interleukin-35

IL-35 is a newly identified inhibitory cytokine produced by T_{reg} cells and is essential for their immunosuppressive function.[42] IL-35-inducible regulatory T (iT$_R$35) cell is a newly recognized subset of induced T_{reg} cells with IL-35$^+$CD4$^+$CD25$^+$FOXP3$^-$ phenotype and potent immune regulatory properties.[43] The role of IL-35 and IL-35-producing iT$_R$35 cells in SLIT has recently been described (see **Fig. 2**). Proliferation and cytokine production of allergen-specific T_H2 effector cells, IL-25- or IL-33-induced IL-5 and IL-13 production of innate lymphoid cells (ILC) 2 cells, and CD40L-, IL-4-, and IL-21-mediated IgE production of B cells can all be inhibited by IL-35, whereas the production of IFN-γ and IL-10 is induced by this cytokine. Moreover, iT$_R$35 cells reduce memory T-cell proliferation and T_H2 cytokine production in an IL-10- and IL-35-dependent manner. Of note, the number of iT$_R$35 cells and allergen-induced IL-35 production is higher in the peripheral blood of patients with allergic rhinitis after successful SLIT than in the blood of untreated patients, and similar to that of healthy control subjects. Both the percentage and the IL-35-producing capacity of the iT$_R$35 cells inversely correlate with rhinitis symptom score.[44] Taken together, IL-35 and its source (iT$_R$35 cell) may represent a new target for biomarker development and for future therapies.[45]

Follicular Helper T Cells

Increasing evidence indicates that the regulation of follicular helper T (T$_{FH}$) cells is also of great importance in the success of AIT (see **Fig. 2**). Circulating T$_{FH}$ cells are divided into subgroups corresponding to T_H1, T_H2, and T_H17 helper cells. IgE antibody production by B cells is supported by type 2 T$_{FH}$ (T$_{FH}$2) cells.[46] T$_{FH}$2 cell numbers are increased in the peripheral blood of patients with allergic rhinitis, and are able to induce IgE production on an IL-4-dependent manner. Moreover, allergen-specific IgE levels correlate only with allergen-specific T$_{FH}$2 cell frequencies, but not with non-follicular T_H2 cells frequencies in patients allergic to HDM. The numbers of T$_{FH}$2 cells reduced more sharply than T_H2 cells in response to AIT. Of note, the combined symptom and medication score improvement in response to SCIT correlated only with the percent reduction of allergen-specific T$_{FH}$2 cell numbers, and not with that of T_H2 cells.[47] T$_{FH}$ activities are modulated by follicular T_{reg} (T$_{FR}$) cells[48] and by regulatory B (B$_{reg}$) cells.[49] T$_{FR}$ cells were first described in human tonsils and differentiate from natural T_{reg} cells.[50] T$_{FR}$ cell frequencies are decreased in tonsils of patients allergic to HDM suffering from allergic rhinitis. Tonsillar and blood T$_{FR}$ cell phenotypes and numbers correlate with each other. Circulating T$_{FR}$ cells of patients with allergic rhinitis fail to suppress IgE production of B cells in vitro. Circulating T$_{FR}$ cell frequencies are increased and their IgE-suppressing function is improved after AIT.[51] Therefore, therapeutic targeting of T$_{FR}$ and T$_{FH}$ cells and their use as a biomarker has been proposed.

INNATE LYMPHOID CELLS IN ALLERGY AND ALLERGEN IMMUNOTHERAPY

Exploration of the diversity of ILCs has substantially changed the understanding of tissue inflammation and immune tolerance in the last few years.[52] ILCs are developmentally related to natural killer cells. Novel members of the ILC family (ILC1s, ILC2s, and ILC3s) show similar biologic characteristics, including transcription factor expression and cytokine production, to the key cellular elements of adaptive immune response, the T_H cell subpopulations: T_H1, T_H2, and T_H17/T_H22, respectively.[53] The whole genome signatures of different ILCs subpopulations and ILC heterogeneity in humans have recently been published.[54,55] Particularly, ILC2s play an important role in allergic airway inflammation.[56] They are dependent on GATA3, and they substantially contribute to IL-5 and IL-13 production in allergic airway responses.[57] ILC3s are RORγt-dependent cells. Their signature-cytokine is IL-22, an important mediator of the mucosal immune defense, tissue repair, and the maintenance of epithelial barrier integrity.[58]

It has recently been demonstrated that seasonal increase in peripheral ILC2s is inhibited by grass pollen extract SCIT.[59] Cross-sectional studies suggest that the relative proportion of circulating ILCs is affected by AIT. The ILC2/ILC1 ratio is increased in patients allergic to HDM suffering from allergic rhinitis[60]; however, it is normalized by a successful AIT. Nonresponders show similar ILC2/ILC1 ratio to untreated patients with allergic rhinitis.[61,62]

Our group demonstrated that IL-10$^+$ regulatory ILCs (ILC$_{reg}$s) are induced from ILC2s by retinoic acid.[63] CRTH-2 and ST2 (hallmarks of ILC2s) are downregulated and CD25 and CTLA-4 are upregulated on ILC$_{reg}$s. These cells are able to suppress T-cell and ILC2 activation. Retinoic acid–producing DCs were found to help peripheral T_{reg} cell differentiation.[64,65] Retinoic acid–induced regulatory DCs have a protective effect on adoptive transfer in a mouse model of food-induced anaphylaxis.[66] Considering the general role of retinoic acid in tolerance-induction, the participation of ILC$_{reg}$s in the mechanisms of AIT-induced tolerance is also possible.

Moreover, we demonstrated recently that activated, CD40L-expressing ILC3s reside on the border of the T cell–B cell areas in tonsils, and are in close contact with B cells in vivo. Furthermore, we showed that CD40L$^+$ ILC3s and B cells are in a mutually beneficial relationship with each other: ILC3s induce IL-15 production in B cells via BAFF-receptor, whereas IL-15, a potent growth factor for ILC3s, upregulates CD40L expression on ILC3s. IL-15-activated CD40L$^+$ ILC3s help B-cell survival, proliferation and differentiation of IL-10 secreting, and functional B$_{reg}$ cells in a CD40L- and BAFF-receptor-dependent manner. Moreover, ILC3-induced B$_{reg}$ cells dominantly have CD27$^-$IgD$^+$IgM$^+$CD24^{high} CD38^{high} CD1d$^+$ immature transitional (itB$_{reg}$) phenotype. This mechanism contributes to the maintenance of immune tolerance to innocuous antigens and becomes insufficient in allergic diseases.[67] Tonsils are important mucosal sites of immune tolerance,[68] where generation of functional allergen-specific T_{reg} cells occurs. We showed that ILC3s and B$_{reg}$ cells colocalize in the interfollicular regions of palatine tonsils, together with T_{reg} cells. These data suggest that there are regulatory niches in tonsils where T_{reg} and B$_{reg}$ cells develop next to each other. CD40L$^+$ ILC3s might be involved in maintenance of immune tolerance in tonsils through induction of functional itB$_{reg}$ cells. These cells can contribute to suppression of T-cell responses through cell-cell contact via programmed cell death-ligand 1 and via secreted IL-10.[67] These mechanisms can also play a role in immune tolerance induction during successful SLIT (see **Fig. 1**).[35,69]

The significant reduction in total and allergen-specific IgE after 3 month of HDM SLIT was not affected by previous tonsillectomy; however, the mitigation of nasal symptoms and wheeze was less pronounced in the tonsillectomy group.[70] In fact, only the palatine tonsils and/or adenoids are removed or reduced during those operations, and the lingual tonsils remained untouched.[69] These data suggest that reduction of the lymphoid tissue mass in Waldeyer ring does not impede systemic tolerance induction by SLIT; however, it may delay the improvement of clinical symptoms. The small-scale study did not reveal reasons for this dichotomy.[70] Neither the cellular infiltration of the affected tissues by T_H2 cells and eosinophils, nor the local IgE levels (entopy) were examined, both of which certainly has an impact on the symptoms and may have been perpetuated in tonsillectomized patients after SLIT. Larger scale, randomized, controlled studies with appropriate blinded design are needed to be able to appreciate the influence of tonsillectomy on AIT efficacy. In addition, it should be considered that lingual tonsil, which has the same structure and cellular composition as palatine tonsils, is a large lymphoid organ that remains intact in tonsillectomy patients. IgE-mediated allergy was found to be associated with substantially lower risk of complicated appendicitis in a cohort of children who underwent surgery for acute appendicitis.[71] However, the influence of appendectomy on development of allergy, and specifically on the response to immunotherapy, has not been investigated thus far.

REGULATORY B CELLS AND ANTIBODY PRODUCTION IN ALLERGEN TOLERANCE AND IMMUNOTHERAPY
Regulatory B Cells

Deficiency of IL-10-producing B_{reg} cells leads to increased inflammation in mouse models of autoimmunity, transplantation, and chronic infection. Absolute numbers of T_{reg} cells and expression levels of FOXP3 in these cells are dependent on IL-10 production by B cells. Modulation of T_{reg} cell frequencies in vivo is exclusively restricted to transitional 2 marginal zone precursor B_{reg} cells in mice.[72] Of note, itB_{reg} cells can prevent and reverse airway inflammation in allergized mice by inducing recruitment of T_{reg} cells to the lung.[73] Adoptive transfer of itB_{reg} cells can ameliorate allergic airway inflammation and hyperresponsiveness in a mouse model of allergic asthma in an IL-10-dependent manner.[74] Human itB_{reg} cells are also able to induce T_{reg} cells in vitro.[75] The relative proportion of B_{reg} cell subsets within B cells was found to be reduced in patients with allergic diseases, such as allergic rhinitis[76] and allergic asthma,[77] and the frequency of IL-10-producing, antigen-specific B cells increased after AIT.[78,79] In vivo evidence for allergen tolerance has been demonstrated: the suppressive B cells and IgG_4-expressing B cells are developed from IL-10$^+$ BR1 cells in human subjects after AIT.[80] Supporting the role of IL-10, solely IL-10-overexpressing B cells acquired an immunoregulatory profile comprising upregulation of suppressor of cytokine signaling 3 (SOCS3), glycoprotein A repetitions predominant (GARP), CD25, and programmed cell death-ligand 1.[81] These cells showed a significant reduction in levels of many proinflammatory cytokines, and augmented the production of anti-inflammatory IL-1 receptor antagonist and vascular endothelial growth factor. In addition, IL-10-overexpressing B cells secreted less IgE and showed a general T-cell and DC suppression.[81] Moreover, a novel mechanism of AIT-induced specific immune tolerance is suggested by our recent data. Increased numbers of IgA- and IgG_4-expressing allergen-specific memory B cells, plasmablasts, and IL-10$^+$ and/or IL-1RA$^+$ B_{reg} cells were found in the peripheral blood over a 2-year period during successful HDM SCIT (see **Fig. 1**).[82]

Modulation of Allergen-Specific IgE and IgG Responses During Allergen Immunotherapy

Specific IgE increases in individuals allergic to pollen during the pollen season and a successful AIT can prevent this increase. AIT itself also induces an early increase in IgE during the up-dosing phase, which rings out in maintenance phase in parallel with the increase in IgA and IgG_4 (see **Fig. 1**).[83]

AIT-induced IgG may be directed against the same epitopes as IgE, resulting in direct competition for allergen binding and a blocking effect.[84] Allergen-specific IgG antibodies can inhibit IgE-mediated basophil and mast cell activation and degranulation with two different mechanisms: allergen neutralization and binding to the inhibitory FcγRIIb. It has been demonstrated recently that although only high-affinity IgG antibodies can have both of these effects, low-affinity IgG antibodies are still able to inhibit mast cell activation via FcγRIIb.[85] IgG$_4$ antibodies have several features that may play a role in their anti-inflammatory effects. Two arms of IgG$_4$ have the ability to separate and repair by dynamic Fab arm exchange, which leads to bispecific antibodies that are functionally monomeric.[86] Furthermore, IgG$_4$ does not fix complement and is capable of inhibiting immune-complex formation by other isotypes.[87] It is likely the decrease in IgE/IgG$_4$ ratio during AIT is a biomarker of skew from allergen-specific T$_H$2 to T$_{reg}$ cell and B$_{reg}$ cell predominance. IL-10 is a potent suppressor of total and allergen-specific IgE, whereas it simultaneously increases IgG$_4$ production.[21,88]

The characteristic changes in the level of IgE and IgG$_4$ during SCIT is mirrored by the local concentrations of those immunoglobulins in nasal secretions[45] and saliva.[89]

The results of some recent studies confirm that the IgG$_4$-mediated inhibition of CD23-dependent IgE-FAB,[90] rather than the serum concentration of IgG$_4$ solely, is a valuable biomarker of the AIT clinical outcome.[29,91] Other investigators evidenced that specific IgG$_4$ and inhibition of IgE-FAB correlates well with clinical efficacy of AIT.[92] Inhibition of IgE-FAB by nasal secretions correlates more closely with clinical outcome than that of serum samples after SCIT.[45]

Regulation of Mast Cells and Basophils by Allergen Immunotherapy

Clinical desensitization starts as early as after the first injection of SCIT. This is mainly linked to decreased mast cell and basophil degranulation, which has been demonstrated in a mouse model.[93] One of the main soluble factors released from mast cells and basophils following allergen challenge is histamine, which mediates its effects via histamine receptors. Immunosilencing of FcεRI-activated basophils by means of selective suppression mediated by H$_2$ receptor might be highly relevant for the early desensitization effect, at least in venom AIT.[94] Although there are individual differences and risks for developing systemic anaphylaxis, the suppression of mast cells and basophils is further increased during the course of AIT. Early reduction in basophil sensitivity predicts symptom relief also in grass pollen immunotherapy.[95] Furthermore, basophil expression of diamine oxidase shows a significant increase after AIT and is suggested as a novel biomarker of AIT responsiveness.[96]

OTHER ASPECTS OF IMMUNOTHERAPY

It has been demonstrated in mouse model of allergic asthma in vivo and human bronchial epithelial cell cultures in vitro that AIT contributes to the restoration of the airway epithelial barrier integrity by the reduction of IL-25 production. IL-25 is one of the main inducers of endoplasmic reticulum stress and tight junction damage.[97] It has been recently shown in a 5-year clinical study that grass pollen SLIT significantly reduces the risk of experiencing asthma symptoms and decreases the need for asthma medications.[98] The systematic meta-analyses of contribution of AIT in allergic asthma[99] and allergic rhinoconjunctivitis[100] have been recently published, supporting the previously mentioned study and confirming that AIT has positive effects on various allergic diseases. The effects of AIT for various phenotypes and endotypes of allergic diseases need to be further elucidated in vivo in animal models and directly in human tissue.[101,102]

SUMMARY

AIT offers an efficient treatment of allergic diseases with a possibility of cure. There is strong evidence for clinical safety and efficacy of AIT. Demonstration of allergen-specific T- and B-cell tolerance, mediated, among others, by the immunosuppressive functions of IL-10, led to a major conceptual change in this area and opened a way to bring AIT from empiricism to a treatment with solid mechanisms of action linked to immune tolerance. The accurate definition of disease endotypes and a correct selection of the responder patients with well-defined biomarkers still remain essential unmet needs in the clinical setting. Therefore, deeper understanding of immuno-pharmaco-metabolo-genomics of allergy and the impact of the environmental exposure and the microbiome on it will probably help improve the AIT to accomplish vaccination strategies that are suitable for whole population-based allergy prevention and cure in the future.

ACKNOWLEDGMENTS

The laboratory of the corresponding author Z.I. Komlósi is supported by Hungarian Pediatric Oncology Network. The laboratories of the authors C.A. Akdis and M. Akdis are supported by the Swiss National Science Foundation.

REFERENCES

1. Hamdi H, Godot V, Maillot MC, et al. Induction of antigen-specific regulatory T lymphocytes by human dendritic cells expressing the glucocorticoid-induced leucine zipper. Blood 2007;110(1):211–9.
2. Karaki S, Garcia G, Tcherakian C, et al. Enhanced glucocorticoid-induced leucine zipper in dendritic cells induces allergen-specific regulatory CD4(+) T-cells in respiratory allergies. Allergy 2014;69(5):624–31.
3. Renand A, Shamji MH, Harris KM, et al. Synchronous immune alterations mirror clinical response during allergen immunotherapy. J Allergy Clin Immunol 2018; 141(5):1750–60.e1.
4. Halken S, Larenas-Linnemann D, Roberts G, et al. EAACI guidelines on allergen immunotherapy: prevention of allergy. Pediatr Allergy Immunol 2017;28(8): 728–45.
5. Bonertz A, Roberts GC, Hoefnagel M, et al. Challenges in the implementation of EAACI guidelines on allergen immunotherapy: a global perspective on the regulation of allergen products. Allergy 2018;73(1):64–76.
6. Larenas-Linnemann DES, Antolin-Amerigo D, Parisi C, et al. National clinical practice guidelines for allergen immunotherapy: an international assessment applying AGREE-II. Allergy 2018;73(3):664–72.
7. Roberts G, Pfaar O, Akdis CA, et al. EAACI guidelines on allergen immunotherapy: allergic rhinoconjunctivitis. Allergy 2018;73(4):765–98.
8. Bonertz A, Roberts G, Slater JE, et al. Allergen manufacturing and quality aspects for allergen immunotherapy in Europe and the United States: an analysis from the EAACI AIT guidelines project. Allergy 2018;73(4):816–26.
9. Ryan D, Gerth van Wijk R, Angier E, et al. Challenges in the implementation of the EAACI AIT guidelines: a situational analysis of current provision of allergen immunotherapy. Allergy 2018;73(4):827–36.
10. Sturm GJ, Varga EM, Roberts G, et al. EAACI guidelines on allergen immunotherapy: hymenoptera venom allergy. Allergy 2018;73(4):744–64.
11. Pajno GB, Fernandez-Rivas M, Arasi S, et al. EAACI Guidelines on allergen immunotherapy: IgE-mediated food allergy. Allergy 2018;73(4):799–815.
12. Agache I, Lau S, Akdis CA, et al. EAACI guidelines on allergen immunotherapy: house dust mite-driven allergic asthma. Allergy 2019;74(5):855–73.
13. Akdis CA, Bachert C, Cingi C, et al. Endotypes and phenotypes of chronic rhinosinusitis: a PRACTALL document of the European Academy of Allergy and

Clinical Immunology and the American Academy of Allergy, Asthma & Immunology. J Allergy Clin Immunol 2013;131(6):1479–90.

14. Wenzel SE. Asthma phenotypes: the evolution from clinical to molecular approaches. Nat Med 2012;18(5):716–25.

15. Sugita K, Sokolowska M, Akdis CA. Key points for moving the endotypes field forward. In: Agache I, Hellings P, editors. Implementing precision medicine in best practices of chronic airway diseases. London: Elsevier; 2018. p. 107–14.

16. Radulovic S, Jacobson MR, Durham SR, et al. Grass pollen immunotherapy induces Foxp3-expressing CD4+ CD25+ cells in the nasal mucosa. J Allergy Clin Immunol 2008;121(6):1467–72, 1472.e1.

17. Kearley J, Barker JE, Robinson DS, et al. Resolution of airway inflammation and hyperreactivity after in vivo transfer of CD4+CD25+ regulatory T cells is interleukin 10 dependent. J Exp Med 2005;202(11):1539–47.

18. Romano M, Fanelli G, Albany CJ, et al. Past, present, and future of regulatory T cell therapy in transplantation and autoimmunity. Front Immunol 2019;10:43.

19. Trzonkowski P, Bacchetta R, Battaglia M, et al. Hurdles in therapy with regulatory T cells. Sci Transl Med 2015;7(304):304ps318.

20. Akdis CA, Akdis M, Blesken T, et al. Epitope specific T cell tolerance to phospholipase A_2 in bee venom immunotherapy and recovery by IL-2 and IL-15 in vitro. J Clin Invest 1996;98:1676–83.

21. Akdis CA, Blesken T, Akdis M, et al. Role of interleukin 10 in specific immunotherapy. J Clin Invest 1998;102(1):98–106.

22. Akdis CA, Akdis M. Mechanisms of immune tolerance to allergens: role of IL-10 and Tregs. J Clin Invest 2014;124(11):4678–80.

23. Suarez-Fueyo A, Ramos T, Galan A, et al. Grass tablet sublingual immunotherapy downregulates the TH2 cytokine response followed by regulatory T-cell generation. J Allergy Clin Immunol 2014;133(1):130–8.e1-2.

24. Boonpiyathad T, Sokolowska M, Morita H, et al. Der p 1-specific regulatory T-cell response during house dust mite allergen immunotherapy. Allergy 2019;74(5):976–85.

25. Meiler F, Zumkehr J, Klunker S, et al. In vivo switch to IL-10-secreting T regulatory cells in high dose allergen exposure. J Exp Med 2008;205(12):2887–98.

26. van de Veen W, Wirz OF, Globinska A, et al. Novel mechanisms in immune tolerance to allergens during natural allergen exposure and allergen-specific immunotherapy. Curr Opin Immunol 2017;48:74–81.

27. Zemmour D, Zilionis R, Kiner E, et al. Publisher correction: single-cell gene expression reveals a landscape of regulatory T cell phenotypes shaped by the TCR. Nat Immunol 2018;19(6):645.

28. Ulges A, Klein M, Reuter S, et al. Protein kinase CK2 enables regulatory T cells to suppress excessive TH2 responses in vivo. Nat Immunol 2015;16(3):267–75.

29. Scadding GW, Shamji MH, Jacobson MR, et al. Sublingual grass pollen immunotherapy is associated with increases in sublingual Foxp3-expressing cells and elevated allergen-specific immunoglobulin G4, immunoglobulin A and serum inhibitory activity for immunoglobulin E-facilitated allergen binding to B cells. Clin Exp Allergy 2010;40(4):598–606.

30. Jutel M, Akdis M, Budak F, et al. IL-10 and TGF-beta cooperate in the regulatory T cell response to mucosal allergens in normal immunity and specific immunotherapy. Eur J Immunol 2003;33(5):1205–14.

31. Berings M, Karaaslan C, Altunbulakli C, et al. Advances and highlights in allergen immunotherapy: on the way to sustained clinical and immunologic tolerance. J Allergy Clin Immunol 2017;140(5):1250–67.

32. Scadding GW, Calderon MA, Shamji MH, et al. Effect of 2 years of treatment with sublingual grass pollen immunotherapy on nasal response to allergen challenge at 3 years among patients with moderate to severe seasonal allergic rhinitis: the GRASS randomized clinical trial. JAMA 2017;317(6):615–25.

33. Ferstl R, Frei R, Barcik W, et al. Histamine receptor 2 modifies iNKT cell activity within the inflamed lung. Allergy 2017;72(12):1925–35.

34. Ferstl R, Frei R, Schiavi E, et al. Histamine receptor 2 is a key influence in immune responses to intestinal histamine-secreting microbes. J Allergy Clin Immunol 2014;134(3):744–6.e3.

35. Palomares O, Martin-Fontecha M, Lauener R, et al. Regulatory T cells and immune regulation of allergic diseases: roles of IL-10 and TGF-beta. Genes Immun 2014;15(8):511–20.

36. Barcik W, Pugin B, Westermann P, et al. Histamine-secreting microbes are increased in the gut of adult asthma patients. J Allergy Clin Immunol 2016; 138(5):1491–4.e7.

37. Lunjani N, Satitsuksanoa P, Lukasik Z, et al. Recent developments and highlights in mechanisms of allergic diseases: microbiome. Allergy 2018;73(12): 2314–27.

38. Barcik W, Pugin B, Bresco MS, et al. Bacterial secretion of histamine within the gut influences immune responses within the lung. Allergy 2019;74(5):899–909.

39. Ihara F, Sakurai D, Yonekura S, et al. Identification of specifically reduced Th2 cell subsets in allergic rhinitis patients after sublingual immunotherapy. Allergy 2018;73(9):1823–32.

40. Wambre E, Bajzik V, DeLong JH, et al. A phenotypically and functionally distinct human TH2 cell subpopulation is associated with allergic disorders. Sci Transl Med 2017;9(401) [pii:eaam9171].

41. Chiang D, Chen X, Jones SM, et al. Single-cell profiling of peanut-responsive T cells in patients with peanut allergy reveals heterogeneous effector TH2 subsets. J Allergy Clin Immunol 2018;141(6):2107–20.

42. Collison LW, Workman CJ, Kuo TT, et al. The inhibitory cytokine IL-35 contributes to regulatory T-cell function. Nature 2007;450(7169):566–9.

43. Collison LW, Chaturvedi V, Henderson AL, et al. IL-35-mediated induction of a potent regulatory T cell population. Nat Immunol 2010;11(12):1093–101.

44. Shamji MH, Layhadi JA, Achkova D, et al. Role of IL-35 in sublingual allergen immunotherapy. J Allergy Clin Immunol 2019;143(3):1131–42.e4.

45. Layhadi JA, Eguiluz-Gracia I, Shamji MH. Role of IL-35 in sublingual allergen immunotherapy. Curr Opin Allergy Clin Immunol 2019;19(1):12–7.

46. Morita R, Schmitt N, Bentebibel SE, et al. Human blood CXCR5(+)CD4(+) T cells are counterparts of T follicular cells and contain specific subsets that differentially support antibody secretion. Immunity 2011;34(1):108–21.

47. Yao Y, Chen CL, Wang N, et al. Correlation of allergen-specific T follicular helper cell counts with specific IgE levels and efficacy of allergen immunotherapy. J Allergy Clin Immunol 2018;142(1):321–4.e10.

48. Lim HW, Hillsamer P, Kim CH. Regulatory T cells can migrate to follicles upon T cell activation and suppress GC-Th cells and GC-Th cell-driven B cell responses. J Clin Invest 2004;114(11):1640–9.

49. Achour A, Simon Q, Mohr A, et al. Human regulatory B cells control the TFH cell response. J Allergy Clin Immunol 2017;140(1):215–22.

50. Varricchi G, Harker J, Borriello F, et al. T follicular helper (Tfh) cells in normal immune responses and in allergic disorders. Allergy 2016;71(8):1086–94.

51. Yao Y, Wang ZC, Wang N, et al. Allergen immunotherapy improves defective follicular regulatory T cells in patients with allergic rhinitis. J Allergy Clin Immunol 2019;144(1):118–28.
52. Kortekaas Krohn I, Shikhagaie MM, Golebski K, et al. Emerging roles of innate lymphoid cells in inflammatory diseases: clinical implications. Allergy 2018; 73(4):837–50.
53. Spits H, Artis D, Colonna M, et al. Innate lymphoid cells: a proposal for uniform nomenclature. Nat Rev Immunol 2013;13(2):145–9.
54. Bjorklund AK, Forkel M, Picelli S, et al. The heterogeneity of human CD127(+) innate lymphoid cells revealed by single-cell RNA sequencing. Nat Immunol 2016;17(4):451–60.
55. Li S, Morita H, Sokolowska M, et al. Gene expression signatures of circulating human type 1, 2, and 3 innate lymphoid cells. J Allergy Clin Immunol 2019;143(6): 2321–5.
56. Bartemes KR, Kephart GM, Fox SJ, et al. Enhanced innate type 2 immune response in peripheral blood from patients with asthma. J Allergy Clin Immunol 2014;134(3):671–8.e4.
57. Mjosberg JM, Trifari S, Crellin NK, et al. Human IL-25- and IL-33-responsive type 2 innate lymphoid cells are defined by expression of CRTH2 and CD161. Nat Immunol 2011;12(11):1055–62.
58. Klose CS, Artis D. Innate lymphoid cells as regulators of immunity, inflammation and tissue homeostasis. Nat Immunol 2016;17(7):765–74.
59. Lao-Araya M, Steveling E, Scadding GW, et al. Seasonal increases in peripheral innate lymphoid type 2 cells are inhibited by subcutaneous grass pollen immunotherapy. J Allergy Clin Immunol 2014;134(5):1193–5.e4.
60. Zhong H, Fan XL, Yu QN, et al. Increased innate type 2 immune response in house dust mite-allergic patients with allergic rhinitis. Clin Immunol 2017;183: 293–9.
61. Fan DC, Wang XD, Wang CS, et al. Suppression of immunotherapy on group 2 innate lymphoid cells in allergic rhinitis. Chin Med J (Engl) 2016;129(23):2824–8.
62. Mitthamsiri W, Pradubpongsa P, Sangasapaviliya A, et al. Decreased CRTH2 expression and response to allergen re-stimulation on innate lymphoid cells in patients with allergen-specific immunotherapy. Allergy Asthma Immunol Res 2018;10(6):662–74.
63. Morita H, Kubo T, Ruckert B, et al. Induction of human regulatory innate lymphoid cells from group 2 innate lymphoid cells by retinoic acid. J Allergy Clin Immunol 2019;143(6):2190–201.e9.
64. Coombes JL, Siddiqui KR, Arancibia-Carcamo CV, et al. A functionally specialized population of mucosal CD103+ DCs induces Foxp3+ regulatory T cells via a TGF-beta and retinoic acid-dependent mechanism. J Exp Med 2007;204(8): 1757–64.
65. Sun CM, Hall JA, Blank RB, et al. Small intestine lamina propria dendritic cells promote de novo generation of Foxp3 T reg cells via retinoic acid. J Exp Med 2007;204(8):1775–85.
66. Dawicki W, Li C, Town J, et al. Therapeutic reversal of food allergen sensitivity by mature retinoic acid-differentiated dendritic cell induction of LAG3(+)CD49b(-) Foxp3(-) regulatory T cells. J Allergy Clin Immunol 2017;139(5):1608–20.e3.
67. Komlosi ZI, Kovacs N, van de Veen W, et al. Human CD40 ligand-expressing type 3 innate lymphoid cells induce IL-10-producing immature transitional regulatory B cells. J Allergy Clin Immunol 2018;142(1):178–94.e11.

68. Palomares O, Ruckert B, Jartti T, et al. Induction and maintenance of allergen-specific FOXP3+ Treg cells in human tonsils as potential first-line organs of oral tolerance. J Allergy Clin Immunol 2012;129(2):510–20, 520.e1-9.

69. Moingeon P. Update on immune mechanisms associated with sublingual immunotherapy: practical implications for the clinician. J Allergy Clin Immunol Pract 2013;1(3):228–41.

70. Refaat M, Ashour ZA, Farres MN, et al. Effect of tonsillectomy on the efficacy of house dust mite sublingual immunotherapy. Allergol Immunopathol (Madr) 2015;43(1):108–11.

71. Salo M, Gudjonsdottir J, Omling E, et al. Association of IgE-mediated allergy with risk of complicated appendicitis in a pediatric population. JAMA Pediatr 2018;172(10):943–8.

72. Carter NA, Vasconcellos R, Rosser EC, et al. Mice lacking endogenous IL-10-producing regulatory B cells develop exacerbated disease and present with an increased frequency of Th1/Th17 but a decrease in regulatory T cells. J Immunol 2011;186(10):5569–79.

73. Amu S, Saunders SP, Kronenberg M, et al. Regulatory B cells prevent and reverse allergic airway inflammation via FoxP3-positive T regulatory cells in a murine model. J Allergy Clin Immunol 2010;125(5):1114–24.e8.

74. Braza F, Chesne J, Durand M, et al. A regulatory CD9(+) B-cell subset inhibits HDM-induced allergic airway inflammation. Allergy 2015;70(11):1421–31.

75. Lemoine S, Morva A, Youinou P, et al. Human T cells induce their own regulation through activation of B cells. J Autoimmun 2011;36(3–4):228–38.

76. Kim AS, Doherty TA, Karta MR, et al. Regulatory B cells and T follicular helper cells are reduced in allergic rhinitis. J Allergy Clin Immunol 2016;138(4):1192–5.e5.

77. Kamekura R, Shigehara K, Miyajima S, et al. Alteration of circulating type 2 follicular helper T cells and regulatory B cells underlies the comorbid association of allergic rhinitis with bronchial asthma. Clin Immunol 2015;158(2):204–11.

78. Boonpiyathad T, Meyer N, Moniuszko M, et al. High-dose bee venom exposure induces similar tolerogenic B-cell responses in allergic patients and healthy beekeepers. Allergy 2017;72(3):407–15.

79. van de Veen W. The role of regulatory B cells in allergen immunotherapy. Curr Opin Allergy Clin Immunol 2017;17(6):447–52.

80. van de Veen W, Stanic B, Yaman G, et al. IgG4 production is confined to human IL-10-producing regulatory B cells that suppress antigen-specific immune responses. J Allergy Clin Immunol 2013;131(4):1204–12.

81. Stanic B, van de Veen W, Wirz OF, et al. IL-10-overexpressing B cells regulate innate and adaptive immune responses. J Allergy Clin Immunol 2015;135(3):771–80.e8.

82. Boonpiyathad T, van de Veen W, Wirz O, et al. Role of Der p 1-specific B cells in immune tolerance during 2 years of house dust mite-specific immunotherapy. J Allergy Clin Immunol 2019;143(3):1077–86.e10.

83. Jimenez-Saiz R, Patil SU. The multifaceted B cell response in allergen immunotherapy. Curr Allergy Asthma Rep 2018;18(12):66.

84. Klunker S, Saggar LR, Seyfert-Margolis V, et al. Combination treatment with omalizumab and rush immunotherapy for ragweed-induced allergic rhinitis: inhibition of IgE-facilitated allergen binding. J Allergy Clin Immunol 2007;120(3):688–95.

85. Zha L, Leoratti FMS, He L, et al. An unexpected protective role of low-affinity allergen-specific IgG through the inhibitory receptor FcgammaRIIb. J Allergy Clin Immunol 2018;142(5):1529–36.e6.

86. van der Neut Kolfschoten M, Schuurman J, Losen M, et al. Anti-inflammatory activity of human IgG4 antibodies by dynamic Fab arm exchange. Science 2007; 317(5844):1554–7.

87. Aalberse RC, Stapel SO, Schuurman J, et al. Immunoglobulin G4: an odd antibody. Clin Exp Allergy 2009;39(4):469–77.

88. Meiler F, Klunker S, Zimmermann M, et al. Distinct regulation of IgE, IgG4 and IgA by T regulatory cells and toll-like receptors. Allergy 2008;63(11):1455–63.

89. Liu Y, Xing Z, Wang J, et al. Salivary immunoglobulin A, E, and G4 levels specific to dermatophagoides pteronyssinus in allergic rhinitis patients treated with subcutaneous immunotherapy. Am J Rhinol Allergy 2018;32(6):458–64.

90. Shamji MH, Wilcock LK, Wachholz PA, et al. The IgE-facilitated allergen binding (FAB) assay: validation of a novel flow-cytometric based method for the detection of inhibitory antibody responses. J Immunol Methods 2006;317(1–2):71–9.

91. Shamji MH, Ljorring C, Francis JN, et al. Functional rather than immunoreactive levels of IgG4 correlate closely with clinical response to grass pollen immunotherapy. Allergy 2012;67(2):217–26.

92. Feng M, Su Q, Lai X, et al. Functional and immunoreactive levels of IgG4 correlate with clinical responses during the maintenance phase of house dust mite immunotherapy. J Immunol 2018;200(12):3897–904.

93. Woo HY, Kim YS, Kang NI, et al. Mechanism for acute oral desensitization to antibiotics. Allergy 2006;61(8):954–8.

94. Novak N, Mete N, Bussmann C, et al. Early suppression of basophil activation during allergen-specific immunotherapy by histamine receptor 2. J Allergy Clin Immunol 2012;130:1153–8.

95. Schmid JM, Wurtzen PA, Dahl R, et al. Early improvement in basophil sensitivity predicts symptom relief with grass pollen immunotherapy. J Allergy Clin Immunol 2014;134(3):741–744 e745.

96. Shamji MH, Layhadi JA, Scadding GW, et al. Basophil expression of diamine oxidase: a novel biomarker of allergen immunotherapy response. J Allergy Clin Immunol 2015;135(4):913–21.e9.

97. Yuan X, Wang J, Li Y, et al. Allergy immunotherapy restores airway epithelial barrier dysfunction through suppressing IL-25 -induced endoplasmic reticulum stress in asthma. Sci Rep 2018;8(1):7950.

98. Valovirta E, Petersen TH, Piotrowska T, et al. Results from the 5-year SQ grass sublingual immunotherapy tablet asthma prevention (GAP) trial in children with grass pollen allergy. J Allergy Clin Immunol 2018;141(2):529–38.e13.

99. Dhami S, Kakourou A, Asamoah F, et al. Allergen immunotherapy for allergic asthma: a systematic review and meta-analysis. Allergy 2017;72(12):1825–48.

100. Dhami S, Nurmatov U, Arasi S, et al. Allergen immunotherapy for allergic rhinoconjunctivitis: a systematic review and meta-analysis. Allergy 2017;72(11): 1597–631.

101. Tan HT, Hagner S, Ruchti F, et al. Tight junction, mucin, and inflammasome-related molecules are differentially expressed in eosinophilic, mixed, and neutrophilic experimental asthma in mice. Allergy 2019;74(2):294–307.

102. Russkamp D, Aguilar-Pimentel A, Alessandrini F, et al. IL-4 receptor alpha blockade prevents sensitization and alters acute and long-lasting effects of allergen-specific immunotherapy of murine allergic asthma. Allergy 2019; 74(8):1549–60.

Highlights of Novel Vaccination Strategies in Allergen Immunotherapy

Zsolt István Komlósi, MD, PhD[a],*, Nóra Kovács, MD[a,b],
Milena Sokolowska, MD, PhD[c,d], Willem van de Veen, PhD[c,d],
Mübeccel Akdis, MD, PhD[c,d], Cezmi A. Akdis, MD[c,d]

KEYWORDS

- Allergy • Allergen immunotherapy • AIT • Adjuvants • Allergoids
- Recombinant allergen peptides • Active immunization • Passive immunization

KEY POINTS

- The current aim is to improve allergen immunotherapy (AIT) to shorten duration of treatment, enhance efficiency, reduce side effects, and, ultimately, significantly increase the utilization of this curative treatment of allergy with high patient adherence and compliance.
- To increase the efficacy of AIT, allergens have been modified to facilitate their uptake and presentation, or have been coupled to innate immunostimulatory substances. New adjuvants have also been introduced recently.
- Hypoallergenic molecules (eg, allergoids and recombinant allergen peptides) have been developed to improve the safety profile of the vaccines.
- Administration of recombinant IgG$_4$ antibodies is a new, quick, passive immunization AIT strategy with remarkable efficiency.
- Recent mouse experiments suggest that it may be possible to develop AIT even for prenatal allergy prevention.

INTRODUCTION

Increasing safety while maintaining or even augmenting efficiency are the main goals of research for novel vaccine development and improvement of treatment schemes in allergen immunotherapy (AIT).[1–4] In spite of encouraging positive experiences,[5] AIT still faces several problems related to worldwide standardization, its limited efficacy,

[a] Department of Genetics, Cell- and Immunobiology, Semmelweis University, Nagyvárad Sqr. 4, Budapest 1089, Hungary; [b] Lung Health Hospital, Munkácsy Mihály Str. 70, Törökbálint 2045, Hungary; [c] Swiss Institute of Allergy and Asthma Research (SIAF), Hermann-Burchard Strasse 9, Davos Wolfgang CH7265, Switzerland; [d] Christine Kühne – Center for Allergy Research and Education, Hermann-Burchard Strasse 1, Davos Wolfgang CH7265, Switzerland
* Corresponding author.
E-mail addresses: komlosi.zsolt@med.semmelweis-univ.hu; drkomlo@yahoo.com

Immunol Allergy Clin N Am 40 (2020) 15–24
https://doi.org/10.1016/j.iac.2019.09.010   **immunology.theclinics.com**

potential severe side effects, low patient adherence, high costs, and long duration (3–5 years) of treatment. There have been many different approaches to improve the standardization, efficacy, and safety of AIT in the past, which have been continuously pursued during the past years.[6–8] Currently, efforts on developing novel vaccines of AIT continue for the treatment of asthma,[9] allergic rhinoconjunctivitis,[10] bee venom allergy,[11] and food allergy.[12] Similar efforts are being undertaken for autoimmune diseases. Studies to offer prophylactic usage are also being performed.[13] Regulatory issues represent an important aspect in this context[14] and global and national strategies are being continuously developed.[15,16] It is essential to develop strong collaborations with the regulatory authorities for extensive preventive usage of AIT vaccines and usage of pollen chambers for outcome evaluations to avoid slowing down of vaccine developments. Here, the authors summarize some current investigations aiming at further improvement of AIT vaccines (**Table 1**).

NOVEL ALLERGEN FORMULATIONS AND ADJUVANTS

Adjuvants are add-on constituents of the vaccines, ideally increase the immunogenicity of the allergens to induce a quicker, stronger, and longer-lasting immune response; meanwhile also modulate the immune response to enhance allergen-specific T regulatory cell differentiation, immunoglobulin (Ig)G_4 antibody production, and, importantly, avoid T_H2-type response as well as anaphylaxis.

Coupling of allergens to innate immunostimulatory substances is primarily aimed at improving vaccine efficiency. These strategies include CpG oligonucleotide-conjugated allergens,[17] allergens coupled to viruslike particles,[18,19] carbohydrate-based particles,[20] and the use of monophosphoryl lipid A formulated with allergoid.[21] Encapsulation of allergens in nanoparticles enables us to design the immunomodulatory and depot effect of a complex vaccine very precisely.[22,23] Nanoparticles can have an adjuvant effect themselves (eg, viruslike particles), or various adjuvant molecules can be conjugated to or packed in the particles (eg, *Vibrio cholerae* neuraminidase on synthetic microparticles), and the physical-chemical characteristics of the particles determine the kinetics of the antigen release (eg, liposomes). Liposomes and microcrystalline tyrosine are promising new alternatives of the widely used aluminum hydroxide (alum) adjuvant.

Sublingual administration of an allergen together with α-galactosylceramide-liposomes increased the therapeutic performance of the vaccine in mouse model of allergic rhinitis.[24] High-affinity glycan ligand of the inhibitory receptor CD33 and the allergen, packed in liposomal nanoparticles, was able to suppress immunoglobulin (Ig)E-mediated activation of mast cells and, thus, was shown to be efficient in preventing anaphylaxis in transgenic mice bearing human CD33-expressing mast cells.[25] Such approaches may help to increase the safety of AIT.

Microcrystalline tyrosine, an alternative depo adjuvant composed of nonessential amino acid L-tyrosine, is a second-generation adjuvant currently used for AIT in humans (eg, Pollinex, Acarovac Plus).[26] It is proven to be safe for human use,[27] and efficiently induces IgG$_4$ production and reduces symptoms in house dust mite (HDM) subcutaneous immunotherapy (SCIT).[26]

Microcrystalline tyrosine-adsorbed grass pollen allergoid (Pollinex quattro) enhanced with monophosphoryl lipid A, a second-generation immunomodulatory adjuvant, had a beneficial long-term effect as well.[28]

Recombinant allergen peptides, selected to have advantageous safety profile are generally less immunogenic. Therefore, various carrier systems, typically of microbial origin, have been developed.[29] Promising new approaches include *Vibrio cholerae*

Table 1
Novel AIT vaccine developmental strategies currently being pursued

Type of the Vaccine/Approach	References
Coupling of allergens to innate immunostimulatory substances	
CpG oligonucleotide-conjugated allergens	17
Allergens coupled to viruslike particles	18,19,32,33
Carbohydrate-based particles	20
Vibrio cholerae neuraminidase on allergen-loaded synthetic microparticles	29
Fusion of nonallergenic peptides and PreS protein from hepatitis B virus	34,35
Fusion of nonallergenic peptides and tetanus toxoid	36
Novel adjuvants	
Monophosphoryl lipid A formulated with allergoid	21
Microcrystalline tyrosine	26,27
Proteoliposome adjuvant from *Neisseria meningitidis*	30
α-Galactosylceramide containing liposomes	24
Encapsulation of allergens in micro-/nanoparticles	
Carbohydrate-based particles	20
α-Galactosylceramide containing liposomes	24
CD33 ligand and the allergen packed in liposomal nanoparticles	25
V cholerae neuraminidase on allergen-loaded synthetic microparticles	29
Allergoids and recombinant allergens	
Monophosphoryl lipid A formulated with allergoid	21
Allergen extracts modified with glutaraldehyde	40
Fusion of nonallergenic peptides and PreS protein from hepatitis B virus	34,35
Fusion of nonallergenic peptides and tetanus toxoid	36
Recombinant T-cell epitope peptides	43
Allergen fragments	44
Recombinant allergen hybrids	45
Conjugation of allergoids to nonoxidized mannan	51,52
Fusion of allergens with other immune response modifiers	
CD33 ligand and the allergen packed in liposomal nanoparticles	25
MAT-vaccine	37,38
Conjugation of allergoids to nonoxidized mannan	51,52
Novel routes of administration	
Intralymphatic AIT	37,38,60
Epicutaneous AIT	59
Combination of AIT with biologicals	
Administration of anti-IgE	55–58
Novel administration protocols	
Passive immunization	69
Prenatal preventive vaccination	68,70

Considering that certain approaches may include different strategies, some of the vaccines are mentioned in multiple categories.

Abbreviations: AIT, allergen immunotherapy; Ig, immunoglobulin; MAT, modular antigen translocation.

neuraminidase, as an immunomodulatory agent, on allergen-loaded synthetic micro-particles[30]; proteoliposome from *Neisseria meningitidis* as an adjuvant for HDM allergy vaccine[31]; and utilization of viruslike particles to enhance uptake of the allergen by antigen-presenting cells.[32] A single dose of allergen Fel d 1-linked virus-like particles is able to prevent type I hypersensitivity response in mice.[33,34] Fusion proteins consisting of nonallergenic peptides from the 4 major timothy grass pollen allergens and the PreS protein from hepatitis B virus as a carrier efficiently reduced T-cell proliferation and proinflammatory cytokine release, while increased blocking IgG activity.[35] Engineered recombinant fusion proteins consisting of nonallergenic peptides of the allergens and microbial components, like hepatitis B PreS protein[36] or partial fragment of a tetanus toxoid molecule,[37] seems to be safe and efficient in model systems.

In a novel approach, the major cat allergen (Fel d 1) was modified in a way that its uptake and presentation by professional antigen-presenting cells was highly improved. Human immunodeficiency virus transacting activator of transcription (TAT)-derived membrane translocation domain was used to enhance entry to cells, and a truncated peptide of the invariant chain was used to increase antigen presentation.[38,39] This modular antigen translocation (MAT)-Fel d 1 vaccine is efficiently internalized and potently presented to T cells by antigen-presenting cells, which stimulated T-cell responses in 100 times lower doses compared with native allergens. In a double-blind, placebo-controlled clinical trial, the MAT-Fel d 1 vaccine was administered in 3 increasing doses into inguinal lymph nodes at 4-week intervals. In addition to a good safety profile, only 3 doses of MAT-Fel d 1 intra-lymph node vaccination induced clinical tolerance to nasal cat allergen challenge in parallel with T-cell tolerance and increased serum IgG_4 and interleukin (IL)-10 levels.[38,39] Currently this approach is being pursued for veterinary vaccine development.

ALLERGOIDS, RECOMBINANT ALLERGENS

Targeting T cells to induce T-cell tolerance and bypassing IgE binding to avoid IgE-mediated side effects is an essential approach in AIT.[40] To improve AIT safety, the primary aim is to use hypoallergenic molecules to prevent severe complications such as anaphylaxis. Currently, there are many modified allergen preparations (allergoids) in the market with decreased IgE binding activity. Chemical modification of allergen extracts (eg, with glutaraldehyde[41]) aims to prevent IgE cross-link with conformational epitopes, while linear epitopes are preserved. To accomplish this aim, several successful new approaches have been developed,[42,43] including mixture of T-cell epitope peptides,[44] allergen fragments,[45] fusion proteins,[36,37] and recombinant allergen hybrids.[46] The prototype of this approach is peptide immunotherapy that uses linear T-cell epitope peptides, and has shown promising results,[47,48] although it still faces challenges in phase III clinical trials.[49–51] All of these allergoid preparations enable the administration of the allergens in higher doses to efficiently induce T-cell tolerance without the risk of anaphylaxis.[40] Conjugation of allergoids to nonoxidized mannan facilitates their uptake by antigen-presenting cells.[52,53]

Some of the clinically significant allergens, however, may be poorly represented in allergen extracts. Development of molecular vaccines, based on recombinant allergen components, helps to overcome the limitations of the vaccines based on natural allergen extracts.[54] Identification of immunodominant molecular components of the allergens is an important initial step of the development of such AIT approaches.[55]

ADD-ON THERAPIES AND NEW PROTOCOLS

Combination of conventional or novel methods of AIT with biological immune response modifiers is a promising new therapeutic approach. Anti-IgE combined with AIT has been evaluated in several studies. Significant decrease in the risk of anaphylaxis and improved rescue medication scores were observed during rush immunotherapy with a quicker dose increment and reach of the maintenance dose.[56,57] Accumulating evidence suggests that anti-IgE treatment is a valuable add-on to AIT for airway allergies, especially to prevent adverse events in the build-up phase and improve safety profile in cases in which the designated maintenance dose is not tolerated by the patient.[58,59] Other possible combinations include anti-IL-4 or anti-IL-13 as well as their receptor antagonists.

Different routes of vaccine administration also have been proposed to improve efficacy and safety. Intralymphatic vaccination and epicutaneous vaccination are recently pursued novel strategies. Both showed similar efficacy to SCIT in grass pollen allergy, however, that has been reached with fewer injections and lower total allergen doses.[60] Intralymphatic administration induces T-cell tolerance or strong T_H1 responses depending on the type of vaccine used.[39,61]

Meta-analysis of the double-blind, placebo-controlled trials has shown that sublingual immunotherapy (SLIT) is safe and clinically efficacious with a treatment benefit approximately half of that achieved with SCIT.[62] Disease-modifying effects of SLIT have been confirmed in large-scale randomized, double-blind, placebo-controlled trials also in children[63–68]; and even its preventive administration has been proposed.[69]

In an exciting, current study, cat-allergic patients were treated with a single dose of 2, fully human, recombinant IgG_4-blocking antibodies specific for Fel d 1, the major cat allergen. This treatment resulted in a rapid and sustained reduction in clinical symptoms after nasal allergen provocation test, suggesting a new, quick, passive AIT strategy for allergies.[70] Treatment-emergent adverse events were closely monitored during the study, and there was neither any difference in the frequency of the adverse events between antibody-treated and placebo group, nor did any severe adverse event occur in relation to the IgG_4 antibody treatment.[70]

In a recent mouse experiment, the administration of anti-IgE antibody during pregnancy caused long-term IgE-class–specific immunosuppression in the offspring that was able to prevent allergic sensitization. These results suggest that it may be possible to develop a vaccination strategy aiming prenatal allergy prevention.[71]

Reduced side-effects
- Chemically modified allergen
- Recombinant allergen peptides
- Conjugation to nonoxidized mannan
- CD33 ligand

Encapsulation
- Liposomes
- Carbohydrate-based particles
- Virus-like particles

Addressing constructs
- MAT vaccine

Improved adjuvants
- Microcrystalline tyrosine

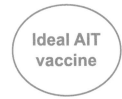

Ideal AIT vaccine

Conjugation to microbial products
- Monophosphoryl lipid A
- GpG oligonucleotide
- Hepatitis B PreS protein
- α-galactosylceramide
- Vibrio cholerae neuraminidase
- Neisseria meningitides proteoliposome
- Tetanus toxoid fragment

New routes and add-ons
- Intralymphatic administration
- Epicutaneous administration
- Single dose recombinant IgG_4
- Add-on anti-IgE

Fig. 1. Strategies for development of a more safe, efficient, and reliable vaccine for AIT.

SUMMARY

Intensive efforts have been invested to improve AIT vaccines by making them more efficient, convenient, and safe[2,16] (**Fig. 1**). Still, fewer than 10% of allergic patients choose to receive AIT.[72] Besides the fear from potential side effects and poor adherence due to long duration of treatment,[73] the possible cause of weak overall, population-wide efficiency of AIT is that not all the potential influencing factors were considered during the development of AIT strategies, because of lack of knowledge. Identification of good biomarkers predicting beneficial vaccine immune response is still an unmet clinical need; however, it is under intensive investigation.[74] Better understanding of the immune response to vaccines will hopefully enable us to develop more efficient AIT strategies specifically tailored to allergic disease endotypes.[75]

ACKNOWLEDGMENTS

The laboratory of Z.I. Komlósi is supported by Hungarian Pediatric Oncology Network. The laboratories of C.A. Akdis and M. Akdis are supported by the Swiss National Science Foundation.

REFERENCES

1. Casale TB, Stokes JR. Immunotherapy: what lies beyond. J Allergy Clin Immunol 2014;133(3):612–9 [quiz: 620].
2. Agache I. EAACI guidelines on allergen immunotherapy—out with the old and in with the new. Allergy 2018;73(4):737–8.
3. Pfaar O, Bonini S, Cardona V, et al. Perspectives in allergen immunotherapy: 2017 and beyond. Allergy 2018;73(Suppl 104):5–23.
4. Pfaar O, Lou H, Zhang Y, et al. Recent developments and highlights in allergen immunotherapy. Allergy 2018;73(12):2274–89.
5. Zielen S, Devillier P, Heinrich J, et al. Sublingual immunotherapy provides long-term relief in allergic rhinitis and reduces the risk of asthma: a retrospective, real-world database analysis. Allergy 2018;73(1):165–77.
6. Passalacqua G, Baena-Cagnani CE, Bousquet J, et al. Grading local side effects of sublingual immunotherapy for respiratory allergy: speaking the same language. J Allergy Clin Immunol 2013;132(1):93–8.
7. Jones SM, Burks AW, Dupont C. State of the art on food allergen immunotherapy: oral, sublingual, and epicutaneous. J Allergy Clin Immunol 2014;133(2):318–23.
8. Vickery BP, Scurlock AM, Kulis M, et al. Sustained unresponsiveness to peanut in subjects who have completed peanut oral immunotherapy. J Allergy Clin Immunol 2014;133(2):468–75.
9. Wahn U, Bachert C, Heinrich J, et al. Real-world benefits of allergen immunotherapy for birch pollen-associated allergic rhinitis and asthma. Allergy 2019; 74(3):594–604.
10. Roberts G, Pfaar O, Akdis CA, et al. EAACI guidelines on allergen immunotherapy: allergic rhinoconjunctivitis. Allergy 2018;73(4):765–98.
11. Sturm GJ, Varga EM, Roberts G, et al. EAACI guidelines on allergen immunotherapy: hymenoptera venom allergy. Allergy 2018;73(4):744–64.
12. Pajno GB, Fernandez-Rivas M, Arasi S, et al. EAACI Guidelines on allergen immunotherapy: IgE-mediated food allergy. Allergy 2018;73(4):799–815.
13. Holt PG, Sly PD, Sampson HA, et al. Prophylactic use of sublingual allergen immunotherapy in high-risk children: a pilot study. J Allergy Clin Immunol 2013; 132(4):991–3.e1.

14. Bonertz A, Roberts GC, Hoefnagel M, et al. Challenges in the implementation of EAACI guidelines on allergen immunotherapy: a global perspective on the regulation of allergen products. Allergy 2018;73(1):64–76.
15. Larenas-Linnemann DES, Antolin-Amerigo D, Parisi C, et al. National clinical practice guidelines for allergen immunotherapy: an international assessment applying AGREE-II. Allergy 2018;73(3):664–72.
16. Muraro A, Roberts G, Halken S, et al. EAACI guidelines on allergen immunotherapy: executive statement. Allergy 2018;73(4):739–43.
17. Creticos PS, Schroeder JT, Hamilton RG, et al. Immunotherapy with a ragweed-toll-like receptor 9 agonist vaccine for allergic rhinitis. N Engl J Med 2006; 355(14):1445–55.
18. Kundig TM, Senti G, Schnetzler G, et al. Der p 1 peptide on virus-like particles is safe and highly immunogenic in healthy adults. J Allergy Clin Immunol 2006; 117(6):1470–6.
19. Engeroff P, Caviezel F, Storni F, et al. Allergens displayed on virus-like particles are highly immunogenic but fail to activate human mast cells. Allergy 2018; 73(2):341–9.
20. Thunberg S, Neimert-Andersson T, Cheng Q, et al. Prolonged antigen-exposure with carbohydrate particle based vaccination prevents allergic immune responses in sensitized mice. Allergy 2009;64(6):919–26.
21. Rosewich M, Schulze J, Eickmeier O, et al. Tolerance induction after specific immunotherapy with pollen allergoids adjuvanted by monophosphoryl lipid A in children. Clin Exp Immunol 2010;160(3):403–10.
22. Di Felice G, Colombo P. Nanoparticle-allergen complexes for allergen immunotherapy. Int J Nanomedicine 2017;12:4493–504.
23. Pohlit H, Bellinghausen I, Frey H, et al. Recent advances in the use of nanoparticles for allergen-specific immunotherapy. Allergy 2017;72(10):1461–74.
24. Suzuki S, Sakurai D, Sakurai T, et al. Sublingual administration of liposomes enclosing alpha-galactosylceramide as an effective adjuvant of allergen immunotherapy in a murine model of allergic rhinitis. Allergol Int 2019;68(3):352–62.
25. Duan S, Koziol-White CJ, Jester WF Jr, et al. CD33 recruitment inhibits IgE-mediated anaphylaxis and desensitizes mast cells to allergen. J Clin Invest 2019;129(3): 1387–401.
26. Roger A, Depreux N, Jurgens Y, et al. A novel microcrystalline tyrosine-adsorbed, mite-allergoid subcutaneous immunotherapy: 1-year follow-up report. Immunotherapy 2016;8(10):1169–74.
27. Baldrick P, Richardson D, Wheeler AW. Review of L-tyrosine confirming its safe human use as an adjuvant. J Appl Toxicol 2002;22(5):333–44.
28. Zielen S, Gabrielpillai J, Herrmann E, et al. Long-term effect of monophosphoryl lipid A adjuvanted specific immunotherapy in patients with grass pollen allergy. Immunotherapy 2018;10(7):529–36.
29. Zahirovic A, Lunder M. Microbial delivery vehicles for allergens and allergen-derived peptides in immunotherapy of allergic diseases. Front Microbiol 2018; 9:1449.
30. Diesner SC, Bergmayr C, Wang XY, et al. Characterization of *Vibrio cholerae* neuraminidase as an immunomodulator for novel formulation of oral allergy immunotherapy. Clin Immunol 2018;192:30–9.
31. Ramirez W, Bourg V, Torralba D, et al. Safety of a proteoliposome from *Neisseria meningitides* as adjuvant for a house dust mite allergy vaccine. J Immunotoxicol 2017;14(1):152–9.

32. Anzaghe M, Schulke S, Scheurer S. Virus-like particles as carrier systems to enhance immunomodulation in allergen immunotherapy. Curr Allergy Asthma Rep 2018;18(12):71.
33. Leb VM, Jahn-Schmid B, Kueng HJ, et al. Modulation of allergen-specific T-lymphocyte function by virus-like particles decorated with HLA class II molecules. J Allergy Clin Immunol 2009;124(1):121–8.
34. Schmitz N, Dietmeier K, Bauer M, et al. Displaying Fel d1 on virus-like particles prevents reactogenicity despite greatly enhanced immunogenicity: a novel therapy for cat allergy. J Exp Med 2009;206(9):1941–55.
35. Focke-Tejkl M, Weber M, Niespodziana K, et al. Development and characterization of a recombinant, hypoallergenic, peptide-based vaccine for grass pollen allergy. J Allergy Clin Immunol 2015;135(5). 1207–7.e1-11.
36. Niederberger V, Neubauer A, Gevaert P, et al. Safety and efficacy of immunotherapy with the recombinant B-cell epitope-based grass pollen vaccine BM32. J Allergy Clin Immunol 2018;142(2):497–509.e9.
37. Fanuel S, Tabesh S, Mokhtarian K, et al. Construction of a recombinant B-cell epitope vaccine based on a Der p1-derived hypoallergen: a bioinformatics approach. Immunotherapy 2018;10(7):537–53.
38. Senti G, Crameri R, Kuster D, et al. Intralymphatic immunotherapy for cat allergy induces tolerance after only 3 injections. J Allergy Clin Immunol 2012;129(5):1290–6.
39. Zaleska A, Eiwegger T, Soyer O, et al. Immune regulation by intralymphatic immunotherapy with modular allergen translocation MAT vaccine. Allergy 2014;69(9):1162–70.
40. Akdis CA, Blaser K. Bypassing IgE and targeting T cells for specific immunotherapy of allergy. Trends Immunol 2001;22:175–8.
41. Rauber MM, Wu HK, Adams B, et al. Birch pollen allergen-specific immunotherapy with glutaraldehyde-modified allergoid induces IL-10 secretion and protective antibody responses. Allergy 2019;74(8):1575–9.
42. Marth K, Focke-Tejkl M, Lupinek C, et al. Allergen peptides, recombinant allergens and hypoallergens for allergen-specific immunotherapy. Curr Treat Options Allergy 2014;1:91–106.
43. Akdis CA. Therapies for allergic inflammation: refining strategies to induce tolerance. Nat Med 2012;18(5):736–49.
44. Prickett SR, Rolland JM, O'Hehir RE. Immunoregulatory T cell epitope peptides: the new frontier in allergy therapy. Clin Exp Allergy 2015;45(6):1015–26.
45. Niederberger V, Horak F, Vrtala S, et al. Vaccination with genetically engineered allergens prevents progression of allergic disease. Proc Natl Acad Sci U S A 2004;101(Suppl 2):14677–82.
46. Asturias JA, Ibarrola I, Arilla MC, et al. Engineering of major house dust mite allergens Der p 1 and Der p 2 for allergen-specific immunotherapy. Clin Exp Allergy 2009;39(7):1088–98.
47. Worm M, Lee HH, Kleine-Tebbe J, et al. Development and preliminary clinical evaluation of a peptide immunotherapy vaccine for cat allergy. J Allergy Clin Immunol 2011;127(1):89–97, 97.e1-14.
48. Spertini F, Perrin Y, Audran R, et al. Safety and immunogenicity of immunotherapy with Bet v 1-derived contiguous overlapping peptides. J Allergy Clin Immunol 2014;134(1):239–40.e13.
49. Mosges R, Bachert C, Panzner P, et al. Short course of grass allergen peptides immunotherapy over 3 weeks reduces seasonal symptoms in allergic

rhinoconjunctivitis with/without asthma: a randomized, multicenter, double-blind, placebo-controlled trial. Allergy 2018;73(9):1842–50.

50. Mosges R, Kasche EM, Raskopf E, et al. A randomized, double-blind, placebo-controlled, dose-finding trial with Lolium perenne peptide immunotherapy. Allergy 2018;73(4):896–904.

51. Mosges R, Koch AF, Raskopf E, et al. Lolium perenne peptide immunotherapy is well tolerated and elicits a protective B-cell response in seasonal allergic rhinitis patients. Allergy 2018;73(6):1254–62.

52. Benito-Villalvilla C, Soria I, Subiza JL, et al. Novel vaccines targeting dendritic cells by coupling allergoids to mannan. Allergo J Int 2018;27(8):256–62.

53. Soria I, Lopez-Relano J, Vinuela M, et al. Oral myeloid cells uptake allergoids coupled to mannan driving Th1/Treg responses upon sublingual delivery in mice. Allergy 2018;73(4):875–84.

54. Hoffmann HJ, Valovirta E, Pfaar O, et al. Novel approaches and perspectives in allergen immunotherapy. Allergy 2017;72(7):1022–34.

55. Curin M, Garmatiuk T, Resch-Marat Y, et al. Similar localization of conformational IgE epitopes on the house dust mite allergens Der p 5 and Der p 21 despite limited IgE cross-reactivity. Allergy 2018;73(8):1653–61.

56. Klunker S, Saggar LR, Seyfert-Margolis V, et al. Combination treatment with omalizumab and rush immunotherapy for ragweed-induced allergic rhinitis: inhibition of IgE-facilitated allergen binding. J Allergy Clin Immunol 2007;120(3):688–95.

57. Larenas-Linnemann D, Wahn U, Kopp M. Use of omalizumab to improve desensitization safety in allergen immunotherapy. J Allergy Clin Immunol 2014;133(3):937–937.e2.

58. Lombardi C, Canonica GW, Passalacqua G. Allergen immunotherapy as add-on to biologic agents. Curr Opin Allergy Clin Immunol 2018;18(6):502–8.

59. Dantzer JA, Wood RA. The use of omalizumab in allergen immunotherapy. Clin Exp Allergy 2018;48(3):232–40.

60. von Moos S, Johansen P, Tay F, et al. Comparing safety of abrasion and tape-stripping as skin preparation in allergen-specific epicutaneous immunotherapy. J Allergy Clin Immunol 2014;134(4):965–7.e4.

61. Kundig TM, Johansen P, Bachmann MF, et al. Intralymphatic immunotherapy: time interval between injections is essential. J Allergy Clin Immunol 2014;133(3):930–1.

62. Devillier P, Dreyfus JF, Demoly P, et al. A meta-analysis of sublingual allergen immunotherapy and pharmacotherapy in pollen-induced seasonal allergic rhinoconjunctivitis. BMC Med 2014;12:71.

63. Matsuoka T, Bernstein DI, Masuyama K, et al. Pooled efficacy and safety data for house dust mite sublingual immunotherapy tablets in adolescents. Pediatr Allergy Immunol 2017;28(7):661–7.

64. Gotoh M, Yonekura S, Imai T, et al. Long-term efficacy and dose-finding trial of japanese cedar pollen sublingual immunotherapy tablet. J Allergy Clin Immunol Pract 2019;7(4):1287–97.e8.

65. Okamoto Y, Fujieda S, Okano M, et al. Efficacy of house dust mite sublingual tablet in the treatment of allergic rhinoconjunctivitis: a randomized trial in a pediatric population. Pediatr Allergy Immunol 2019;30(1):66–73.

66. Masuyama K, Okamoto Y, Okamiya K, et al. Efficacy and safety of SQ house dust mite sublingual immunotherapy-tablet in Japanese children. Allergy 2018;73(12):2352–63.

67. Demoly P, Kleine-Tebbe J, Rehm D. Clinical benefits of treatment with SQ house dust mite sublingual tablet in house dust mite allergic rhinitis. Allergy 2017;72(10):1576–8.

68. Okamoto Y, Fujieda S, Okano M, et al. House dust mite sublingual tablet is effective and safe in patients with allergic rhinitis. Allergy 2017;72(3):435–43.
69. Ponce M, Schroeder F, Bannert C, et al. Preventive sublingual immunotherapy with House Dust Mite extract modulates epitope diversity in pre-school children. Allergy 2019;74(4):780–7.
70. Orengo JM, Radin AR, Kamat V, et al. Treating cat allergy with monoclonal IgG antibodies that bind allergen and prevent IgE engagement. Nat Commun 2018; 9(1):1421.
71. Morita H, Tamari M, Fujiwara M, et al. IgE-class-specific immunosuppression in offspring by administration of anti-IgE to pregnant mice. J Allergy Clin Immunol 2019;143(3):1261–4.e6.
72. Leuthard DS, Duda A, Freiberger SN, et al. Microcrystalline tyrosine and aluminum as adjuvants in allergen-specific immunotherapy protect from IgE-mediated reactivity in mouse models and act independently of inflammasome and TLR signaling. J Immunol 2018;200(9):3151–9.
73. Mao J, Heithoff KA, Koep E, et al. Cost of subcutaneous immunotherapy in a large insured population in the United States. Curr Med Res Opin 2019;35(2): 351–8.
74. Shamji MH, Kappen JH, Akdis M, et al. Biomarkers for monitoring clinical efficacy of allergen immunotherapy for allergic rhinoconjunctivitis and allergic asthma: an EAACI Position Paper. Allergy 2017;72(8):1156–73.
75. Sugita K, Sokolowska M, Akdis CA. Key points for moving the endotypes field forward. In: Agache I, Hellings P, editors. Implementing precision medicine in best practices of chronic airway diseases. London: Elsevier; 2018. p. 107–14.

Subcutaneous Immunotherapy Safety
Incidence per Surveys and Risk Factors

Mario Sánchez-Borges, MD[a],*, David I. Bernstein, MD[b,c],
Chris Calabria, MD[d]

KEYWORDS

- Allergen immunotherapy • Anaphylaxis • Immunotherapy
- Subcutaneous immunotherapy • Venom immunotherapy

KEY POINTS

- Subcutaneous immunotherapy (SCIT) is effective in children and adults suffering allergic rhinitis, asthma, and insect venom hypersensitivity.
- The treatment is based on the clinical relevance of allergens as assessed by a detailed allergologic evaluation and the availability of standardized or good-quality allergenic extracts.
- SCIT is indicated in patients with persistent symptoms despite appropriate medications.
- Physicians should be aware of the possibility of severe adverse reactions from SCIT.
- Risk assessment should be performed for each patient before initiating SCIT and measures should be implemented to prevent untoward reactions to SCIT.

INTRODUCTION

Allergic rhinitis is the fifth most common chronic disease in the United States. Allergen-specific immunotherapy is currently the only therapeutic modality able to modify Th2 immune responses and reduce symptoms elicited by environmental exposure to aeroallergens. Although subcutaneous immunotherapy (SCIT) is generally safe and effective for treating allergic rhinoconjunctivitis, asthma, and Hymenoptera venom

Conflicts of Interest: None.
Funding: Supported by investigator's funds.
[a] Allergy and Clinical Immunology Department, Centro Médico Docente La Trinidad and Clínica El Avila, 6a transversal Urb. Altamira, piso 8, consultorio 803, Caracas 1060, Venezuela; [b] Division of Immunology, Allergy and Rheumatology, Department of Medicine, University of Cincinnati College of Medicine, 231 Albert Sabin Way, Cincinnati, OH 45267-0563, USA; [c] Bernstein Clinical Research Center, Cincinnati, OH, USA; [d] Department of Allergy and Immunology, Wilford Hall Medical Center, Lackland Air Force Base, 1100 Wilford Hall Loop, San Antonio, TX 78236, USA
* Corresponding author.
E-mail address: sanchezbmario@gmail.com

hypersensitivity and the risk of systemic allergic reactions (SRs) remains low, near-fatal and fatal anaphylaxis may occur. Therefore, optimizing safety remains an important goal for both allergists and patients.

Clinical indications that have been established for SCIT are presented in **Box 1**.

There are some medical conditions that contraindicate the administration of allergen-specific SCIT (**Box 2**).

Factors that contribute to adverse reactions to SCIT include the type of allergen, patient selection, schedule of treatment, and the use of pretreatment. Studies done between 1980 and 1989 established the safety of SCIT when performed on carefully selected patients by experienced physicians who exercised caution and provided adequate monitoring.

In a survey done in the period 1990 to 2001 the incidence of fatal reactions was one in every 2.5 million injection visits or approximately 3.4 fatal reactions per year.[1]

This article summarizes the epidemiologic data currently available on SRs induced by SCIT, risk factors for severe reactions, preventive measures recommended to avoid morbidity and mortality from this type of treatment, and patient management in various clinical settings.

EPIDEMIOLOGY OF SYSTEMIC REACTIONS INDUCED BY SUBCUTANEOUS IMMUNOTHERAPY
Nonfatal Reactions

Different surveys to ascertain the incidence of nonfatal SRs to SCIT have varied (**Table 1**). From 1981 to 1990, one hundred fifteen SRs occurred (5.2% of patients and 0.06% of injections).[2] From 1991 to 2000 there were 26 SRs reported in Italy (1.08% of patients and 0.01% of injections).[3] There were 23 unconfirmed reactions per year reported between 1990 and 2001 or 5.4 events per million injections.[4]

Another study by Phillips and colleagues[5] reported SRs in 4% of patients, with no late-phase or protracted phase reactions. In the US surveillance study among practicing allergists, there were approximately 10 SRs per 10,000 injection visits or 0.1% of allergy injection visits reported between 2008 and 2011, and 3 of every 100,000 were graded as severe anaphylaxis (0.003%) with similar rates in years 2 and 3 of the same survey.[6]

Between 2008 and 2016, SRs were observed in 80% to 85% of allergy practices in the United States and during 0.1% of injection visits.[7] When the World Allergy Organization grading system, which includes 4 severity grades (grade 1, Mild; grade 2, moderate; grade3, severe; and grade 4, very severe) was applied, it was observed that annually there were 8.7 SRs per 10,000 injection visits (grade 1: 5.6; grade 2: 2.7; grade 3: 0.35 SRs per 10,000 injection visits) and one grade 4 reaction in every 160,000 injection visits from 2012 to 2016.[7]

Box 1
Indications for allergen-specific immunotherapy

- Allergic rhinitis and asthma symptoms induced by prolonged intermittent or persistent allergen exposure.
- Hymenoptera venom hypersensitivity.
- Atopic dermatitis.
- Patients inadequately controlled with pharmacologic therapy.
- Patients who do not wish to take constant or prolonged pharmacotherapy.
- Patients who experience adverse effects from pharmacotherapy.

Box 2
Relative contraindications for allergen-specific immunotherapy

- Severe asthma.
- Uncontrolled asthma at the time of the injection.
- Autoimmune diseases that are not well controlled.
- Malignancies undergoing active treatment.
- Concomitant treatment with β-blockers.
- Pregnancy (may continue on maintenance).

SRs occurred in 0.6% of patients receiving SCIT injections from 2013 to 2016, with grade 4 life-threatening reactions in 0.005% of patients (1 in 20,000 treated patients). Overall nonfatal SRs did not increase from 2008 to 2016 and grade 1 SRs (mild) showed a tendency to decline. In general, SR rates from SCIT have remained stable, but there has been an increase in reported fatalities in recent years.

Fatal Reactions

The first report of a fatal reaction (FR) from SCIT was published by Lamson in 1924 (**Table 2**).[8] Six additional cases were observed between 1932 and 1980.[9] In a study in which more than one million injections were given to 8700 patients between 1935 and 1955, no fatalities were found.[10] Also, no fatalities were observed in a second study in which there were SRs in 25 out of 2989 patients.[11]

In 1988, 13 fatalities from SCIT were reported.[12] At that time there was another study reporting 40 fatalities in the United States,[13] with a total number of 46 FRs between 1945 and 1984, and 26 in the United Kingdom between 1957 and 1986.[14] Mean age was 34 years and there was no gender predilection. In Germany 40 fatalities occurred between 1977 and 1994.[15] Another survey found 17 deaths between 1985 and 1989.[16] Mean age was 36 years, including 5 men and 11 women. The survey

---

Table 1
Incidence of nonfatal systemic reactions to subcutaneous immunotherapy

Author, Year of Publication	Period of Study	Incidence
Ragusa et al,[2] 1997	1981–1990	N = 115 (5.2% of patients and 0.06% of injections)
Ragusa & Massolo,[3] 2004	1991–2000	N = 26 (1.08% of patients and 0.01% of injections)
Amin et al,[4] 2006	1990–2001	N = 23 per y; 5.4 per million injections
Bernstein et al,[19] 2010	2008–2016	80%–85% of allergy practices; 0.1% of injection visits; 8.7 per 10,000 injections
Phillips et al,[5] 2011	NA	4% of patients
Epstein et al,[6] 2013	2008–2011	10.2 per 10,000 injection visits (0.1% of injection visits); 3% severe (3 per 100000 injection visits)
Epstein et al,[20] 2019	2013–2016	0.6%

Abbreviation: NA, not available.

Table 2
Incidence of fatal reactions to subcutaneous immunotherapy

Author, Year of Publication	Period of Study	Incidence
Lamson,[8] 1924	1924	1 case report
Van Arsdel & Sherman,[10] 1957	1935–1955	0 FRs
CSM update, U.K.,[14] 1986	1957–1980	26 FRs
Hepner et al,[11] 1987	-	0 FRs 25 SRs out of 2989 patients
Rawlins et al,[12] 1988	1988	13 FRs
Rieckenberg et al,[13] 1990	1945–1984	46 FRs
Reid et al,[16] 1993	1985–1989	17 FRs
Lüderitz-Puchel et al,[15] 1996	1977–1994	40 FRs
Reid & Gurka,[17] 1996	1990–1995	27 FRs
Bernstein et al,[1] 2004	1990–2001	41 FRs 1 in every 2.5 million injection visits
Bernstein et al,[19] 2010	2001–2007	6 FRs
Bagg & Lockey,[9] 2014	1932–1980	6 cases
Epstein et al,[7] 2016	2008–2013	4 FRs
Epstein et al,[20] 2019	2008–2017	7 FRs 0.8 FRs per year 6 per 54.4 million injection visits 1 in every 9.1 million injection visits

for 1990 to 1995 reported 27 deaths (5 deaths per year).[17] Annual rates of FRs in the United States were estimated at 3.4 per year in the period 1990 to 2001 or 1 per 2.5 million injections with 41 confirmed FRs and near-fatal reactions in that period of time.[1,18] From 2001 to 2007, six FRs from SCIT were confirmed.[19] In 2008 to 2013, four FR to SCIT occurred, a decrease when compared with the incidence in 1990 to 2001. In this survey 14% of reactions began 30 minutes after the injection, most being mild or moderate and none fatal. Incidence of grade 4 SRs was 1 in every 100000 injection visits.[7]

In a study of 54.4 million injection visits between 2008 and 2017, seven fatalities from SCIT were observed or 0.8 FR per year. Fifteen percent of all reported SRs occurred 30 minutes or more after the injection.[20] Between 2008 and 2016 the rate of FRs from SCIT was calculated in 6 per 54.4 million injection visits or 1 fatality in every 9.1 million injection visits.

The rate of SCIT-associated SRs with conventional nonaccelerated buildup protocols is low, 0.1% to 0.2% (1 in 500–1 in 1000 injections),[21] although it is higher if accelerated cluster or rush buildup regimens are used.[22,23]

Delayed Reactions

These are defined as SRs occurring more than 30 minutes after injections. Incidences of delayed reactions in North American clinics have been estimated to be 14% of all SRs and 15% of SRs identified from 2014 to 2016.[24] Only 0.5% of SRs occur after 60 minutes.[20]

Pediatric Data

Data on SRs and fatalities from SCIT in children are scarce. In a European study that included 1500 patients, 1.53% (24 patients) experienced 29 SRs, and only 3 reactions were identified as anaphylaxis. In this study the risk of SRs was lower in dust mite–sensitized patients when compared with pollen-allergic patients.[25] The incidence of SR was 0.017 per patient year and 72.4% were late-phase reactions.

Venom Immunotherapy

Of 1410 patients who received SCIT with Hymenoptera venoms, 171 experienced 323 SRs, 28 of them (9%) severe but not fatal.[26] For immunotherapy with Hymenoptera venoms it has been observed that honeybee venom injections present a relatively higher risk of SRs. Among factors that predict severe SRs to these vaccines, basophil activation assay (CD63 expression), and a short interval between the insect sting and onset of symptoms (<5 minutes), have been proposed as risk factors.[27]

RISKS OF SUBCUTANEOUS ALLERGEN IMMUNOTHERAPY

Allergen immunotherapy is a proven, highly effective treatment of patients with allergic rhinitis, immunoglobulin E–dependent asthma, and prevention of stinging insect anaphylaxis.[21] It is not surprising, however, that systemic exposure to potent allergens during SCIT can elicit SRs and rarely, life-threatening anaphylaxis in highly sensitized patients. SCIT injections are generally well tolerated and those patients likely to benefit are relatively easy to identify. Recognition of those patients who may be at higher risk for SRs is an essential part of making the decision to recommend SCIT. Once started, it is important to continuously reassess the risk versus benefit as treated patients progress from build-up to maintenance injections. For example, a patient who experiences recurrent SRs after achieving maintenance SCIT doses should be reassessed and a decision on whether to continue treatment is appropriate. This section reviews available evidence pertaining to recognized risk factors for injection-related SRs and fatal anaphylaxis.

Over the last 50 years, our understanding of risk factors for SCIT SRs has been enhanced by retrospective evaluation of reported cases of fatal anaphylaxis. Between 1973 and 2001, the American Academy of Allergy, Asthma, & Immunology (AAAAI) sponsored data collection of fatal SCIT reactions voluntarily reported by treating allergists.[1,16,20,28] During this period 89 FRs were identified, yielding important clues from detailed physician reports regarding contributing risk factors. Between 1990 and 2001 during which the numbers of injections were collected, one FR was estimated to have occurred in every 2.5 million injection visits.[1] From 2008 to 2016, the estimated rate of FRs was 1 in 9,000,000 injection visits.[20] The latter incidence rates are estimates and subject to reporting bias. Circumstances presumed to contribute to these fatal events according to the treating physicians have been very helpful in identifying important risk factors for injection-related anaphylaxis. As shown in **Box 3**, these include administration of injections to patients with uncontrolled and severe asthma; prior history of SRs to injections; administration of injections during the height of pollen season when patients are symptomatic; failure or delay in timely administration of epinephrine; allergen dosing errors; inadequate observation time after injections; and administration of injections in an inadequately supervised or suboptimal setting (eg, at home or outside clinic).

To enhance information provided by retrospective surveys of fatal reactions, the annual North American Surveillance Survey of SCIT-related SRs was initiated among practicing member allergists in 2008, cosponsored by the AAAAI and American College of Allergy, Asthma, and Immunology.[19] This survey has gathered data to assess annual incidence of nonfatal SRs of varying severity. During this period, 7 confirmed FRs have been confirmed. Overall, one SR of any severity was reported

Box 3
Risk factors identified by reporting physicians for fatal allergic reactions to subcutaneous immunotherapy in 2 retrospective surveys

1. Uncontrolled asthma.
2. History of prior injection-related systemic allergic reactions.
3. Administration during the peak pollen seasons.
4. Emergency epinephrine not given or delayed.
5. Dosing or administration errors of therapeutic allergens.
6. No contributing factor was identified.
7. Inadequate postinjection observation time.
8. Reactions began 30 minutes after administration.
9. Fatal injections given at home or unsupervised setting.
10. Administration of β-blockers and angiotensin converting enzyme inhibitors.

Data from Bernstein DI, Wanner M, Borish L, et al. Twelve-year survey of fatal reactions to allergen injections and skin testing: 1990-2001. J Allergy Clin Immunol 2004;113:1129-36; and Reid MJ, Lockey RF, Turkeltaub PC, et al. Survey of fatalities from skin testing and immunotherapy 1985-1989. J Allergy Clin Immunol 1993;92(1 Pt 1):6-15.

to occur every 1000 injection visits. The survey has also investigated many specific questions regarding clinical SCIT practices and how these may or may not affect risk of SRs, including delayed onset SRs (>30 minutes); routine administration of epinephrine autoinjectors to all treated patients; accelerated build-up protocols; administration of injections during peak pollen seasons; and the impact of higher therapeutic allergen doses. Evidence supporting specific contributing factors to fatal and nonfatal reactions is discussed in the following section.

Risk of Uncontrolled Asthma

Uncontrolled asthma remains the most frequently identified factor contributing to fatal SCIT SRs. In a survey of confirmed fatal reactions that occurred between 1990 and 2001, most patients had poor asthma control as well as prior emergency department visits or hospitalizations for asthma.[1] Most fatal reactions were characterized with acute bronchospasm (50%) and/or respiratory failure (94%). In a retrospective survey of treating allergists reporting near-fatal anaphylactic reactions, administration during the height of pollen season (46%) and dosing errors (25%) were cited as the most frequent contributing factors, with uncontrolled asthma implicated in just 10% of cases.[4] In 2 published reviews of fatal SCIT reactions (1985–2001), 62% of all fatal SCIT reactions were associated with uncontrolled asthma.[1,16] Four of seven fatal SRs identified between 2009 and 2017 were diagnosed with either persistent or severe asthma.[2] Analysis of a special survey conducted in Year 5 (2012–13) suggested that allergy practices that always avoided the administration of SCIT injections to patients with uncontrolled asthma (ie, an Asthma Control test score <20) experienced fewer severe Grade 3 and 4 SRs (WAO Grading Criteria) than practices not following this protocol.[7,29]

Prior Systemic Reactions

A history of prior SRs seems to enhance the risk of severe fatal and near-fatal SRs after SCIT injections.[1,4,16] The North American survey data in Year 2 (2009–10) also identified that 26% of all SRs of any severity was preceded by a prior SR and that 36% of severe anaphylactic reactions to SCIT had been preceeded by prior reported SRs (Epstein TG, 2013, personal communication). Thus, those patients receiving SCIT with prior histories of SRs seem to be worthy of intensive efforts to prevent future reactions (eg, adjusting dosages).

Postinjection Observation Period and Late-Onset Systemic Reactions

Because most fatal allergic reactions after SCIT injections have occurred within the first 30 minutes, the Allergy Immunotherapy Practice Parameter recommends all patients be observed for 30 minutes. The latest survey data indicated that 73% of clinical practices follow this recommendation and 24% observe patients for less than 30 minutes after injections.[20] The need to observe for 30 minutes has been questioned by data from single practices suggesting that as many as 50% of SRs began after 30 minutes.[30] In the data collected in the North American Survey representing hundreds of practices during 2 separate annual surveys, approximately 15% of SRs were reported to have begun after 30 minutes.[20,24] Nearly all late-onset reactions were Grade 1 and 2 and no FRs were identified supporting the Practice Parameter recommendation.[21]

It is noteworthy that about 30% of all allergists routinely prescribe emergency epinephrine autoinjectors to all patients on SCIT. In the most recent annual survey only one-third of patients who experienced severe delayed Grade 3 and 4 reactions (10 of 30) and were prescribed epinephrine autoinjectors used the device during the SR. Practices that prescribed epinephrine to greater than90% of patients receiving SCIT were no less likely to experience delayed severe SRs than those who did not follow this practice.[20] Because of poor adherence with epinephrine self-administration, prescribing autoinjectors for all patients is not an effective alternative to observing patients for at least 30 minutes following SCIT injections.

Peak Pollen Season

As mentioned, the administration of injections during patients' peak symptomatic pollen seasons has been consistently implicated in fatal and near-fatal injection–related anaphylaxis.[4] A study comparing relative severity of SRs in patients receiving single-allergen SCIT reported that grass pollen elicited more severe SRs than other single therapeutic aeroallergens, suggesting that certain allergens may be more problematic.[31] The Year 4 North American survey identified those practices who never adjust allergen doses during peak pollen season; such clinics reported more Grade 3 and 4 SRs compared with practices that sometimes, often, or always adjust doses.[23] Further analysis of survey data revealed that lowering doses during pollen seasons for patients with highly positive skin tests reduced SRs of all severity grades.[7]

Accelerated Buildup Schedules

In Year 5 of the North American Survey, 31% of 453 respondents reported using cluster buildup for initiating at least some of their patients on SCIT.[7] There was an increased risk of Grade 1, 2, and 3 SRs reported in practices using cluster buildup protocols. Rush buildup carried a much higher risk of SRs versus cluster or slow-buildup regimens.[32] In a substudy of the North American Survey, a trend was detected suggesting that lower target doses at end of cluster before transitioning to maintenance doses was associated with lower risk of severe SRs ($P = .07$).[23]

Injection Errors

As mentioned, retrospective surveys up to 2001 indicated that dosing error or inappropriate dose adjustments were implicated in about one-third of fatal reactions.[1,16] Aaronson and colleagues[33] conducted a survey among practicing allergists and found that 58% respondents reported an event where a patient received an injection meant for another patient and 74% knew of patients receiving an incorrect amount of allergen extract. Specific circumstances resulting in an incorrect dose included patients responding to a same or similar sounding name or an incorrect name check.

Allergen Doses

A post hoc analysis compared allergen dose ranges used by clinical practices reporting severe versus mild SRs with SCIT. Those clinical practices reporting severe SRs were significantly more likely to use house dust mite standardized extracts (ie, 1000–1999 AU per injection) in a higher dose range versus practices reporting mild SRs ($P = .0225$).[34] This does not prove a causal association but raises a question that higher doses within the therapeutic ranges might enhance risk in certain patients receiving SCIT. **Table 2** summarizes the risk factors identified by reporting physicians for fatal allergic reactions to SCIT in 2 retrospective surveys.[1,16]

PREVENTION OF SUBCUTANEOUS IMMUNOTHERAPY SYSTEMIC REACTIONS
Preinjection Health Assessment

Patients should be queried about their general health status before receiving an injection, to ensure immunotherapy is given under optimal conditions. First, they should be asked about recent respiratory infections, antibiotics, fevers, and about lower respiratory tract symptoms to include cough, wheeze, chest tightness, dyspnea, or recent rescue inhaler use. Next, they should be asked about new health problems or new medications. Finally, patients should be questioned about delayed SRs or large local reactions (LLRs) after their previous injection, in order to determine if dosage adjustment is indicated.

Asthmatics should undergo a screening questionnaire and either peak flow or spirometric evaluation before injections. Low measurements should preclude them receiving an injection. Recent data demonstrated 86% of US practices prescreened asthmatics for symptoms and 33% of practices performed routine peak flow or lung function measurements[6]; ideally all practices would do both.

Avoid Dosing Errors

Another critical way to prevent SRs is to avoid dosing errors. The first element in preventing dosing errors is to link the correct patient (2 identifiers including name and date of birth) with the correct vials. Individual vials should also have 2 patient identifiers, consistent with one goal of the Joint Commission of National Patient Safety Goals.[35] Using technology for this means can enhance patient safety, such as using patient ID cards with bar codes that link to their specific vials.

Next, review injection records to ensure the correct dose is given. Dosages may need to be adjusted for new vials or missed doses. The nurse/medical assistant needs to have good attention to detail and minimal distractions in order to avoid errors. After the dose is administered, documenting the correct dose and whether any LLR or SR occurred is critical to preventing an error next visit.

Dose Adjustments

Missed doses/late injections

There is no standardized protocol for missed doses due to late injections. Decreasing the dose for late injections will presumably lower SR risk. Dose adjustment schedules are highly variable, as some dose adjust based on number of days since last injection and some dose adjust based on number of days late. The practice parameter includes a sample protocol.[21] One observational review documented marked practice variation among Allergists at their institution with 16 different late injection dose-adjustment protocols; they argued for standardizing protocols to lessen medical error risk.[36] A retrospective cohort analysis reviewed a standardized dosage adjustment schedule over a 4-year period where doses were advanced (during buildup) if less than 14 days since last injection, repeated (during either buildup or maintenance) if 14 to 28 days since last injection, decreased by 1 dose if 29 to 35 days (4–5 weeks) since last injection, and decreased by 1 additional dose for each additional week late. Dose adjustments using this schedule were not associated with increased SR risk.[37] Further studies are needed to find optimal dose adjustment protocols.

Refills

Dose adjustments for refills/new maintenance vials are routinely performed due to nonstandardized allergens and potency differences between extract lots. The practice parameters on Allergen Immunotherapy from the American Academy of Allergy, Asthma and Immunology, the American College of Allergy, Asthma and Immunology, and the Joint Council of Allergy, Asthma and Immunology recommends reducing the dose 50% to 90% with manufacturer lot changes.[21] One study found no SRs when reducing the dose 50% with maintenance vial refills.[37] A recent investigation performed cluster dosing for refills (0.25 mL followed by 0.25 mL 30 minutes later) in patients on 1:1 v/v 0.5 mL maintenance dosing and found no SR increase.[38]

Large local reactions

Routine dose adjustments for LLR are not recommended, as they have not been shown to predict LLR or predict SR at the next injection.[39] Frequent LLR have been associated with an overall increased SR risk at some point during the immunotherapy course, but this risk was present regardless of whether routine dosage adjustments for LLR were made.[40,41] Dose adjustments solely for LLR should be made on an individual basis if the LLR is bothersome to the patient.

Peak Pollen Seasons

As previously mentioned, injections given during peak pollen seasons might be associated with increased SR risk, especially if patients are very symptomatic. However, 2 prospective studies found no increase in SRs during peak pollen seasons.[42,43] A recent study found that in-season pollen exposure did not increase SR rates in mountain cedar allergic patients.[44] A retrospective review of two 3-year time periods (one with and one without seasonal dose adjustments) found SRs were similar in pediatric subjects regardless of whether seasonal dose adjustments were made.[45] Finally, a meta-analysis suggested no increase in SRs with coseasonal SCIT initiation.[46] Therefore, although individual highly sensitive patients may experience an SR during their pollen season, most patients do well without seasonal dose adjustments; individualized dose adjustment for highly sensitive patients seems warranted.

Highly Sensitive/Reactive Patients

A retrospective study found highly reactive individuals on skin testing, defined as greater than 33% 3+ and 4+ skin test responses, had a nearly 6-fold increased rate of SRs.[47] Initial fatality survey data found that a large proportion of fatalities to immunotherapy and skin testing occurred in patients who were "extremely sensitive" on testing.[16,28] For "highly sensitive" individuals, one may start SCIT at the 1:10,000 v/v (silver) versus 1:1000 v/v (red) vial and using slower buildup dosing (ie, by 0.05 mL vs 0.1 mL).

Premedication

Historically there was concern antihistamines may mask early signs of an SR. This concern seems to have lessened, as recent national survey data reported antihistamine premedication was used by 84% of physician respondents.[6] One randomized controlled study showed fexofenadine premedication reduced the frequency of severe SRs (0% vs 9% control group) caused by conventional immunotherapy.[48] However, more data are needed on this topic, as no other study has reported the effect of antihistamines on LLRs or SRs during conventional inhalant SCIT buildup or maintenance injections. Because many SCIT patients take antihistamines as part of their treatment plan, it is important to determine whether they have taken it on the day of their injection and recommend they either consistently take it or avoid it on SCIT days.

Cluster Schedules

Several studies evaluated antihistamine use during cluster protocols. Premedication with loratadine 2 hours before visits reduced the number and frequency of SRs during cluster SCIT with grass or birch pollen versus placebo (33 vs 79%).[49] A cat cluster immunotherapy study using loratadine pretreatment of all 28 subjects showed no SRs.[50] A grass cluster immunotherapy study using loratadine pretreatment (no placebo) showed no immediate SRs but 18% of patients had delayed SRs.[51] Overall, the weight of evidence supports antihistamine premedication in cluster immunotherapy.

Rush Schedules

Multiple rush immunotherapy (RIT) studies have demonstrated lower SR rates with premedication. One group demonstrated that premedication with methylprednisolone, ketotifen, and long-acting theophylline reduced the SR rate during RIT in both dust mite and pollen-allergic patients.[52,53] After an initial RIT study without premedication resulted in 55% SRs, a pediatric group implemented premedication with astemizole, ranitidine, and prednisone for 2-day RIT, which reduced the SR rate to 27% (vs 73% placebo).[54,55] A subsequent 1-day RIT protocol with similar premedication demonstrated a 23% SR rate, all at 1:1000 wt/vol (1:10 v/v) or higher.[56] Finally, a 1-day RIT up to 0.05 mL concentrate found a 38% SR rate with 72% of SRs occurring after the final dose.[57] Therefore, premedication may modify RIT risk, but there is increased risk in the 1:10 and 1:1 v/v vials.

Of note, one should consider premedicating aggressively for 2 visits after RIT. An RIT study using premedication with Cetirizine, 10 mg; Ranitidine, 150 mg; Montelukast, 10 mg; and Prednisone, 50 mg evaluated SR rates after RIT to 1:10 v/v 0.1 mL.[58] They noted an SR peak during the second injection after RIT (1:10 v/v 0.3 mL), which was the first injection given with only Cetirizine, 10 mg.

MANAGEMENT AFTER A SYSTEMIC REACTION
Immediate Management

Epinephrine is the first-line treatment of SRs and early administration is critical. Fatalities during anaphylaxis usually result from delayed epinephrine administration, severe respiratory complications, or cardiovascular complications. Epinephrine dosage (aqueous epinephrine 1:1000 dilution) should be 0.3 to 0.5 mL in adults (>or = 30 kg) and 0.15 mL (15–30 kg) to 0.3 mL (>or = 30 kg) in children (0.01 mg/ kg) depending on weight. Epinephrine may be repeated every 5 minutes for severe reactions not responding to the initial dose. Epinephrine should be administered intramuscularly (IM), as plasma levels reach higher levels more rapidly.[21] Studies in children and adults not experiencing anaphylaxis demonstrated IM epinephrine in the thigh produced higher peak plasma concentrations more rapidly than when injected in the arm,[59,60] although a recent SCIT SR study showed epinephrine IM in the deltoid was clinically effective.[61] For patients with more subcutaneous tissue, use a longer needle (up to 1 inch especially in the thigh) to make sure epinephrine gets IM. There are no studies evaluating outcomes in immunotherapy-induced anaphylaxis directly comparing administration sites.

Concurrent with epinephrine administration, obtain vital signs and administer oxygen. Position patients in a recumbent (supine) position with lower extremities elevated to help increase blood flow to the heart and brain (unless precluded by vomiting).[62] Second-line supportive treatments include administering H1 and H2 antihistamines to relieve cutaneous (itch, hives) and gastrointestinal symptoms and inhaled beta-agonists to relieve bronchospasm/chest symptoms. These should never replace epinephrine as first-line therapy.[62,63] Corticosteroids may be administered to help protracted or biphasic symptoms, but they do not provide rapid relief of acute upper or lower airway obstruction or anaphylaxis. Glucagon can be administered to patients on β-blockers to overcome epinephrine resistance.

For patients not responding to multiple epinephrine doses or for those with significant lower respiratory/cardiovascular symptoms, one should activate emergency response systems and arrange transfer to the emergency department. For patients who respond to epinephrine administration, they should be observed generally for at least 60 minutes.

Biphasic Systemic Reactions

Before discharge, patients should be counseled on the possibility of a biphasic reaction. Biphasic reactions from SCIT SRs occur in 10% to 23% of patients and at a median time of 5.5 hours and are typically milder.[64,65]

Management for Rest of Subcutaneous Immunotherapy Course

It is customary to decrease the patient's dose after an SR. The optimal dosage adjustment has not been formally studied, but one may decrease by 1 vial (10-fold), by 50%, or to a previously tolerated dose depending on reaction severity and clinical situation.[21] After the dosage adjustment for a first SR, in most cases patients may build back up to goal maintenance dose. However, for patients who have experienced 2 SRs at higher doses or at maintenance dosing (ie, 1:1 v/v 0.5 mL), it would be advisable to lower their goal maintenance dose to a dose previously tolerated. For one severe SR or for patients with 3 or more SRs, one should strongly consider stopping immunotherapy altogether.

In addition to the dosage adjustment, if the SR occurs during buildup, one may slow down their buildup from a 0.1 mL to 0.05 mL increase per visit. If the SR occurs very early in buildup, one may add an additional dilution (ie, drop them from 1:1000 v/v to 1:10,000 v/v).

For patients with delayed SR (onset >30 minutes), it would be advisable to consider increasing their wait time to 45 to 60 minutes or longer. It would also be warranted to prescribe epinephrine autoinjectors to have available for any future SR.[66] Initiating (starting antihistamines) or changing the current premedication regimen (change antihistamine or add leukotriene blocker) may help modify future SR risk. Finally, all practices should routinely evaluate their treatment responses to SRs via practice anaphylaxis drills and make adjustments to ensure they are in line with best practices.[18]

SUMMARY

SCIT is effective for common allergic diseases such as rhinitis and conjunctivitis, asthma, and insect venom hypersensitivity. The risk of severe allergic reactions induced by SCIT seems to be relatively low and apparently is declining in recent years, probably because allergists are better prepared to prevent risky situations associated with the occurrence of severe reactions to SCIT and especially due to compliance with the recommendation for patient observation after each vaccine injection. There is also an increased awareness on early detection and treatment of reactions when they occur. There is an unmet need for new biomarkers that permit the identification of patients who will show a better response and those who have higher risk for developing severe adverse reactions to SCIT.

REFERENCES

1. Bernstein DI, Wanner M, Borish L, et al. Immunotherapy Committee AAAAI. Twelve-year survey of fatal reactions to allergen injections and skin testing: 1990-2001. J Allergy Clin Immunol 2004;113:1129–36.
2. Ragusa FV, Passalacqua G, Gambardella R, et al. Nonfatal systemic reactions to subcutaneous immunotherapy: a 10-year experience. J Investig Allergol Clin Immunol 1997;7:151–4.
3. Ragusa VF, Massolo A. Non-fatal systemic reactions to subcutaneous immunotherapy: a 20-year experience comparison of two 10-year periods. Allerg Immunol (Paris) 2004;36:52–5.
4. Amin HS, Liss GM, Bernstein DI. Evaluation of near-fatal reactions to allergen immunotherapy injections. J Allergy Clin Immunol 2006;117:169–75.
5. Phillips JF, Lockey RF, Fox RW, et al. Systemic reactions to subcutaneous allergen immunotherapy and the response to epinephrine. Allergy Asthma Proc 2011;32:288–94.
6. Epstein TG, Liss GM, Murphy-Berendts K, et al. AAAAI and ACAAI surveillance study of subcutaneous immunotherapy, year 3: what practices modify the risk of systemic reactions? Ann Allergy Asthma Immunol 2013;110:274–8.
7. Epstein TG, Liss GM, Murphy-Berendts K, et al. Risk factors for fatal and nonfatal reactions to subcutaneous immunotherapy: National surveillance study on allergen immunotherapy (2008-2013). Ann Allergy Asthma Immunol 2016;116:354–9.
8. Lamson R. Death associated with injection of foreign substances. J Am Med Assoc 1924;82:1090.
9. Bagg AS, Lockey RF. Adverse effects and fatalities associated with allergen skin testing and subcutaneous allergen immunotherapy [Chapter: 33]. In: Lockey RF,

Ledford DK, editors. Allergens and allergy immunotherapy. Subcutaneous, sublingual and oral. Boca Raton (FL): CRC Press; 2014. p. 447–59.

10. Van Arsdel PP, Sherman WB. Risk of inducing constitutional reactions in allergic patients. J Allergy 1957;28:251–61.

11. Hepner M, Ownby D, Mac Kechnie H, et al. The safety of immunotherapy – A prospective study. J Allergy Clin Immunol 1987;79:135.

12. Rawlins MD, Wood SM, Mann RD. Hazards with desensitizing vaccines. Arb Paul Ehrlich Inst Bundesamt Sera Impfstoffe Frankf A M 1988;(82):147–51.

13. Rieckenberg MR, Kahn RH, Day JH. Physician reported patient response to immunotherapy: a retrospective study of factors affecting the response. Ann Allergy 1990;64:364–7.

14. CSM update: desensitising vaccines. Br Med J (Clin Res Ed) 1986;293:948.

15. Lüderitz-Puchel U, May S, Haussein D. Incidents following hyposensitization. Munch Med Wochenschr 1996;138:1–7.

16. Reid MJ, Lockey RF, Turkeltaub PC, et al. Survey of fatalities from skin testing and immunotherapy 1985-1989. J Allergy Clin Immunol 1993;92(1 Pt 1):6–15.

17. Reid M, Gurka G. Deaths associated with skin testing and immunotherapy. J Allergy Clin Immunol 1996;97:231.

18. Rank MA, Bernstein DI. Improving the safety of immunotherapy. J Allergy Clin Immunol Pract 2014;2:131–5.

19. Bernstein DI, Epstein T, Murphy-Berendts K, et al. Surveillance of systemic reactions to subcutaneous immunotherapy injections: year 1 outcomes of the ACAAI and AAAAI collaborative study. Ann Allergy Asthma Immunol 2010;104:530–5.

20. Epstein TG, Liss GM, Murphy-Berendts K, et al. AAAAI/ACAAI subcutaneous immunotherapy (SCIT) surveillance study (2013-2017): fatalities, infections, delayed reactions, and use of epinephrine autoinjectors. J Allergy Clin Immunol Pract 2019;7(6):1996–2003.e1.

21. Cox L, Nelson H, Lockey RF. Allergen immunotherapy: a practice parameter third update. J Allergy Clin Immunol 2011;127:S1–55.

22. Copenhaver CC, Parker A, Patch S, et al. Systemic reactions with aeroallergen cluster immunotherapy in a clinical practice. Ann Allergy Asthma Immunol 2011;107:441–7.

23. Epstein TG, Liss GM, Murphy-Berendts K, et al. ACAAI/AAAAI surveillance study of subcutaneous immunotherapy, years 2008-2011: an update on fatal and nonfatal systemic allergic reactions. J Allergy Clin Immunol Pract 2014;2:161–7.

24. Epstein TG, Liss GM, Murphy-Berendts K, et al. Immediate and delayed-onset systemic reactions after subcutaneous immunotherapy injections: ACAAI/AAAAI surveillance study of subcutaneous immunotherapy: year 2. Ann Allergy Asthma Immunol 2011;107:426–31.

25. Rodriguez Del Rio P, Vidal C, Just J, et al. The European survey on adverse systemic reactions in allergen immunotherapy (EASSI): a pediatric assessment. Pediatr Allergy Immunol 2017;28:60–70.

26. Lockey RF, Turkeltaub PC, Olive ES, et al. The Hymenoptera venom study, III, Safety of venom immunotherapy. J Allergy Clin Immunol 1990;86:775.

27. Korosec P, Ziberna K, Silar M, et al. Immunological and clinical factors associated with adverse systemic reactions during the build-up phase of honeybee venom immunotherapy. Clin Exp Allergy 2015;45:1579–89.

28. Lockey RF, Benedict LM, Turkeltaub PC, et al. Fatalities from immunotherapy (IT) and skin testing (ST). J Allergy Clin Immunol 1987;79:660–77.

29. Cox L, Larenas-Linnemann D, Lockey RF, et al. Speaking the same language: the World Allergy Organization Subcutaneous Immunotherapy Systemic Reaction Grading System. J Allergy Clin Immunol 2010;125:569–74, 574.e1-574.e7.
30. Cook KA, Ford CM, Leyvas EA, et al. Half of systemic reactions to allergen immunotherapy are delayed, majority require treatment with epinephrine. J Allergy Clin Immunol Pract 2017;5:1415–7.
31. Winther L, Arnved J, Malling HJ, et al. Side-effects of allergen-specific immunotherapy: a prospective multi-centre study. Clin Exp Allergy 2006;36:254–60.
32. Winslow AW, Turbyville JC, Sublett JW, et al. Comparison of systemic reactions in rush, cluster, and standard-build aeroallergen immunotherapy. Ann Allergy Asthma Immunol 2016;117:542–5.
33. Aaronson DW, Gandhi TK. Incorrect allergy injections: allergists' experiences and recommendations for prevention. J Allergy Clin Immunol 2004;113:1117–21.
34. Liss GM, Murphy-Berendts K, Epstein T, et al. Factors associated with severe versus mild immunotherapy-related systemic reactions: a case-referent study. J Allergy Clin Immunol 2011;127:1298–300.
35. The Joint Commission on Accreditation of Healthcare Organizations 2010 National Patient Safety Goals. Available at: https://www.jointcommission.org/assets/1/6/NPSG_Chapter_AHC_Jan2019.pdf. Accessed May 26, 2019.
36. Montgomery JR. The need for standardizing the aeroallergen immunotherapy missed-dose adjustment protocol. Allergy Asthma Proc 2008;29:425–6.
37. Webber C, Calabria C. Assessing the safety of subcutaneous immunotherapy dose adjustments. Ann Allergy Asthma Immunol 2010;105:369–75.
38. Waibel K, Owens T, Crips H, et al. Clinical and immunologic assessment of a cluster method during allergen immunotherapy refill dosing. J Allergy Clin Immunol Pract 2014;2:793–4.
39. Tankersley MS, Butler KK, Butler WK, et al. Local reactions during allergen immunotherapy do not require dose adjustment. J Allergy Clin Immunol 2000;106:840–3.
40. Calabria CW, Stolfi A, Tankersley MS. The REPEAT study: recognizing and evaluating periodic local reactions in allergen immunotherapy and associated systemic reactions. Ann Allergy Asthma Immunol 2011;106:49–53.
41. Roy S, Sigmon JR, Oliver J, et al. Increased frequency of large local reactions among systemic reacgtors during subcutaneous allergen immunotherapy. Ann Allergy Asthma Immunol 2007;99:82–6.
42. Tinkelman DG, Cole WQ 3rd, Tunno J. Immunotherapy: a one-year prospective study to evaluate risk factors of systemic reactions. J Allergy Clin Immunol 1995;95:8–14.
43. Lin MS, Tanner E, Lynn J, et al. Nonfatal systemic allergic reactions induced by skin testing and immunotherapy. Ann Allergy 1993;71:557–62.
44. Wong P, Quinn J, Gomez R, et al. Systemic reactions to immunotherapy during mountain cedar season: implications for seasonal dose adjustment. J Allergy Clin Immunol Pract 2017;5(5):1438–9.
45. Albuhairi S, Sare T, Lakin P, et al. Systemic reactions in pediatric patients receiving standardized allergen subcutaneous immunotherapy with and without seasonal dose adjustment. J Allergy Clin Immunol Pract 2018;6:1711–6.
46. Creticos P, Bernstein D, Casale T, et al. Coseasonal initiation of allergen immunotherapy: a systematic review. J Allergy Clin Immunol Pract 2016;4:1194–204.
47. DaVeiga SP, Liu X, Caruso K, et al. Systemic reactions associated with subcutaneous allergen immunotherapy: timing and risk assessment. Ann Allergy Asthma Immunol 2011;106:533–7.

48. Ohashi Y, Nakai Y, Murata K. Effect of pretreatment with fexofenadine on the safety of immunotherapy in patients with allergic rhinitis. Ann Allergy Asthma Immunol 2006;96:600–5.
49. Neilsen L, Johnsen CR, Mosbech H, et al. Antihistamine premedication in specific cluster immunotherapy: a double-blind, placebo-controlled study. J Allergy Clin Immunol 1996;97:1207–13.
50. Ewbank PA, Murray J, Sanders K, et al. A double-blind, placebo-controlled immunotherapy dose-response study with standardized cat extract. J Allergy Clin Immunol 2003;111:155–61.
51. Walker SM, Pajno GB, Lima MT, et al. Grass pollen immunotherapy for seasonal rhinitis and asthma: a randomized, controlled trial. J Allergy Clin Immunol 2001; 107:87–93.
52. Heijaioui A, Dhivert H, Michel FB, et al. Immuntoherapy with a standardized Dermatophagoides pteronyssinus extract. IV. Systemic reactions according to the immunotherapy schedule. J Allergy Clin Immunol 1990;85:473–9.
53. Heijaioui A, Ferrando R, Dhivert H, et al. Systemic reactions occurring during immunotherapy with standardized pollen extracts. J Allergy Clin Immunol 1992; 89:925–33.
54. Portnoy J, King K, Kanarek H, et al. Incidence of systemic reactions during rush immunotherapy. Ann Allergy Asthma Immunol 1992;68:493–8.
55. Portnoy J, Bagstad K, Kanarek H, et al. Premedication reduces the indicence of systemic reactions during inhalant rush immunotherapy with mixtures of allergenic extracts. Ann Allergy Asthma Immunol 1994;73:409–18.
56. Sharkey P, Portnoy J. Rush immunotherapy: experience with a one-day schedule. Ann Allergy Asthma Immunol 1996;76:175–80.
57. Harvey SM. Safety of rush immunotherapy to multiple aeroallergens in an adult population. Ann Allergy Asthma Immunol 2004;92:414–9.
58. Cook KA, Kelso JM, White AA. Increased risk of systemic reactions extends beyond completion of rush immunotherapy. J Allergy Clin Immunol Pract 2017; 5:1773–5.
59. Simons FE, Roberts JR, Gu X, et al. Epinephrine absorption in children with a history of anaphylaxis. J Allergy Clin Immunol 1998;101:33–7.
60. Simons FE, Gu X, Simons KJ. Epinephrine absorption in adults: intramuscular versus subcutaneous injection. J Allergy Clin Immunol 2001;108:871–3.
61. Wong PH, Adams KE, Carlson GS, et al. Experience with epinephrine delivery in immunotherapy-associated systemic reactions. Ann Allergy Asthma Immunol 2016;116:166–8.
62. Kim H, Fischer D. Anaphylaxis. Allergy Asthma Clin Immunol 2011;7(Suppl 1):S6.
63. Simons FE. Anaphylaxis: recent advances in assessment and treatment. J Allergy Clin Immunol 2009;124:625–36.
64. Scranton S Gonzalez EG, Waibel KH. Incidence and chaaracteristics of biphasic reactions after allergen immunotherapy. J Allergy Clin Immunol 2009;123:493–8.
65. Confino Cohen R, Goldberg A. Allergen immunotherapy-induced biphasic systemic reactions: incidence, characteristics, and outcome: a prospective study. Ann Allergy Asthma Immunol 2010;104:73–8.
66. Fitzhugh DJ, Bernstein DI. Should epinephrine autoinjectors be prescribed to all patients on subcutaneous immunotherapy? J Allergy Clin Immunol Pract 2016;4: 862–7.

Sublingual Immunotherapy for Other Indications

Venom Large Local, Latex, Atopic Dermatitis, and Food

Derek M. Smith, MD[a],*, Theodore M. Freeman, MD[b]

KEYWORDS

- Sublingual immunotherapy • Food allergy • Latex allergy • Venom allergy
- Atopic dermatitis • Dust mite

KEY POINTS

- Latex sublingual immunotherapy trials have produced evidence for efficacy, but safety concerns exist. In addition, latex extracts are not available in the United States.
- Evidence to support the use of venom sublingual immunotherapy for large local reactions is lacking.
- Dust mite sublingual immunotherapy for atopic dermatitis has produced promising results, but trials using the available US tablet are lacking.
- Food sublingual immunotherapy trials have shown modest efficacy with minimal local reactions, but dose and duration trials are lacking.

INTRODUCTION

With the United States Food and Drug Administration's (FDA) recent approval of standardized sublingual tablets for grasses, ragweed, and dust mites, the scientific data to support the safe and efficacious use of sublingual immunotherapy (SLIT) for allergic rhinitis and asthma are accumulating. These tablets are ideal for furthering SLIT research because they are standardized and reproducibly manufactured, much like medications; however, their FDA indications of use are currently limited. Nevertheless, there are decades of international data regarding less well-known applications of less

Disclaimer: The opinions or assertions herein are the private views of the authors and are not to be construed as reflecting the views of the Department of the Air Force or the Department of Defense.
[a] Department of Allergy/Immunology, Wilford Hall Ambulatory Surgical Center, 1100 Wilford Hall Loop, JBSA- Lackland, San Antonio, TX 78236, USA; [b] San Antonio Asthma and Allergy Clinic, 2833 Babcock Road, Suite 304, San Antonio, TX 78229, USA
* Corresponding author.
E-mail address: derek.m.smith34.mil@mail.mil

standardized, liquid SLIT drops. This article is a thorough attempt to analyze the prospective clinical trial data regarding these alternative applications of SLIT in order to provide an evidence-based review of the efficacy, safety, and potential indications or limitations of their use for practicing clinicians.

VENOM SUBLINGUAL IMMUNOTHERAPY

The concept of SLIT for venom allergy has a small amount of published data. Two Italian studies regarding the use of SLIT for venom immunotherapy were published in 2008 with optimistic views of this treatment modality.

Severino and colleagues[1] performed a randomized, double-blind, placebo-controlled trial in 30 adult patients with large local reactions to honeybee stings. Patients' local reactions were confirmed via sting challenge and then randomized to honeybee venom SLIT or placebo for 6 months of therapy. Patients in the SLIT group rapidly built up to 35 μg of venom every other day for a total dose of 535 μg monthly. Of the 26 patients who completed the study, a statistically significant reduction in median peak diameter of local reaction was observed in the SLIT group (20.5–8.5 cm), whereas no difference was noted in the placebo group. No adverse reactions to SLIT were reported. The investigators concluded that this study provided a proof of concept regarding the possible utility of SLIT in venom hypersensitivity and admitted that this end point may not be the most clinically important. They suggested this concept warranted further dosing trials and trials regarding patients with systemic reactions to venom stings. This interpretation of the results was debated by Rueff and colleagues,[2] who cited several methodological flaws in the trial to include differing characteristics of groups, unclear determination of SLIT dosing, and differing interpretation of the same end-point results.

Patriarca and colleagues[3] published a case-control study of venom SLIT versus subcutaneous immunotherapy (SCIT) the same year. Forty-one patients with a history of systemic reactions to wasp stings were randomized to receive standard-of-care SCIT (100 μg monthly) versus SLIT (100 μg weekly) via ultrarush buildup protocols. No baseline sting challenges were performed, but immunoglobulin (Ig) E and IgG4 levels were drawn at enrollment and at 6, 12, and 24 months of therapy. Two (9.5%) patients in the SLIT group experienced mild side effects (dysphagia with spontaneous remission and diffuse itching, which resolved with oral antihistamine), whereas 3 (15%) patients in the SCIT group experienced adverse reactions to the same ultrarush buildup protocol. In the SLIT group, no significant changes in IgE and IgG4 levels were observed. In contrast, in the SCIT group, serum-specific IgE levels initially increased, but returned to baseline. IgG4 levels increased significantly at 6 months and remained increased throughout the trial. Four patients had field stings in the SLIT group; each patient experienced a milder reaction than before therapy and only 1 person experienced a systemic reaction (isolated throat constriction). In the SCIT group, 9 patients had field stings, resulting in 8 large local reactions and 1 systemic reaction (dizziness). The investigators argue that this study reveals similar safety and efficacy between venom SCIT and SLIT, but admit that larger randomized controlled trials with standardized sting challenges are needed before venom SLIT can be considered for treatment.

Further research trials into venom SLIT could not be found and no trials seem to be ongoing. Given the lack of data, SLIT for venom allergy cannot currently be recommended. In addition, in an era of flying Hymenoptera venom shortage, it remains difficult to even recommend continuing research into a therapy that would require the use of 4 to 5 times more venom per month compared with SCIT.

LATEX SUBLINGUAL IMMUNOTHERAPY

As researchers began to expand the potential uses of SLIT in the early 2000s, its applicability to latex allergy became interesting to researchers as well. The published literature regarding latex SLIT began in 2001 when Nucera and colleagues[4] described a case report of a 23-year-old patient with latex allergy who became able to tolerate 1-hour mucosal and 6-hour cutaneous latex challenge tests after a 3-day rush buildup with latex SLIT. This case was a proof of concept and suggested further research into the treatment modality.[4]

The scientific evidence regarding the topic was advanced in 2002 by Patriarca and colleagues.[5] Their trial randomized 24 children (8 years old at the youngest) and adult patients into a latex extract versus placebo group in a double-blinded fashion after baseline laboratory tests were drawn and latex hypersensitivity was confirmed via latex-specific challenges (cutaneous, mucosal, conjunctival, and sublingual).[5] Both groups of 12 patients underwent a 4-day rush protocol followed by daily SLIT maintenance for 3 months. After maintenance, all patients in the latex SLIT group were able to tolerate the maximal cutaneous, mucosal, and sublingual latex exposure challenge times (statistically significantly improved compared with placebo group). No systemic reactions and only mild local reactions were noted. Although this was a small trial, these data suggested that SLIT could be safe and efficacious for the treatment of latex allergy.

In 2004, Cistero Bahima and colleagues[6] published the results of a case series of 26 latex-allergic patients. These patients followed the ALK-Abello sublingual rush protocol with the European commercially available SLIT-LATEX product. Patients were rushed to 100 µg of latex protein and then continued every other day (300 µg weekly) for 9 weeks. After this maintenance phase, the skin prick tests did not significantly reduce in size, but the tolerance of cutaneous exposure did significantly improve, although less drastically than the previous study by Patriarca and colleagues.[5] This trial also highlighted the potential safety risks of latex SLIT, because 12 of 26 patients (46.2%) experienced at least 1 systemic reaction and 23 of 26 patients (88.5%) reported at least 1 local reaction, predominantly lip itching. Systemic reactions resolved without treatment in 44.7%, with antihistamines alone in 26.3%, with beta-2 agonists alone in 5.3%, and with antihistamines and corticosteroids in 18.4% of patients. One patient was treated with epinephrine twice for separate reactions (immediate dyspnea in 1 case and abdominal pain, headache, cough, dyspnea, rhinitis, and chest tightness in the other). Although these rates were concerning, they could also be at least partially attributed to trial design because all patients were being openly exposed to known allergen.

Bernardini and colleagues[7] published the robust results of their randomized, double-blind, placebo-controlled trial with 20 latex-allergic pediatric patients (4 to 15 years old) in 2006 after 1 year of SLIT-LATEX treatment and again in 2008 after 3 years of immunotherapy. After randomization, 12 children received 40 µg of latex extract daily after a 4-day rush protocol. After the first year, this active group was allowed to continue SLIT in an open fashion for the remaining 2 years. At the termination of the blinded trial period, cutaneous exposure tolerance significantly improved, but skin prick testing results and IgE levels remained similar to the placebo group. However, cutaneous tolerance continued to improve after 2 years of SLIT and all patients could complete the latex glove use test after 3 years of therapy. No systemic or local side effects were reported and these data supported the long-term safe and efficacious use of latex SLIT, but the duration of this tolerance after the cessation of SLIT was not evaluated.

After Tabar and colleagues'[8] latex study was published in 2006, latex SCIT was largely abandoned for safety concerns because 81.8% of patients receiving latex immunotherapy experienced systemic reactions. Although the tolerability of SLIT allowed it to remain as a potential immunotherapy modality, its safety continued to be closely monitored. Meanwhile, continued SLIT trails in Europe began to accumulate safety and efficacy of the SLIT-LATEX product.

Nettis and colleagues[9] published an additional randomized, double-blind, placebo-controlled latex SLIT study in 2007. Patients with asthma or urticaria on latex exposure were randomized to the ultrarush protocol with the SLIT-LATEX extract followed by every-other-day administration of 100 μg of extract. After 12 months, patients underwent cutaneous challenge and statistically significant improvement was again noted compared with the placebo group. Skin prick testing and reduction of medication use also significantly improved, but IgE levels remained similar to placebo. Three of the 18 patients (17%) reported local oral reactions during the induction phase of the active group, which was similar to the placebo group, and no side effects were noted in the maintenance phase.

Buyukozturk and colleagues[10] published their experiences in 2011 with latex SLIT in health care workers that remained symptomatic despite attempted avoidance. Of the 12 people that agreed to participate in this blinded trial, 8 were randomized in the SLIT group and 4 to placebo. However, 3 of these 8 patients (37.5%) experienced severe systemic reactions (anaphylaxis or severe bronchoconstriction) and withdrew from the trial. The remaining people in the SLIT group again showed improved glove use and decreased skin prick responses compared with placebo, but these results perpetuated safety concerns, especially in health care workers.

Curiously, conflicting efficacy results were published by Gastaminza and colleagues[11] in 2011. This double-blind, placebo-controlled study of 28 latex-allergic patients found no significant difference in specific provocation tests or in vitro testing after a year of SLIT-LATEX. This study stopped at the lower dose of SLIT at 40 μg daily, but still reported 4 patients with mild adverse events (similar to the control group's rate of side effects). This dose of SLIT-LATEX was also the dose used in the Bernardini and colleagues[7] trial. Because trial designs have differed beyond just SLIT dose, no clear association could be made between tolerability and efficacy of a 210-μg weekly dose compared with a 300-μg weekly dose.

Lasa Luaces and colleagues[12] furthered the concept of latex SLIT in 2012 when they published the results of their 12-month open, case-control study of 23 children who were allergic to latex. This trial was the first to argue that the previous randomized, double-blind, placebo-controlled trials had already established the safety and efficacy of latex SLIT. Therefore, this trial was designed to use the known data regarding latex component sensitization patterns to further refine the immunologic changes of SLIT to attempt to find correlations to predict clinical efficacy or safety outcomes. Patients were again rapidly built up to 100 μg of SLIT-LATEX and continued every other day for 12 months. In summary, although some serologic changes were observed, this trial failed to show consistent significant changes in IgE, IgG4, and basophil activation test, which could help predict patients' safety or efficacy outcomes.

The most recent and largest study regarding latex SLIT was published by Nucera and colleagues[13] in 2018. This observational (nonblinded) case series of 76 latex-allergic adults again used SLIT-LATEX via standard 4-day rush to 100 μg of latex protein every other day for 3 years of treatment. Latex IgE, mean wheal diameters of skin prick testing, and provocation tests again significantly improved, but IgG4 levels did not change. The investigators supported the clinical use of SLIT-LATEX for patients with latex allergy.

Rush protocols used in these trials and 2 additional independent trials[14,15] have provided reasonable evidence to suggest that effective doses of latex SLIT can be safely and rapidly achieved. Regrettably, there are several limitations to these studies. The complexity of the clinical manifestation of latex allergy continues to limit the power of these studies because patients with differing symptoms are often grouped together when exposed to specific challenge tests, but the validity of this assumption could be challenged. In addition, sample sizes remained small, with 20 patients as the largest active arm of a randomized, placebo-controlled trial. There is also a lack of long-term data (1 case report) to suggest sustained efficacy after cessation of SLIT. No ongoing trials were discovered. In addition, although there are reasonable data to support the use latex SLIT, there is no commercially available latex extract in the United States, and therefore it is not yet a viable treatment option.

SUBLINGUAL IMMUNOTHERAPY FOR ATOPIC DERMATITIS

The concept of specific immunotherapy as a treatment of atopic dermatitis has gained popularity specifically for the treatment of dust mite–allergic patients. As such, the investigation of SLIT for the treatment of atopic dermatitis also increased for dust mite–sensitized patients and was the first application of SLIT among the topics of this article.

The first prospective trial investigating the effect of dust mite SLIT was published in 1994. Galli and colleagues[16] divided 60 dust mite–allergic children, aged 6 months to 12 years, into separate groups of atopic dermatitis with allergic comorbidities (rhinitis or asthma) and solely atopic dermatitis. The group of children with atopic dermatitis with comorbidities and half of the children with just atopic dermatitis received thrice-weekly dust mite SLIT for up to 3 years. The remaining children with atopic dermatitis served as a control group. Of the 26 children with atopic dermatitis and other comorbidities receiving dust mite SLIT, 21 had significant improvement in dermatitis scores. Ten of 16 children with atopic dermatitis alone receiving SLIT also experienced significant improvement. Eleven of 18 children in the control group similarly experienced significant improvement ($P<.05$) in atopic dermatitis scores before and after the trial period without treatment. As such, the treatment groups did not improve compared with the control group.

The best evidence supporting the use of SLIT for atopic dermatitis originates from a double-blind, placebo-controlled trial published by Pajno and colleagues[17] in 2007. This trial enrolled 56 children that were 5 to 16 years old with atopic dermatitis with a Scoring Atopic Dermatitis (SCORAD) score greater than 7 and evidence of mono-sensitization to dust mites via skin prick testing or serum-specific IgE. Patients with asthma and food allergy were excluded to attempt to limit confounders. Children were stratified based on their atopic dermatitis severity and randomized to SLIT (approximately 3 µg each of Der p 1 and Der f 1 weekly) or placebo for 18 months of continuous therapy. This method allowed for blinding, but not true randomization. Data regarding the change in SCORAD, rescue medication use, and visual analog score were collected every 3 months and at the end of therapy. Forty-eight (85%) of the children completed the trial, with the 8 dropouts occurring in the first 6 months (2 active and 6 in the placebo group), with the 2 dropouts from the active group citing worsening dermatitis as their motivation to stop participation. After 9 months of therapy, mean SCORAD improved (10 points) in the SLIT group compared with placebo, and they maintained this improvement for the remaining months. This improvement was statistically significant but also likely clinically significant, as shown by the subsequent first publication of a minimal clinically important difference for the SCORAD as

8.7 in 2012.[18] Medication use was also significantly less in the SLIT group. When patients with mild to moderate dermatitis (SCORAD<40) were analyzed separately from severe dermatitis, this effect was noted to be greater for the mild to moderate group and nonsignificant for the severe group. The investigators concluded that SLIT was a safe and effective option to consider in the treatment of patients with mild to moderate atopic dermatitis with dust mite sensitization.

In 2013, Qin and colleagues[19] published the results of their trial of 107 adults with atopic dermatitis with or without atopic comorbidities who were randomized (but not blinded) to receive dust mite SLIT plus medical therapy (levocetirizine and topical mometasone cream) or medical therapy alone for 12 months. Only 84 patients completed the trial and most of the dropouts occurred in the first 6 months at a similar rate between groups. Of the participants who withdrew from the treatment group, the reasons cited were primarily failure to adhere to the protocol and cost. Among the control group, the major reason cited was lack of efficacy. Two patients withdrew from each group because of unspecified adverse events. The statistics were not analyzed on an intention-to-treat basis; however, the trial reported a statistically significant ($P<.05$) higher rate of greater than 60% improvement in SCORAD in the SLIT group (77.8%) compared with the standard-of-care medical therapy group (53.9%). Raw SCORAD scores were not provided, so this improvement could not be compared with the previously mentioned minimal clinically important difference for SCORAD.[18]

In 2014, Di Rienzo and colleagues[20] published the results of an open, randomized controlled (but again not blinded) study of 27 children aged 5 to 18 years with atopic dermatitis and dust mite sensitization who were treated with dust mite SLIT or medical therapy for 72 weeks. Again, a statistically and clinically significant improvement SCORAD score (mean reduction of −11.9) was noted in the treatment group between baseline and week 72 and between groups at 48 and 72 weeks. No difference was noted in the control group throughout the trial. Although the results are again promising, the lack of blinding continued to introduce possible bias into these studies.

Most recently, in 2017, You and colleagues[21] published their results of their open trial of SLIT in Korean children and young adults. They treated dust mite–allergic patients with 12 months of SLIT and noted that 19 of 23 (82.6%) had a least 30% decrease in Eczema Area and Severity Index (EASI) score. The mean EASI reduction during the 12 months of SLIT was 6.88, just higher than the minimal clinically important difference of 6.6 determined in 2012.[18] Two patients experienced lip and tongue swelling, which resolved with temporarily withholding SLIT. No systemic reactions were noted. Despite the inherent biases in nonrandomized, nonblinded studies, these data did reveal similar efficacy in patients who were monosensitized to dust mite as well as polysensitized to other aeroallergens and broadened the supportive data to additional ethnic groups as well.

There is an ongoing Brazilian randomized, double-blind, placebo-controlled trial (NCT03388866) continuing to evaluate the efficacy and safety of dust mite SLIT drops. With the FDA approval of a standardized dust mite sublingual tablet, well-designed trials using this product should now be conducted to confirm these optimistic results in the treatment of atopic dermatitis before its widespread use for this indication in the United States.

FOOD-SPECIFIC SUBLINGUAL IMMUNOTHERAPY

Case reports and case series of successful applications of SLIT to food allergy also began receiving attention in the early 2000s.[22–24] At that time, investigators were also evaluating the use of SLIT for oral allergy syndrome and the first blinded and controlled trial was published regarding this potential indication. In 2004, Hansen and colleagues[25] published their results from a double-blind, double-dummy, placebo-controlled trial of subcutaneous versus sublingual immunotherapy with birch pollen extracts in 40 patients with oral symptoms to apple ingestion. Neither the SCIT nor the SLIT group reported significant symptomatic improvement to an open apple challenge after 2 years of immunotherapy, but unexpectedly the placebo group did have significant improvement. This trial was limited by disease-specific design constraints because subjective symptom scores were the only way to evaluate the results of food challenges, but the lack of blinded challenges likely also biased results. The results argued that neither SCIT nor SLIT improved oral allergy symptoms to apples.

A subsequent study published by Mauro and colleagues[26] in 2011 also failed to find significant benefit in either birch SCIT or SLIT for apple oral allergy syndrome. As such, recombinant Mal d 1 extracts were created and initial studies found the antigen could induce immunologic effects in vivo.[27] More recently, in 2018 a clinical trial by Kinaciyan and colleagues[28] showed the efficacy of recombinant Mal d 1 for the treatment of birch pollen–related food allergy, suggesting that further investigations using recombinant allergens may improve clinical efficacy.

The first trial to show clinical efficacy for SLIT in the treatment of systemic food allergy was published in 2005 by Enrique and colleagues.[29] This was a multicenter, randomized, double-blind, placebo-controlled trial evaluated the safety and efficacy of hazelnut sublingual extracts in the treatment of hazelnut allergy. A total of 23 patients with a clinical history of hazelnut allergy, positive hazelnut skin prick testing, and a positive double-blind hazelnut oral challenge were randomized to receive hazelnut extract or placebo for 12 weeks after a 4-day rush buildup protocol. Three cutaneous systemic reactions were observed (0.2% of doses) and all resolved with oral antihistamines alone. Local reactions (oral itching) were noted in 7.4% of doses. After completion, the mean dose of hazelnut that provoked objective symptoms increased significantly from 2.29 g to 11.56 g in the SLIT group. No significant changes were noted in the placebo group. In addition, 5 of 11 patients (45%) tolerated the maximum dose of 20 g of hazelnut challenge in the SLIT group, but only 1 of 11 patients (9%) in the placebo group could tolerate this dose.

The same research group then published a follow-up study in 2008 in which patients in the hazelnut group had the opportunity to undergo another food challenge 1 year after the previous study officially ended.[30] Seven of the 11 patients consented to and underwent this additional challenge. In the interim, 2 patients remained on SLIT as prescribed, 3 stopped maintenance drops 3 to 4 months after study completion, and 2 reported intermittent compliance with drops. The mean provoking dose increased again to 14.57 g, which was significantly increased from baseline and the initial trial's exit food challenge. Five of the 7 (71%) patients could tolerate the maximal dose of 20 g of hazelnut, but 1 patient who could previously tolerate this dose lost immunologic protection. The study established SLIT as a safe and effective potential long-term tool for the treatment food allergy even without rigorous dosing controls used in clinical trials.

Soon afterward, in 2009, Fernandez-Rivas and colleagues[31] published their results for the use of SLIT for peach allergy. Fifty-six adult patients with IgE-mediated peach allergy confirmed by peach skin testing or serum-specific IgE testing and positive double-blind, placebo-controlled oral peach challenges were randomized to receive 6 months of SLIT or matching placebo. A total of 4944 doses were given during the trial and 1356 adverse reactions were deemed potentially related to the trial; 1344 were in the active group and 12 in the placebo group, and they were overwhelmingly local reactions (1328 or 98.8%). Nineteen systemic reactions were noted (16 in active and 3 in placebo groups) and 15 were in the buildup phase of the trial. All of the systemic reactions were considered mild and none required epinephrine for treatment. Sublingual immunotherapy resulted in the tolerance of greater than 3-fold more peach at the end of the trial compared with beforehand. No change was noted in the placebo group. This improvement did not translate to a statistically significant difference between groups ($P = .21$). However, secondary end points of skin test reactivity and IgG4 levels did reach significant improvement levels. The therapy's safety profile and modest improvements in various outcomes motivated an optimistic view that SLIT could have a potential role for the treatment of food allergy and that SLIT would be possible for a variety of foods.

This concept was advanced by a trial by Gomez and colleagues,[32] who evaluated the effect of 12 months of peach SLIT on peanut allergy given the cross reactivity of Pru p 3 with Ara h 9. In this case-control trial, 48 peach-allergic patients were divided into groups of 12 based on their peanut allergy status (allergic, sensitized, or tolerant) as well as a control group. In this Mediterranean population, peach SLIT seemed to protect against peach reactions as well as peanut reactions because a significant increase in oral tolerance of peanut protein was observed in those patients with concomitant peanut allergy. This trial was limited by its lack of blinding, and questions remain regarding the extrapolation of this effect to other geographic locations given the varying sensitization profiles to peanut components, but the concept of improving tolerance using cross-reactive allergens is intriguing.

The application of SLIT to the treatment of peanut allergy was first published in 2011 by Kim and colleagues.[33] This randomized, double-blind, placebo-controlled trial of 18 children entailed a 6-month buildup phase followed by 6 months of maintenance-dose immunotherapy. Peanut protein tolerance and immunologic end points were evaluated. The most notable result was that the treatment group could tolerate statistically significant, 20-times more protein than the placebo group (median, 1710 vs 85 mg) during the final food challenge. Entry food challenges were not performed so comparison with baseline levels of tolerance was not possible. Adverse reactions were reported in 11.5% of peanut doses, most commonly oral itching, and 8.6% of placebo doses, most commonly skin itching. No epinephrine was required to treat reactions. The investigators used these data to argue that SLIT for peanut allergy was safe and efficacious and deserved further investigation.

The same group of researchers published a follow-up study in 2019, which evaluated the long-term outcomes of peanut SLIT.[34] This open-label cohort study evaluated 48 children who consumed 2 mg/d of peanut SLIT for 3 to 5 years by means of double-blind, placebo-controlled food challenge of up to 5 g of peanut protein. On completion, 32 (67%) of the 48 children could tolerate 750 mg of peanut protein, 12 (25%) of the 48 could tolerate the entire 5-g peanut challenge, and 10 (21%) could tolerate the 5-g peanut challenge again 2 to 4 weeks after cessation of SLIT, showing sustained unresponsiveness. The therapy was associated with side effects, mostly oropharyngeal itching, in 4.8% of doses (representing 94% of patients), which required antihistamines after 0.21% of doses, and no epinephrine was required. The investigators again argued that this trial showed meaningful desensitization in most children.

Fleischer and colleagues[35] published the initial findings and Burks and colleagues[36] published the long-term and most convincing data to support peanut SLIT in 2015. This multicenter, randomized, double-blind, placebo-controlled trial evaluating the safety and efficacy of peanut SLIT found that 14 of 20 (70%) patients in the treatment group (of up to 1386 μg of peanut protein) could tolerate 5 g of peanut powder or a 10-fold increase in the amount of protein at 44 weeks of therapy compared with their baseline oral challenge. Only 3 of 20 (15%) patients in the placebo group could tolerate this level of peanut protein. Data were promising that longer duration would provide additional benefit, so the trial was opened and the placebo group was started on peanut SLIT at a higher dose of 3696 μg. Both groups continued for a total of 3 years of active therapy. Patients subsequently underwent oral challenge at 2 and 3 years of active therapy. Patients who could tolerate a full 10-g oral peanut challenge at 3 years discontinued SLIT for 8 weeks and then underwent an additional oral peanut challenge. Four patients were able to complete this entire protocol and were determined to show sustained unresponsiveness to peanut. Adverse reactions were noted in 18.3% of doses, but typically were mild oral symptoms. No epinephrine was required. Significant differences in oral peanut tolerance were not noted between the 1386-μg and the 3696-μg dose SLIT groups at the end of the trial. This fact suggests that more than a 2.3-mg increase in daily protein exposure is needed to suggest that a higher dose of SLIT will provide additional clinical protective benefit. Although only 4 of the original 40 patients achieved sustained unresponsiveness, all patients who completed the trial experienced modest levels of desensitization. However, the high rate of dropout, with the most common reason being participant decision, suggested that SLIT patients were not finding the clinical benefit worth the daily drops and oral side effects.

Two additional clinical trials provided data regarding the use of SLIT for food allergy by comparing the safety and efficacy of SLIT with oral immunotherapy (OIT) in the treatment of cow's milk allergy[37] and peanut allergy.[38] Both trials made the same general conclusions that OIT could be more effective than SLIT, but this benefit comes at the expense of a higher rate of systemic reactions. Despite many controlled OIT trials, randomized controlled trials using SLIT could not be found for patients with hen's egg allergy. There is an ongoing trial evaluating the safety and efficacy of a peanut SLIT product with adjuvant (NCT03463135) as well as an ongoing trial of early intervention with peanut SLIT in peanut-allergic patients less than 4 years old (NCT02304991). The trials discussed earlier suggest that some immunologic tolerance can be created given sublingual exposures to known allergens with minimal side effects.

SUMMARY

Because this is a summation of the available prospective controlled clinical trials (**Table 1**), there is a clear lack of long-term outcome data, and few foods have been studied. At present, there are no commercially available food SLIT extracts approved by the FDA, making any food SLIT an off-label therapy. Most importantly, the SLIT dose required to prevent systemic reactions to accidental exposures remains unknown. Until these issues are resolved, the use of this modality cannot be recommended in the United States beyond research settings.

With the accumulating data supporting the use of SLIT for allergic rhinitis and asthma, it is only natural to evaluate how this treatment modality could be used in different allergic diseases. To summarize, there are several randomized, double-blind, placebo-controlled trials to support the use of SLIT in food allergy (hazelnut, peach, and peanut specifically) with acceptable tolerability and modest efficacy. The role of this therapy in the future treatment of food allergy remains unclear given its limited efficacy and the availability of other modalities undergoing research. There is 1 randomized, double-blind, placebo-controlled trial to support the safe and efficacious use of dust mite SLIT in children with mild to moderate atopic dermatitis, but these data have not been confirmed with the current FDA-approved dust mite tablet. Although there are several randomized, double-blind, placebo-controlled trials to

Table 1
Clinical trials for sublingual allergen immunotherapy

Investigators, Year	Patients (Age in Years)	Allergen (Dose)	Design/ Duration (mo)	Outcome Assessed	Efficacy	Safety
Severino et al,[1] 2008	30 (44 mean)	Honeybee venom (535 µg monthly)	RDBPC (6)	Mean peak local reaction to sting challenge, specific IgE, specific IgG	Treatment: mean reduction from 20.5 to 8.5 cm 9 (P = .014) NS change in IgE. IgG increased (P = .03) Placebo: mean reduction from 23.0 to 20.5 (P = NS) NS change in IgE or IgG	Treatment: no reactions to treatment or sting Placebo: no reactions to treatment. One episode of isolated systemic urticaria to sting
Patriarca et al,[3] 2008	41 (14–71)	Wasp venom (SLIT 100 µg weekly vs SCIT 100 µg monthly)	Case control (24)	SPT size, specific IgE, specific IgG4, rate of SR to field sting	SLIT: NS change in SPT IgE or IgG4 SCIT: NS change in SPT or IgE, but IgG4 increased (P = .001)	AR to therapy: SLIT 9.5%, SCIT 15% SR rate to field sting: SLIT 25%, SCIT 11%
Patriarca et al,[5] 2002	24 (8–64)	Latex (300 µg weekly)	RDBPC (3)	Glove use, conjunctival challenge, sublingual challenge, specific IgE, specific IgG4	Treatment: all could tolerate specific challenges. NS change in IgE Placebo: NS change in specific challenges, IgE, and IgG4	Treatment: no side effects to therapy or challenges Placebo: no side effects to therapy or challenges
Bernardini et al,[7] 2006	20 (4–15)	Latex (210 µg weekly)	RDBPC (12)	Glove use, rubbing test, SPT, specific IgE	Treatment: significant improvement in glove use (P<.0005) and rubbing test (P<.0005). NS change in SPT or IgE Placebo: NS change in glove use, rubbing test, SPT, or IgE	No side effects were reported in either group

Nettis et al,[9] 2007	35 (18–47)	RDBPC (12)	Latex (300 μg weekly)	Glove use, specific bronchial provocation, symptom/medication score, SPT, specific IgE	Treatment: significant improvement in glove use, specific bronchial provocation, symptom/medication score, SPT results at 12 mo. NS change in specific IgE Placebo: NS changes at 12 mo	Treatment: AR rate 17% of patients (mouth itching/burning, angioedema) Placebo: AR rate 6% (asthma exacerbation)
Buyukozturk et al,[10] 2010	12 (26–32)	RDBPC (12)	Latex (300 μg weekly)	Glove use, symptom/medication score	Treatment: significant improvement in glove use ($P = .01$) and symptom/medication scores ($P = .035$) Placebo: NS change in glove use or symptom/medication score	Treatment: 2 patients experienced serious SRs prompting trial discontinuation. One patient experienced dyspnea, which improved with beta agonist but also stopped the trial Placebo: no ARs reported
Gastaminza et al,[11] 2011	28 (24–57)	RDBPC (12 + 12)	Latex (210 μg weekly)	Glove use, conjunctival challenge, SPT, specific IgE, basophil activation test	NS difference in any of the measured outcomes	Treatment: 4 mild reactions during buildup Placebo: 5 mild reactions during buildup; 2 patients withdrew because of ARs
Lasa-Luaces et al,[12] 2012	23 (5–18)	Case control (12)	Latex (300 μg weekly)	Conjunctival challenge, SPT, specific IgE and IgG4, BAT	Treatment: NS change in IgE or BAT at 12 mo. Significant improvement in SPT ($P<.05$), conjunctival challenge ($P = .05$), IgG4 levels ($P<.05$) at 12 mo	Treatment: AR rate 33% of patients during buildup and 28% during maintenance reported local symptoms Placebo: none reported

(continued on next page)

Table 1
(continued)

Investigators, Year	Patients (Age in Years)	Allergen (Dose)	Design/Duration (mo)	Outcome Assessed	Efficacy	Safety
Galli et al,[16] 1994	60 (0.5–12)	HDM (?)	RCT (36)	Physician-assessed dermatitis score	All groups improved. NS difference between the groups	No side effects to treatment were reported
Pajno et al,[17] 2007	58 (5–16)	HDM (3.2 μg Der p1 and 2.6 μg Der f1 weekly)	*RDBPC (18)*	SCORAD, VAS	Significant improvement in SCORAD between groups beginning at 9 mo of SLIT (P = .025), which was most pronounced in mild-moderate AD. NS change in VAS	Treatment: AR rate of 14% reporting local reaction. SR rate of 7% (2 patients) who experienced itching and flares and were ultimately excluded Placebo: no reported AR
Qin et al,[19] 2014	107 (18–46)	HDM (50 μg Df protein daily)	RCT (12)	Compliance rate, drug scores, SCORAD, VAS, IgG4	Treatment: significantly less drug score after 6 mo (P<.01), improved total efficacy at 12 mo (P ≤ 0.05), improved VAS at 12 mo (P<.05), and higher IgG4 (P<.01) at 6 mo. NS difference in compliance rates	Treatment: 4 patients reported mild events, 2 patients withdrew because of AR Placebo: 3 patients reported mild events, 2 patients withdrew because of AR. No severe adverse effects were reported
Di Rienzo et al,[20] 2014	27 (5–18)	HDM (50% Df/50% Dp)	RCT (18)	SCORAD, VAS	Treatment: Mean SCORAD improved compared with baseline and placebo group (P = .02) at 12 and 18 mo	Treatment: AR rate 17% of patients Placebo: AR rate 7% of patients

Study	N (age)	Allergen (dose)	Type (no.)	Outcomes measured	Immunologic results	Reaction results
Enrique et al,[29] 2005	23 (19–53)	Hazelnut (38 µg Cor a1 and 24 µg Cor a8 daily)	RDBPC (3)	Oral challenge, specific IgE, IgG4 and IL-10	Treatment: significant improvement in oral tolerance ($P = .02$), IL-10 ($P<.05$), and IgG4 ($P<.05$). NS difference in placebo group outcomes. Oral tolerance was significantly more in treatment compared with placebo group ($P<.05$)	Treatment: SR rate 8% of patients Placebo: SR rate 9%. NS difference SR rate between groups. Local reactions observed in 7.4% of doses, but not specified from which groups
Fernandez-Rivas et al,[31] 2009	56 (29 mean)	Peach (30 µg Pru p3 weekly)	RDBPC (6)	Oral challenge, SPT, specific IgE and IgG4	Treatment: significant improvement in oral tolerance ($P = .005$), SPT ($P<.05$), IgE ($P = .001$), and IgG4 ($P = .01$). Placebo: significant increase in IgE only ($P = .03$). Only SPT ($P<.05$) and IgG4 ($P = .02$) levels were significantly different between groups	Treatment: local reaction rate of 89% and SR rate 13% of patients Placebo: local reaction rate of 28% and SR rate 17%. NS difference SR rate between groups
Kim et al,[33] 2011	18 (1.6–10.5)	Peanut (2000 µg weekly)	RDBPC (12)	Oral challenge dose, SPT, BAT, specific IgE and IgG4, IL-5, IL-13, IL-10, IFN-γ and regulatory T cells	Between groups, there were significant improvements in oral tolerance ($P = .011$), SPT ($P<.02$), BAT (0.009), IL-5 ($P = .015$), peanut IgE ($P = .02$), and IgG4 levels ($P = .014$). NS change in IL-13, IL-10, IFN-γ levels, or Treg numbers between groups	Treatment: local reaction rate of 11.5% and 0.28% of doses required treatment Placebo: local reaction rate of 8.6% and none required treatment. No epinephrine was required for either group

(continued on next page)

Table 1
(continued)

Investigators, Year	Patients (Age in Years)	Allergen (Dose)	Design/ Duration (mo)	Outcome Assessed	Efficacy	Safety
Fleischer et al,[35] 2013	40 (12–37)	Peanut (1386 μg daily)	RDBPC (11)	Oral challenge dose, SPT, BAT, specific IgE and IgG4	Significant increase in oral tolerance in treatment group ($P<.01$), but NS different than placebo at 44 wk. Also a decrease in BAT ($P<.008$), increase in IgG4 ($P<.001$) in treatment group. NS difference in peanut IgE levels or SPT response	Treatment: local reaction rate of 40.1% Placebo: local reaction rate of 0.6%. Only 1.1% of doses required treatment, including 1 dose of epinephrine for the study during this blinded stage (SLIT group)

Abbreviations: AR, adverse reaction; BAT, basophil activation test; Df, *Dermatophagoides farinae*; Dp, *Dermatophagoides pteronyssinus*; HDM, house dust mite; IFN, interferon; IL, interleukin; NS, nonsignificant; RCT, randomized controlled trial; RDBPC, randomized, double-blind, placebo-controlled; SPT, skin prick test; SR, systemic reaction; Treg, regulatory T cell; VAS, visual analog scale.

support the use of SLIT-LATEX, this product is not available in the United States and extrapolation of these effects to "homemade" latex extracts is unsubstantiated. In addition, there is insufficient evidence to support the use of SLIT for venom hypersensitivity at this time.

DISCLOSURE STATEMENT

The authors have nothing to disclose.

REFERENCES

1. Severino MG, Cortellini G, Bonadonna P, et al. Sublingual immunotherapy for large local reactions caused by honeybee sting: a double-blind, placebo-controlled trial. J Allergy Clin Immunol 2008;122:44–8.
2. Rueff F, Bilo MB, Jutel M, et al. Sublingual immunotherapy with venom is not recommended for patients with Hymenoptera venom allergy. J Allergy Clin Immunol 2009;123:272–3.
3. Patriarca G, Nucera E, Roncallo C, et al. Sublingual desensitization in patients with wasp venom allergy: preliminary results. Int J Immunopathol Pharmacol 2008;21:669–77.
4. Nucera E, Schiavino D, Buonomo A, et al. Latex rush desensitization. Allergy 2001;56:86–7.
5. Patriarca G, Nucera E, Pollastrini E, et al. Sublingual desensitization: a new approach to latex allergy problem. Anesth Analg 2002;95:956–60.
6. Cistero Bahima A, Sastre J, Enrique E, et al. Tolerance and effects on skin reactivity to latex of sublingual rush immunotherapy with a latex extract. J Investig Allergol Clin Immunol 2004;14:17–25.
7. Bernardini R, Campodonico P, Burastero S, et al. Sublingual immunotherapy with a latex extract in paediatric patients: a double-blind, placebo-controlled study. Curr Med Res Opin 2006;22:1515–22.
8. Tabar AI, Anda M, Bonifazi F, et al. Specific immunotherapy with standardized latex extract versus placebo in latex-allergic patients. Int Arch Allergy Immunol 2006;141:369–76.
9. Nettis E, Colanardi MC, Soccio AL, et al. Double-blind, placebo-controlled study of sublingual immunotherapy in patients with latex-induced urticaria: a 12-month study. Br J Dermatol 2007;156:674–81.
10. Buyukozturk S, Gelincik A, Ferhan İ, et al. Latex sublingual immunotherapy: can its safety be predicted? Ann Allergy Asthma Immunol 2010;104:339–42.
11. Gastaminza G, Algorta J, Uriel O, et al. Randomized, double-blind, placebo controlled clinical trial of sublingual immunotherapy in natural rubber latex allergic patients. Trials 2011;12:191.
12. Lasa Luaces EM, Tabar Purroy AI, Garcia Figueroa BE, et al. Component resolved immunologic modifications, efficacy, and tolerance of latex sublingual immunotherapy in children. Ann Allergy Asthma Immunol 2012;108:367–72.
13. Nucera E, Mezzacappa S, Buonomo A, et al. Latex immunotherapy: evidence of effectiveness. Postepy Dermatol Alergol 2018;35(2):145–50.
14. Nucera E, Schiavino D, Sabato V, et al. Sublingual immunotherapy for latex allergy: tolerability and safety profile of rush build-up phase. Curr Med Res Opin 2008;24:1147–54.
15. Nettis E, Di Leo E, Calogiuri G, et al. The safety of a novel sublingual rush induction phase for latex desensitization. Curr Med Res Opin 2010;26:1855–9.

16. Galli E, Chini L, Nardi S, et al. Use of a specific oral hyposensitization therapy to *Dermatophagoides pteronyssinus* in children with atopic dermatitis. Allergol Immunopathol (Madr) 1994;22:18–22.

17. Pajno GB, Caminiti L, Vita D, et al. Sublingual immunotherapy in mite-sensitized children with atopic dermatitis: a randomized, double-blind, placebo-controlled study. J Allergy Clin Immunol 2007;120:164–70.

18. Schram ME, Spuls PI, Leeflang MM, et al. EASI, (objective) SCORAD and POEM for atopic eczema: responsiveness and minimal clinically important difference. Allergy 2012;67(1):99–106.

19. Qin YE, Mao JR, Sang YC, et al. Clinical efficacy and compliance of sublingual immunotherapy with *Dermatophagoides farinae* drops in patients with atopic dermatitis. Int J Dermatol 2014;53(5):650–5.

20. Di Rienzo V, Cadario G, Grieco T, et al. Sublingual immunotherapy in mite-sensitized children with atopic dermatitis: a randomized, open, parallel-group study. Ann Allergy Asthma Immunol 2014;113(6):671–3.

21. You HS, Yang MY, Kim GW, et al. Effectiveness of specific sublingual immunotherapy in Korean patients with atopic dermatitis. Ann Dermatol 2017;29(1):1–5.

22. Mempel M, Rakoski J, Ring J, et al. Severe anaphylaxis to kiwi fruit: immunologic changes related to successful sublingual allergen immunotherapy. J Allergy Clin Immunol 2003;111:1406–9.

23. Kerzl R, Simonowa A, Ring J, et al. Life-threatening anaphylaxis to kiwi fruit: protective sublingual allergen immunotherapy effect persists even after discontinuation. J Allergy Clin Immunol 2007;119(2):507–8.

24. de Boissieu D, Dupont C. Sublingual immunotherapy for cow's milk protein allergy: a preliminary report. Allergy 2006;61(10):1238–9.

25. Hansen KS, Khinchi MS, Skov PS, et al. Food allergy to apple and specific immunotherapy with birch pollen. Mol Nutr Food Res 2004;48(6):441–8.

26. Mauro M, Russello M, Incorvaia C, et al. Birch-Apple syndrome treated with birch pollen immunotherapy. Int Arch Allergy Immunol 2011;156(4):416–22.

27. Geroldinger-Simic M, Kinaciyan T, Nagl B, et al. Oral exposure to Mal d 1 affects the immune response in patients with birch pollen allergy. J Allergy Clin Immunol 2013;131(1):94–102.

28. Kinaciyan T, Nagl B, Faustmann S, et al. Efficacy and safety of 4 months of sublingual immunotherapy with recombinant Mal d 1 and Bet v 1 in patients with birch pollen–related apple allergy. J Allergy Clin Immunol 2018;141(3):1002–8.

29. Enrique E, Pineda F, Malek T, et al. Sublingual immunotherapy for hazelnut food allergy: a randomized, double-blind, placebo-controlled study with a standardized hazelnut extract. J Allergy Clin Immunol 2005;116(5):1073–9.

30. Enrique E, Malek T, Pineda F, et al. Sublingual immunotherapy for hazelnut food allergy: a follow-up study. Ann Allergy Asthma Immunol 2008;100:283–4.

31. Fernandez-Rivas M, Garrido Fernandez S, Nadal JA, et al. Randomized double blind, placebo-controlled trial of sublingual immunotherapy with a Pru p 3 quantified peach extract. Allergy 2009;64:876–83.

32. Gomez F, Bogas G, Gonzalez M, et al. The clinical and immunological effects of Pru p 3 sublingual immunotherapy on peach and peanut allergy in patients with systemic reactions. Clin Exp Allergy 2017;47(3):339–50.

33. Kim EH, Bird JA, Kulis M, et al. Sublingual immunotherapy for peanut allergy: clinical and immunologic evidence of desensitization. J Allergy Clin Immunol 2011;127:640–6.e1.

34. Kim EH, Yang L, Ye P, et al. Long-term sublingual immunotherapy for peanut allergy in children: clinician and immunologic evidence of desensitization. J Allergy Clin Immunol 2019 [pii:S0091-6749(19)31020-6].
35. Fleischer DM, Burks AW, Vickery BP, et al. Sublingual immunotherapy for peanut allergy: a randomized, double-blind, placebo-controlled multicenter trial. J Allergy Clin Immunol 2013;131:119–27.e1-7.
36. Burks AW, Wood RA, Jones SM, et al. Sublingual immunotherapy for peanut allergy: long-term follow-up of a randomized multicenter trial. J Allergy Clin Immunol 2015;135(5):1240–8.
37. Keet CA, Frischmeyer-Guerrerio PA, Thyagarajan A, et al. The safety and efficacy of sublingual and oral immunotherapy for milk allergy. J Allergy Clin Immunol 2012;129(2):448–55.
38. Narisety SD, Frischmeyer-Guerrerio PA, Keet CA, et al. A randomized, double blind, placebo-controlled pilot study of sublingual versus oral immunotherapy for the treatment of peanut allergy. J Allergy Clin Immunol 2015;135(5):1275–82.e6.

Venom Immunotherapy
Questions and Controversies

David B.K. Golden, MD

KEYWORDS

- Venom immunotherapy • Insect sting • Venom allergy • Anaphylaxis • Epinephrine

KEY POINTS

- It is important to recognize high-risk factors that identify patients who require VIT and pre-scription of EAI.
- Adverse reactions to VIT are managed with a variety of measures including rush VIT.
- The risk of β-blockers and ACE inhibitors during VIT is small and should not deter treatment.
- The choice of venoms, regimen, and dose for VIT is individualized.
- The decision to stop VIT after 5 years rests on the history and known risk factors rather than any diagnostic tests.

Venom immunotherapy (VIT) has changed little in the four decades since it was approved in the United States. There are excellent chapters, review articles, guidelines, and practice parameters on VIT.[1–4] Yet, there are always questions and problems that arise with patients with insect allergy that seem to eclipse all those publications and cause great vexation to clinicians. Allergists commonly address their questions and problems to experts in the field and to the Joint Task Force on Practice Parameters of the American Academy of Allergy Asthma and Immunology (AAAAI) and American College of Allergy Asthma and Immunology (ACAAI), which have often brought them to my attention. Rather than review VIT and the few recent developments, I review the frequently asked questions of VIT, including questions, problems, and controversies. Most of the things I discuss fall into the category of "what do I do now," and some represent ongoing controversies that remain unresolved even with the availability of new evidence.

The frequent uncertainty surrounding patients with insect allergy is partly caused by knowledge gaps that remain after years of research, and by the low threshold of risk in

Disclosure Statement: Dr D.B.K. Golden discloses the following potential conflicts of interest: Speaker Bureau (honoraria): Genentech. Clinical trials (research grants): Genentech and Stallergenes/Greer. Consultant: ALK-Abello. Editor (royalties): UpToDate.
Department of Medicine, Division of Allergy-Immunology, Johns Hopkins University, 20 Crossroads Drive, Owings Mills, MD 21117, USA
E-mail address: dbkgolden@gmail.com

Immunol Allergy Clin N Am 40 (2020) 59–68
https://doi.org/10.1016/j.iac.2019.09.002
0889-8561/20/© 2019 Elsevier Inc. All rights reserved.

the arena of anaphylaxis. If the chance of a runny nose was 5%, extreme precautions (carrying an emergency treatment, years of immunotherapy) would be judged to be unnecessary. But if the chance of anaphylaxis is even 1%, the level of concern seems to rise exponentially. This paradigm underlies many of the decisions that are made regarding the testing and treatment of patients who present with a history of reaction to an insect sting. It is also important to distinguish between those patients at high risk for anaphylaxis, and those at low risk despite showing evidence of venom sensitivity. This focus on risk stratification was emphasized in the most recent update of the Practice Parameters of Insect Allergy.[3] Many of the frequently asked questions I review revolve around this understanding of the relative risk of anaphylaxis.

WHAT DO I DO NOW?
Does This Patient Need Venom Immunotherapy?

In this review on VIT, I am not directly addressing the diagnosis of insect sting allergy. In basic terms, the indication for VIT is a history of sting anaphylaxis and a positive test (skin or serum) for venom-IgE. The strength or level of the test result suggests, but does not reliably predict, the severity of a reaction to a future sting.[5,6] The severity of a sting reaction is, however, highly correlated with the severity of previous reactions, and the level of basal serum tryptase.[5,7] As with all allergies, there are three types of individuals with positive results for allergen-IgE: (1) those with a history of immediate severe reaction, (2) those who have never had a severe reaction to despite known exposure, and (3) those with no known exposure. In the patient with insect allergy, any of these three presentations could be difficult to assess.

A patient with an incidental history of remote anaphylaxis to a sting may have presented for hay fever. Questions arise about the relative risk when decades have elapsed, either with no stings, or with known stings but no reaction. Venom allergy can persist for decades and the risk does not necessarily decline with time.[5,6] In some children who did not receive VIT, sting anaphylaxis recurred even 20 years after initial diagnosis.[8] The risk is present even when there have been intervening stings without reaction. This is because of the known variability in reactions to stings, which is caused by differences in the insects. For example, yellow jackets can deliver between 2 and 20 μg of venom per sting, a 10-fold variation that could easily explain why a reaction would happen to some stings and not others. There is also a significant difference in the potency of stings from different yellow jackets, even though they look alike.[5] A sting could also be tolerated because it was a species to which the patient is not allergic (it is easy to mistake one species of insect for another). It is recommended that a patient with a history of sting anaphylaxis should be tested (and treated if positive) even if it occurred in the remote past. If there have been several intervening stings with no reaction, there is evidence that the patient may no longer be reactive.[9]

A patient who had no severe reaction, but had generalized urticaria and facial swelling, or progressive large local reactions (LLR), may still avoid outdoor activities because of a fear of anaphylaxis. Because their risk of more severe anaphylaxis to a future sting is low, VIT is not required. However, those with frequent exposure and reactions, or those with marked impairment of quality of life, may clearly benefit from a course of VIT.[3,10]

A patient who has never been stung may present because of a relative (or news report) with a severe (or fatal) reaction. It is recommended not to test individuals for venom sensitivity if they are not candidates for VIT. This is because a positive test is more likely to increase anxiety and impair quality of life, even when there is little increased risk of anaphylaxis. As with other allergens, there are many people with asymptomatic sensitization. About 20% of the adult population, and up to 40% of those who have been stung in the past 3 months, will have positive venom allergy tests, and yet only 3% of the adult population has a history of systemic reaction to a sting.[11] Venom sensitivity is transient or asymptomatic in most cases, and clinically significant only in those with a history of sting anaphylaxis. Nevertheless, many such individuals are not satisfied with these explanations, and find someone to do the test. For this reason, it is sometimes better to do the test so that an experienced allergist can explain what the results do or do not mean. However, it is important to explain to the patient before doing any tests what you will or will not recommend if the test is positive.

Systemic Reaction to Venom Immunotherapy

One of the most common dilemmas is what to do when the patient cannot build up the venom dose because of recurrent adverse reactions. Problems may arise early with reactions to venom skin tests, creating obvious concerns about initiating VIT, or can occur during up-dosing or maintenance VIT. LLR have caused some patients to undergo much slower build-up regimens or to be held at doses lower than 100 µg. These measures are usually unnecessary and counterproductive. LLR are generally not predictive of later systemic reactions to VIT. Patients should be encouraged to tolerate moderate LLR in the hope that the sooner they achieve the maintenance dose, the sooner the reactions will lessen.

It is generally recommended for patients to take a second-generation antihistamine before each VIT treatment during the build-up phase. This has been shown to reduce the occurrence of LLR and mild systemic reactions.[12] Antihistamines may even increase the efficacy of treatment, through their effects on histamine receptors on immune-regulatory cells.[13,14] There is a single report of leukotriene modifier giving significant reduction of LLR, greater than the effect of antihistamines.[15]

When LLR are excessive and the discomfort is unacceptable and prolonged, some measures are tried to work around the problem. The dose can be split between two sites, although this is difficult when the patent is receiving multiple venoms. Some patients tolerate the injection better if it is a smaller volume of a more concentrated extract: the venom can be reconstituted to 200 µg/mL, with a maintenance dose of 0.5 mL. Occasionally, it is reasonable to reduce the dose temporarily and build it up again in the hope that the reactions lessen. Keeping the dose lower for extended periods not only gives suboptimal protection, but very low doses (<25 µg) can even increase the venom-IgE levels.

Systemic reactions require immediate treatment and adjustment of the subsequent treatment dose and regimen. As with any immunotherapy, the first step after a systemic reaction is to reduce the dose by about 50% and then resume the build-up schedule. In most cases there is not another reaction. When there are repeated systemic reactions, it is not recommended to continue administering progressively lower doses, nor to keep the dose low enough to avoid reactions (for the same reasons described previously for LLR). Before deciding to take any further action, it is important to clarify the nature of the systemic reaction. Although one should have great respect for the risks of anaphylaxis, one may be too hasty to diagnose and treat anaphylaxis in a patient who has just received a venom injection. Some patients have systemic reactions that are entirely subjective (eg, throat or chest discomfort, slight light-headedness, itching, nausea) without objective signs (eg, hives, reduced peak flow or oxygen saturation, reduced blood pressure).[5] Despite the chance that this represents a mild systemic reaction, such patients may be approached with reassurance and patient observation rather than immediate epinephrine and changes in treatment dose. In many cases, the dose is advanced with no objective signs of anaphylaxis. Another example of this problem is the patient who has a subjective systemic reaction to venom skin tests, but the tests themselves are negative. This should raise suspicion about whether the reaction is truly allergic. In both scenarios, it is often necessary to begin treatment with a series of negative and positive control injections to clarify whether the symptoms might be nonspecific and not truly allergic. The rationale can be explained to patients in a way that is perceived as reassuring rather than accusatory or reproachful.

When there are repeated anaphylactic reactions to VIT, specific measures are taken. Initial measures can include reducing the number of venoms to a single species (or give different ones on different days); trying a cluster regimen of three smaller doses at 30-minute intervals on each weekly visit; and premedication with H_1 and H_2 blockers, montelukast, and sometimes prednisone. Paradoxically, the best solution to repeated systemic reactions is a rush regimen (usually with premedication), because it rarely causes reactions even in these "high-risk" patients.[16] An alternative or supplemental approach to rush VIT is the use of omalizumab because it generally reduces or eliminates the systemic reactions, enabling the patient to achieve the maintenance dose.[17,18] Occasionally this is not adequately effective, and in a few cases the reactions recurred when omalizumab was discontinued.[19]

There are some misconceptions that must be identified. When patients have a history of very severe anaphylaxis to a sting, there is often a feeling that VIT should be started at a very low dose and increased only slowly. Again, paradoxically, the exact opposite is true (discussed later in relation to rush regimens). This is important because using extra cautious slow regimens may just increase the occurrence of systemic reactions, and only delays achieving the level of immunity that reduces the occurrence of adverse reactions.

In patients who have had very severe reactions to stings or systemic reactions to VIT either repeatedly or at the maintenance dose, it is important to measure the basal serum tryptase because underlying mast cell disorders are a common reason for these problems. It is important to identify patients with mast cell disorders because there are significant increased risks for these patients even during and after VIT.[20]

Venom Dose

The starting dose varies by orders of magnitude in different reports and recommendations. A typical suggestion is to begin with doses in the range of 0.001 µg and proceed with incremental doubling doses. However, a dose of 1 µg was shown to be equally safe 40 years ago, and confirmed in a recent and much larger study.[21,22] Paradoxically, an initial dose of 100 µg was given in two different studies, with no severe reactions in either study.[23,24]

The recommended maintenance dose for VIT is 100 µg of each venom. This was originally determined empirically to be double the known amount of venom protein in a honeybee sting (50 µg). Yellow jacket stings may contain 2 to 20 µg of venom protein per sting. For many years there was controversy about whether 50 µg was an effective maintenance dose. One study showed reduced efficacy, whereas another showed it to be fully effective.[25,26]

We have long wished we could give smaller doses to young children because of the difficulty with local reactions, but the recommended dose has been 100 µg for all ages since the introduction of venom extracts for VIT. Only recently have studies been designed to test the safety and efficacy of a 50-µg dose in children during and after finishing a course of VIT.[27,28] These studies lead to further questions because they included children up to 18 years old. If the 50-µg dose is effective in 16 to 18 year olds, then should it not also be adequate for adults? An early study of dosing regimens for VIT showed that the 50-μg dose could induce the same IgG response as the 100-μg dose but it took a few weeks longer.[21] This led the investigators to try giving 50 μg as a maintenance dose, but they reported an inadequate clinical response.[25]

Higher maintenance doses (200 μg) are required for full protection in some patients. This is primarily true in patients who have had systemic reactions during VIT (discussed later in the section on systemic reactions to VIT) and in others with less than optimal protection (eg, beekeepers).[29]

When to Stop Venom Immunotherapy

When to recommend discontinuing VIT remains a difficult question for many clinicians and their patients, although there are no new studies and no changes in the guidelines. The problem usually centers around the reluctance to take any chance of the patient having a systemic reaction to a future sting. In adults it is clear that 5 years of VIT gives better immunologic and clinical outcomes than 3 years.[30,31] In children, 3.5 years was the mean duration of treatment in a long-term study that found 95% of children developed long-term tolerance after finishing a course of VIT.[8] The early studies of stopping VIT revealed several risk factors associated with relapse. Patients with none of these factors rarely have problems after completing 5 years of VIT. These factors include very severe (near fatal) pre-VIT sting reaction (eg, hypotensive shock), abnormal basal serum tryptase, older age and underlying medical conditions, use of β-blockers and angiotensin-converting enzyme inhibitors (ACEI), honeybee anaphylaxis, and frequent unavoidable exposure.[3] There is no test that is useful in deciding whether to stop VIT except for the basal serum tryptase. There are reports of patients who had negative venom skin tests and borderline serum IgE when they stopped VIT but still had recurrence of sting anaphylaxis.[32] Extending VIT beyond 5 years may also be justified because of impaired quality of life. For patients in whom stopping VIT will cause psychological distress and avoidance of outdoor activities, continued VIT is reasonable. When VIT is continued beyond 5 years, the maintenance interval can generally be increased to 12 weeks.

For patients who continue VIT beyond 5 years, it is not known how long is long enough. In studies of discontinuing VIT, it was observed that reactions to stings could occur even 12 to 13 years after stopping treatment in some patients.[32] Therefore treatment for 15 to 20 years in some cases may seem reasonable. However, some patients who started treatment 20 to 30 years ago have now eclipsed knowledge of the natural history of insect sting anaphylaxis and VIT. It is not yet known whether even high-risk patients can safely stop treatment eventually. The one case that seems to truly require indefinite VIT is mastocytosis, because of the reported risk of fatal anaphylaxis in such patients who stop treatment.

CONTROVERSIES
To Rush or Not to Rush?

There are surprising paradoxes related to rush VIT. The common belief in the United States remains that rush VIT is dangerous or experimental, but evidence, experience, and guidelines say the opposite. One problem has been terminology. Reviewing the literature on VIT is a confusing experience. There are published rush regimens that achieve the 100-μg maintenance dose more rapidly than certain reported ultrarush regimens. It is suggested that regimens should be described as conventional (traditional) when they reach maintenance dose in months, semirush (or cluster) in weeks, rush in days, and ultrarush in hours.[33]

Traditional regimens for allergen immunotherapy are most widely accepted in the United States, usually involving weekly or twice a week dosing for about 6 months to reach the maintenance dose. This is the regimen recommended in the Food and Drug Administration–approved product package insert for the only venom extract products remaining on the market in the United States. In the most severely allergic patients, many allergists begin treatment with even lower doses and proceed even more cautiously over a period of up to 12 months. However, even early studies showed that systemic reactions did not occur more often with rush regimens, and that the reaction rate (reactions per 100 injections) is actually the same with rush, semirush, and traditional regimens.[21] Although a plethora of rapid regimens has been described, mostly in the European literature, one of the most widely used is a 2- to 3-day regimen described by Bernstein and colleagues,[34] and modified by Goldberg and Confino-Cohen.[16] Goldberg and his group have reported the safety and efficacy of this regimen in a wide range of high-risk patients including those with repeated systemic reactions, patients allergic to honeybee, and children.[16,35,36] Brown and colleagues[37] compared several regimens and found that the semirush regimen had comparable safety with the traditional regimen, but there was a higher reaction rate with an ultrarush regimen. The US Practice Parameters and the European Academy of Allergy and Clinical Immunology (EAACI) guidelines advise that the risk of systemic reactions is higher with ultrarush (and perhaps some rush) regimens.[3,4]

One Venom or All Venoms?

Another frequently asked question is whether to include in the patient's VIT regimen only the venom that was the culprit in the patient's anaphylactic reaction, or also other venoms to which the patient demonstrates IgE by skin or serum test. It is possible in most cases to determine from a detailed history and venom IgE tests whether the sting was caused by a honeybee, a yellow jacket, or a paper wasp. Hornet stings are least common and hornet venoms are highly cross reactive with yellow jacket venom. Most patients with vespid allergy should receive mixed vespid venom for optimal protection and for the convenience of a single injection. When a vespid allergic patient also has a positive test for honeybee venom (but no history of anaphylaxis to a honeybee sting), the decision on treatment must consider the degree of exposure, the degree of cross reactivity, and the risk tolerance of the patient. If the patient is certain to not walk in the grass barefoot or in sandals, or garden without gloves, then a honeybee sting is highly unlikely. But for the patient who wants absolute certainty of not reacting to any sting, addition of honeybee venom to the treatment regimen may be considered.

Although concerns about the need for dual therapy with honeybee and yellow jacket venoms predominate in Europe, there is greater concern in the United States about the need for dual therapy with yellow jacket and wasp (Polistes) venom, which have about 50% cross reactivity. It is possible to distinguish cross reactivity from dual sensitization by a venom-IgE immunoassay inhibition test, but this is not widely available.[38] The use of recombinant component allergens for immunoassays can more accurately identify true sensitization, but these are not yet approved for commercial use in the United States. There is great promise for such recombinant allergen-based component-resolved diagnosis to improve the diagnostic accuracy and specificity of insect allergy testing.[39]

Epinephrine Autoinjector for All or Few?

Does this patient need an epinephrine autoinjector (EAI)? When this question comes up, it is obviously because the risk is not so high as to make the question unnecessary. Like the question of "does this patient need VIT," the answer is either obvious or requires discussion and shared decision making with the patient or family. The risk of anaphylaxis is low (<3%) in people with a history of LLR or cutaneous systemic reactions. It is confusing when we tell them they do not need VIT but should carry an EAI, leaving them still fearful of having a reaction if they get stung. Prescription of an EAI can cause impairment of quality of life, and is a burden in many ways.[40,41] This dilemma is best addressed by discussion and shared decision-making, to determine if this individual/family will feel much more secure having an EAI, or will they feel even more fearful thinking they might have to use it? There is no consensus on how much risk is too much, or how much is acceptable (eg, 10%, 5%, 1%, or 0.1% chance of anaphylaxis). There is no such thing as zero risk, but there is certainly a cost and a burden that may not justify too low a threshold. The same principles apply to the relative need for EAI in patients on maintenance VIT or after discontinuing VIT (in patients with no high-risk factors).

Angiotensin-Converting Enzyme Inhibitor and β-Blockers: Too Risky or No Problem?

The product package insert for venom extracts in the United States clearly states, as with all immunotherapy extracts, that there is a contraindication to immunotherapy in patients taking β-blockers or ACEI. There is reason for concern that these medications may increase the severity of anaphylactic reactions.[7,42] However, there have been conflicting reports on the relative risk associated with these medications during VIT.[43,44] The EAACI guidelines advise that anaphylaxis does not occur more frequently in patients receiving β-blockers, and that "based on the risk/benefit profile there is no contraindication for VIT in patients treated with β-blockers."[4]

There are studies that find no safety problems with VIT in patients on ACEI, and others that show no increased risk for severe systemic reaction in untreated patients with insect sting allergy.[44,45] There are also studies that found a higher chance of severe systemic reactions in treated or untreated patients taking ACEI.[7,43] As with β-blockers, the calculation of risk is often confounded by the close relation of these medications to older age and underlying medical conditions. The EAACI guidelines suggest that "ACEI therapy may be continued during VIT, but the patient should be informed about possible risks."[4]

The US practice parameters on anaphylaxis state that "the benefits of allergen immunotherapy with Hymenoptera venoms clearly outweigh the potential risks associated with b-blockers or ACEIs in those patients with anaphylaxis to stinging insects who also have cardiovascular disease that requires these medications" and that "consideration should be given to the discontinuation of any drug treatment that may worsen an episode of anaphylaxis or complicate its treatment."[46] The US practice parameters on insect allergy summarize the published evidence but give no specific guidance to the clinician. They state that "the incidence of systemic reactions to VIT is not significantly affected by these medications. The possibility that the severity of such reactions, should they occur, might be increased by the medications is supported by some studies and not by others."[3] The likelihood is that age and underlying medical conditions are the true risk factors for severe reactions to stings or VIT, and that the protection from anaphylaxis to stings in the field that is provided by VIT outweighs the small chance of a severe reaction to VIT in the clinic.

SUMMARY

VIT presents some puzzling paradoxes that inevitably contribute to uncertainty and confusion in the diagnosis and management of the insect-allergic patient. We assume that VIT is riskier than grass or cat immunotherapy, and yet we do not have more systemic reactions with VIT. We assume that rush VIT is more risky than slower traditional regimens (as it is with inhalant allergens), and yet the opposite is true. We tend to extreme caution in recommending epinephrine injectors or VIT to patients with any form of venom sensitivity, but we often do not distinguish those with low risk from those with high risk. This review is oriented to the clinician with an insect-allergic patient who presents a dilemma not easily resolved by existing guidelines and reviews. These problems and questions seem to come up surprisingly often with insect-allergic patients.

There are also significant knowledge gaps that remain and limit confidence in clinical recommendations. It is not yet known with certainty whether β-blockers or ACEI create unacceptable risk in certain patients, or how to best use recombinant venom allergens for more accurate section of patients and venoms for treatment. The optimal duration of VIT is still not fully understood. For those who are recommended to have extended or indefinite treatment, it is not known whether there is any benefit to VIT beyond 15 to 20 years. Further research studies should be designed to address these questions.

REFERENCES

1. Dhami S, Zaman H, Varga EM, et al. Allergen immunotherapy for insect venom allergy: a systematic review and meta-analysis. Allergy 2017;72:342–65.
2. Golden DBK. Insect allergy. In: Adkinson NFYJ, Bochner BS, Busse WW, et al, editors. Middleton's allergy: principles and practice. 8th edition. Philadelphia: Elsevier; 2014. p. 1260–73.
3. Golden DBK, Demain J, Freeman T, et al. Stinging insect hypersensitivity: a practice parameter update 2016. Ann Allergy Asthma Immunol 2017;118:28–54.
4. Sturm GJ, Varga EM, Roberts G, et al. EAACI guidelines on allergen immunotherapy: Hymenoptera venom allergy. Allergy 2018;73:744–64.
5. Golden DBK, Breisch NL, Hamilton RG, et al. Clinical and entomological factors influence the outcome of sting challenge studies. J Allergy Clin Immunol 2006;117:670–5.
6. Reisman RE. Natural history of insect sting allergy: relationship of severity of symptoms of initial sting anaphylaxis to re-sting reactions. J Allergy Clin Immunol 1992;90:335–9.
7. Rueff F, Przybilla B, Bilo MB, et al. Predictors of severe systemic anaphylactic reactions in patients with Hymenoptera venom allergy: importance of baseline serum tryptase. A study of the EAACI Interest Group on Insect Venom Hypersensitivity. J Allergy Clin Immunol 2009;124:1047–54.
8. Golden DBK, Kagey-Sobotka A, Norman PS, et al. Outcomes of allergy to insect stings in children with and without venom immunotherapy. N Engl J Med 2004;351:668–74.
9. Hauk P, Friedl K, Kaufmehl K, et al. Subsequent insect stings in children with hypersensitivity to Hymenoptera. J Pediatr 1995;126:185–90.
10. Golden DBK, Kelly D, Hamilton RG, et al. Venom immunotherapy reduces large local reactions to insect stings. J Allergy Clin Immunol 2009;123:1371–5.
11. Golden DBK, Marsh DG, Kagey-Sobotka A, et al. Epidemiology of insect venom sensitivity. JAMA 1989;262:240–4.
12. Brockow K, Kiehn M, Riethmuller C, et al. Efficacy of antihistamine pretreatment in the prevention of adverse reactions to Hymenoptera immunotherapy: a

prospective, randomized, placebo-controlled trial. J Allergy Clin Immunol 1997; 100:458–63.

13. Muller U, Hari Y, Berchtold E. Premedication with antihistamines may enhance efficacy of specific allergen immunotherapy. J Allergy Clin Immunol 2001;107:81–6.

14. Muller UR, Jutel M, Reimers A, et al. Clinical and immunologic effects of H1 antihistamine preventive medication during honeybee venom immunotherapy. J Allergy Clin Immunol 2008;122:1001–7.

15. Wohrl S, Gamper S, Hemmer W, et al. Premedication with montelukast reduces large local reactions of allergen immunotherapy. Int Arch Allergy Immunol 2007;144:137–42.

16. Goldberg A, Confino-Cohen R. Rush venom immunotherapy in patients experiencing recurrent systemic reactions to conventional venom immunotherapy. Ann Allergy 2003;91:405–10.

17. Galera C, Soohun N, Zankar N, et al. Severe anaphylaxis to bee venom immunotherapy: efficacy of pretreatment with omalizumab. J Investig Allergol Clin Immunol 2009;19:225–9.

18. Kontou-Fili K. High omalizumab dose controls recurrent reactions to venom immunotherapy in indolent systemic mastocytosis. Allergy 2008;63:376–8.

19. Gomis VS, Delgado PG, Hernandez EN. Failure of omalizumab treatment after recurrent systemic reactions to bee-venom immunotherapy. J Investig Allergol Clin Immunol 2008;18:225–6.

20. Niedoszytko M, Bonadonna P, Oude-Elberink JNG, Golden DBK. Epidemiology, diagnosis, and treatment of Hymenoptera venom allergy in mastocytosis patients. Immunol Allergy Clin North Am 2014;34:365–81.

21. Golden DBK, Valentine MD, Kagey-Sobotka A, et al. Regimens of Hymenoptera venom immunotherapy. Ann Intern Med 1980;92:620–4.

22. Roumana A, Pitsios C, S Vartholomaios EK, et al. The safety of initiating Hymenoptera immunotherapy at 1 microgram of venom extract. J Allergy Clin Immunol 2009;124:379–81.

23. Hunt KJ, Valentine MD, Sobotka AK, et al. A controlled trial of immunotherapy in insect hypersensitivity. N Engl J Med 1978;299:157–61.

24. Vos B, Dubois A, Rauber M, et al. Initiating yellow jacket venom immunotherapy with a 100 mcg dose: a challenge? J Allergy Clin Immunol Pract 2019;7:1332–4.

25. Golden DBK, Kagey-Sobotka A, Valentine MD, et al. Dose dependence of Hymenoptera venom immunotherapy. J Allergy Clin Immunol 1981;67:370–4.

26. Reisman RE, Livingston A. Venom immunotherapy: 10 years of experience with administration of single venoms and 50 micrograms maintenance dose. J Allergy Clin Immunol 1992;89:1189–95.

27. Houliston L, Nolan R, Noble V, et al. Honeybee venom immunotherapy in children using a 50-mcg maintenance dose. J Allergy Clin Immunol 2011;127:98–9.

28. Konstantinou GN, Manoussakis E, Douladiris N, et al. A 5-year venom immunotherapy protocol with 50 mcg maintenance dose: safety and efficacy in school children. Pediatr Allergy Immunol 2011;22:393–7.

29. Rueff F, Wenderoth A, Przybilla B. Patients still reacting to a sting challenge while receiving conventional Hymenoptera venom immunotherapy are protected by increased venom doses. J Allergy Clin Immunol 2001;108:1027–32.

30. Keating MU, Kagey-Sobotka A, Hamilton RG, et al. Clinical and immunologic follow-up of patients who stop venom immunotherapy. J Allergy Clin Immunol 1991;88:339–48.

31. Lerch E, Muller U. Long-term protection after stopping venom immunotherapy. J Allergy Clin Immunol 1998;101:606–12.

32. Golden DBK, Kagey-Sobotka A, Lichtenstein LM. Survey of patients after discontinuing venom immunotherapy. J Allergy Clin Immunol 2000;105:385–90.

33. Golden DBK. Rush venom immunotherapy: ready for prime time? J Allergy Clin Immunol Pract 2017;5:804–5.

34. Bernstein JA, Kagan SL, Bernstein DI, et al. Rapid venom immunotherapy is safe for routine use in the treatment of patients with Hymenoptera anaphylaxis. Ann Allergy 1994;73:423–8.

35. Confino-Cohen R, Rosman Y, Goldberg A. Rush venom immunotherapy in children. J Allergy Clin Immunol Pract 2017;5:799–803.

36. Goldberg A, Yogev A, Confino-Cohen R. Three days rush venom immunotherapy in bee allergy: safe, inexpensive, and instantaneously effective. Int Arch Allergy Immunol 2011;156:90–8.

37. Brown SG, Wiese MD, vanEeden P, et al. Ultrarush versus semirush initiation of insect venom immunotherapy: a randomized controlled trial. J Allergy Clin Immunol 2012;130:162–8.

38. Hamilton RH, Wisenauer JA, Golden DBK, et al. Selection of Hymenoptera venoms for immunotherapy based on patients' IgE antibody cross-reactivity. J Allergy Clin Immunol 1993;92:651–9.

39. Muller UR, Schmid-Grendelmeier P, Hausmann O, et al. IgE to recombinant allergens Api m 1, Ves v 1, and Ves v 5 distinguish double sensitization from cross reaction in venom allergy. Allergy 2012;67:1069–73.

40. Oude-Elberink JNG, deMonchy JGR, vanderHeide S, et al. Venom immunotherapy improves health-related quality of life in yellow jacket allergic patients. J Allergy Clin Immunol 2002;110:174–82.

41. Oude-Elberink JN, vanderHeide S, Guyatt GH, et al. Analysis of the burden of treatment in patients receiving an Epi-Pen for yellow jacket anaphylaxis. J Allergy Clin Immunol 2006;118:699–704.

42. Nassiri M, Babina M, Dolle S, et al. Ramipril and metoprolol intake aggravate human and murine anaphylaxis: evidence for direct mast cell priming. J Allergy Clin Immunol 2015;135:491–9.

43. Rueff F, Vos B, Oude-Elberink J, et al. Predictors of clinical effectiveness of Hymenoptera venom immunotherapy. Clin Exp Allergy 2014;44:736–46.

44. Stoevesandt J, Hain J, Stolze I, et al. Angiotensin-converting enzyme inhibitors do not impair the safety of Hymenoptera venom immunotherapy build-up phase. Clin Exp Allergy 2014;44:747–55.

45. Stoevesandt J, Hain J, Kerstan A, et al. Over- and underestimated parameters in severe Hymenoptera venom-induced anaphylaxis: cardiovascular medication and absence of urticaria/angioedema. J Allergy Clin Immunol 2012;130:698–704.

46. Lieberman P, Nicklas RA, Randolph C, et al. Anaphylaxis: a practice parameter update 2015. Ann Allergy Asthma Immunol 2015;115:341–84.

The Cost-Effectiveness of Allergen Immunotherapy Compared with Pharmacotherapy for Treatment of Allergic Rhinitis and Asthma

Linda S. Cox, MD[a],*, Andrew Murphey, MD[b], Cheryl Hankin, PhD[c]

KEYWORDS

- Allergen immunotherapy • Asthma • Allergic rhinitis • Subcutaneous immunotherapy
- Sublingual immunotherapy • Atopic dermatitis • Pharmacoeconomics

KEY POINTS

- After an extensive search of the PubMed and Medline databases was performed, the authors concluded that SCIT and SLIT were cost-effective compared with SDT from around 6 years after treatment initiation (with most treatments being 3 years). There was no strong evidence indicating superior cost-efficacy of SCIT or SLIT over SDT in either of these systematic reviews.
- There is strong evidence in the collective literature, which included individual studies and systematic reviews, that AIT is cost-effective in the management of allergic rhinitis and asthma as compared with SDT alone.
- The magnitude of AIT's cost-effectiveness is likely underestimated because most of the studies considered during-treatment costs and not AIT's long-term benefits or preventive/prophylactic effects.

INTRODUCTION

Allergic rhinitis (AR) affects approximately 20% to 30% of the United States and European populations.[1–4] Symptoms include rhinorrhea, sneezing, congestion, and nasal pruritis.[5] According to the American Academy of Allergy, Asthma and Immunology and American College of Allergy, Asthma and Immunology's Joint Task Force on Practice Parameters, Allergen Immunotherapy, AR treatment may include appropriate environmental control measures directed at reducing the allergen load,[6–9]

[a] Nova Southeastern University, 1108 S. Wolcott Street, Casper, Wyoming 82601, USA;
[b] Asthma Allergy and Sinus Center, 1965 Andrew Drive, West Chester, PA 19380, USA;
[c] BioMedEcon, PO Box 129, Moss Beach, CA 94038, USA
* Corresponding author.
E-mail address: lscoxmd@gmail.com

Immunol Allergy Clin N Am 40 (2020) 69–85
https://doi.org/10.1016/j.iac.2019.09.003
0889-8561/20/© 2019 Elsevier Inc. All rights reserved.

immunology.theclinics.com

pharmacotherapy,[5] and allergen immunotherapy (AIT).[10] Among these treatments, only AIT induces immunologic tolerance to the specific allergens responsible for allergy symptoms.[11]

There is a tendency toward underdiagnosis and undertreatment of AR by health care professionals.[12–15] The burden of poorly controlled AR is borne by patients, caregivers, employers, and health care systems.[16,17] Patients whose AR is poorly controlled are at increased risk for asthma, recurrent otitis media, chronic rhinosinusitis, and other comorbid conditions.[1,18,19] These patients also face decrements in health-related quality of life, which can manifest as disturbed sleep, poor school and work performance, decreased energy, depressed mood, and low frustration tolerance.[20–25]

The economic costs of poorly controlled AR include those for over-the-counter medications to treat symptoms; prescription medications; and medical care for treatment of comorbid complications, such as asthma and acute sinusitis.[16,26–29] The indirect costs of poorly controlled AR include absenteeism and "presenteeism" from work or school, reduced productivity, lost wages, and fatigue-related injuries.[4,17,20,26,30] This article examines published literature regarding the pharmacoeconomics of AIT versus standard drug treatment (SDT) for the treatment of AR. Where possible, we also considered studies that examined outcomes of AIT versus SDT for the treatment of allergic asthma, atopic dermatitis, and other allergic conditions.[31] The review includes research specifically designed to evaluate the pharmacoeconomics of AIT and studies that provided sufficient secondary data for pharmacoeconomic analyses.

BACKGROUND: THE ECONOMIC IMPACT OF POORLY CONTROLLED ALLERGIC RHINITIS

In addition to pharmacotherapy, management of AR must include allergy diagnostic testing to identify the specific causative allergens so that appropriate avoidance measures are recommended and initiated.[6,8,9,32] Pharmacotherapy includes topical nasal and oral antihistamines, topical nasal corticosteroids, nasal ipratropium, and leukotriene modifiers.[5] These medications are used regularly to control symptoms or on an as-needed basis. It is worth noting that pharmacotherapy generally provides only partial symptomatic relief: approximately 33% of children and 60% of adults report a suboptimal response to medications.[33] Furthermore, none of these medications have a disease-modifying effect.

AIT is distinguished from avoidance measures and pharmacotherapy because it modifies the allergic disease.[11,34] AIT has also has been shown to mitigate the development of asthma and the development of new allergen sensitivities.[35–38] Furthermore, AIT can induce long-term tolerance, which translates into clinical efficacy and cost savings that persist years after AIT is discontinued.[4,39,40] According to US and international guidelines, AIT is indicated as a treatment option for patients with AR and/or asthma with[10,41,42]

- Symptoms unresponsive to pharmacotherapy
- Troublesome medication side effects
- Patient preference, that is, patients who are reluctant to take medications indefinitely to control or "mask" rather than cure their allergic disease

There are currently two Food and Drug Administration–approved forms of AIT that are commercially available in the United States: subcutaneous immunotherapy (SCIT) and sublingual immunotherapy (SLIT). Each route has its advantage and disadvantages.[34] Although SCIT is a well-established effective treatment of seasonal and perennial allergic diseases,[25,35–37] its disadvantage is that it must be administered in a physician's office or clinic with appropriate emergency equipment and personnel equipped to recognize and manage serious allergic reactions, such as anaphylaxis.[25,38] SLIT has emerged as an alternative form of effective AIT that provides the advantage of home administration because of its superior safety compared with SCIT.[39]

SUBCUTANEOUS IMMUNOTHERAPY PHARMACOECONOMIC STUDIES

In 2005, estimated total direct US costs of AR exceeded $11 billion, with 60% of expenditures for prescription medications.[17,18,26] Treatment of the comorbid conditions associated with AR (eg, asthma, otitis media, and recurrent sinusitis) are estimated in the billions of dollars.[1,19,20] Several studies have examined the cost-effectiveness of AIT versus pharmacotherapy alone. In general, most of these studies found the AIT was associated with significant cost-savings either during treatment or after treatment completion. The explanation for the delayed cost-effectiveness related to the AIT treatment costs being offset by AIT's post-treatment clinical efficacy, which translated into reduced health care utilization and costs, medications, and so forth.

In the most compelling study demonstrating the cost-effectiveness of AIT, Ariano and colleagues[40] examined the pharmacoeconomics of SCIT with SDT compared with SDT alone among 30 patients with an at least 2-year history of *Parietaria*-induced AR and asthma. Patients were treated for 3 years and followed for an additional 3 years after treatment discontinuation. In addition to tracking symptom scores and medication use, the investigators calculated patients' health care costs, which included scheduled and unscheduled clinic visits and prescription medications. Within the first year of the study, those receiving SCIT experienced significant improvements in symptoms and reductions in medication use compared with patients receiving SDT alone. In the second year of treatment, SCIT conferred a 48% cost savings compared with SDT alone. At study end, researchers reported that SCIT conferred a net per patient annual savings of $830, which represented an 80% cost reduction compared with the SDT group. Although this was a small study, it was well designed because it captured not only the direct costs of SCIT, but also the total health care costs (ie, all prescribed medications, scheduled and unscheduled medical clinic visits, and so forth). This study provides strong support for AIT in terms of reduction in direct and indirect costs compared with SDT alone.

In a 2-year double blind placebo-controlled trial (DBPC) comparing ragweed allergen extract administered by SCIT with placebo for the treatment of 77 adolescents and adults with ragweed-induced asthma, researchers reported a significant improvement in clinical and economic outcomes in the patient population receiving SCIT compared with the placebo group.[43] The costs of asthma medication and allergen extracts used over the 2-year study period were considered. Over the course of the study, asthma medication costs for those receiving SCIT were $840 versus $1194 for those receiving placebo; this represented a 30% cost savings benefit conferred by SCIT. However, these cost savings were offset by the $527 expended for SCIT-related supplies and administration costs. Of note, the study did not examine costs of AR-associated comorbid conditions, nor did investigators consider the long-term efficacy of AIT after discontinuation.

A 2005 Danish study that examined the direct and indirect costs of AIT for seasonal grass pollen allergic and house dust mite (HDM) allergic patients revealed significant savings associated with AIT.[44] Before AIT initiation, the direct per patient annual costs of allergy treatment were 2580 Danish Krone (DKK). In the years following AIT discontinuation, direct per patient annual costs fell to DKK 1072, representing a 60% savings. When direct and indirect cost were considered, the per patient annual costs were significantly less form SCIT than SDT. This study further supports the cost savings benefits of SCIT for patients with allergic respiratory conditions.

In a multinational study that included Austria, Denmark, Finland, Germany, the Netherlands, and Sweden, Keiding and Jorgensen[45] evaluated the pharmacoeconomics of SCIT versus SDT among adult patients with grass pollen–induced seasonal AR that was not controlled by SDT (oral antihistamines, topical steroids, or sodium cromoglycate). This analysis was based on the UK Immunotherapy Study Group's (UKIS) 1-year randomized multinational European randomized, DBPC, parallel-group trial, which included an economic analysis evaluating 3 years of SCIT treatment and 6 years of follow-up after SCIT discontinuation.[46] From the health care system perspective, SCIT was found to be cost-effective in comparison with SDT with the estimated cost savings to be €10,000 to €25,000 per quality-adjusted life year (QALY). A QALY is a generic measure of disease burden, which includes the quality and the quantity of life lived. It is used in economic evaluations to assess the value of medical interventions. One QALY is equal to 1 year in perfect health.[2] If an individual's health is lower than this maximum, QALYs are accrued at a rate of less than 1 per year. To be dead is associated with 0 QALY. From a societal and patient perspective and the indirect costs, which included days lost from work, productivity, lost wages, and other factors, SCIT was found to be considerably more cost-effective than SDT.

A 2008 study examined 15 years of German health care systems claims. Investigators found that compared with SDT alone, SCIT was associated with a significant reduction in new cases of asthma.[47] Furthermore, the total per-patient costs in the SDT-alone group were approximately €2100 higher than costs among those receiving SCIT (€26,100 SDT vs €24,000 SCIT). Investigators estimated that the annual per-patient cost benefit for SCIT was approximately €140. From a societal point of view the SCIT reached an incremental cost-effectiveness ratio (ICER) of -€19,787 per additional QALY, which implies that SCIT and standard treatment were more effective and less costly that symptomatic treatment alone. The ICER is a statistical figure for determining the value of a health care intervention. It is defined by the difference in cost between two possible interventions, divided by the difference in their effect. It represents the average incremental cost associated with one additional unit of the measure of effect. There was variation in the ICER with adults being the largest beneficiary most likely reflecting a more significant reduction in indirect costs.

In a claims-based analysis of Florida Medicaid patients, Hankin and associates[48] compared direct costs (pharmacy, outpatient and inpatient services for any reason) incurred by pediatric patients newly diagnosed with AR in the 6 months before SCIT initiation with parallel direct costs these patients incurred in the 6 months following SCIT discontinuation. Investigators found significant (P<.001) cost reductions in the 6-month period following SCIT, even after the costs of SCIT were included. In an extension of the previously mentioned data, Hankin and colleagues[49] conducted a retrospective, matched-cohort analysis of 10 years of claims data (1997–2007) to examine whether children with newly diagnosed AR who received SCIT incurred less health care utilization and fewer costs during an 18-month follow-up period compared with a matched group of children with AR who did not receive SCIT. Children treated with SCIT incurred significantly lower 18-month median per-patient total health care costs even after including the costs associated with allergen immunotherapy (IT) ($3247 vs $4872), outpatient costs exclusive of SCIT-related care ($1107 vs $2626), and pharmacy costs ($1108 vs $1316) compared with the matched control subjects (P<.001 for all). Consistent with the previous study, the significant difference in total health care costs was evident within the first 3 months of initiating immunotherapy. This study demonstrated that the early cost savings associated with SCIT persisted and, more importantly, increased through the 18-month study period.

In a large-scale retrospective, matched cohort, claims analysis that evaluated 12 years of Florida Medicaid data, Hankin and colleagues[16] found comparable cost savings in adults with newly diagnosed AR treated with SCIT. In this study, investigators compared the mean 18-month health care costs (pharmacy, outpatient and inpatient services) of adult and pediatric patients with newly diagnosed AR who received SCIT with those who did not. Overall, SCIT-treated patients demonstrated a 38% reduction in 18-month total (pharmacy, outpatient and inpatient services, including costs associated with SCIT) mean health care costs ($6637 vs $10,644; P<.0001). Specifically, SCIT treatment was associated with the following cost savings:

- Adults: 30% total 18-month health care cost reduction ($10,457 SCIT vs $14,854 matched control subjects; P<.0001)
- Children: 30% total 18-month health care cost reduction (42%; $5253 AIT vs matched $9118 control subjects; P<.0001)

These health care cost savings, which included costs associated with SCIT, were evident within the first 3 months of treatment and continued throughout the 18 months of follow-up. Together, these three studies provide strong support for the cost saving benefits of AIT for adults and pediatric patients with AR.

A 2000 German study compared the cost-effectiveness of SCIT in addition to standard therapy versus the use of SCIT alone.[50] The combination of SCIT with SDT was associated with a cost-savings of €140 per patient. From a society perspective, the ICER for SCI was €19,787 per additional QALY, indicating that SCIT plus SDT was more effective and less costly compared with SDT only. In some European countries, an ICER up to €50,000 per QALY is considered cost-effective. Against this background SCIT was again reported to be a cost-effective treatment.

A study investigated the cost-effectiveness of SCIT in children with allergic asthma.[51] In this study, patients were treated with HDM SCIT for 3 years or pharmacotherapy alone. In the first year of treatment, the investigators found no difference between the two groups in terms of medication costs. However, they found a significant reduction in total medications cost in the SCIT-treated group versus the SDT group after 3 years of SCIT (€193 vs €498, respectively; P<.001). This included a reduction in allergy medication costs (€168 vs €453, respectively; P<.002). The study was not powered to evaluate the effect of SCIT on outpatient visit costs or hospitalizations This cost-effectiveness analysis (CEA) study provides further support that SCIT provides significant cost savings compared with SDT alone. Presumably, this is because of SCIT's disease modifying effect.

PHARMACOECONOMICS OF SUBLINGUAL IMMUNOTHERAPY

One of the initial studies analyzing the cost-effectiveness of SLIT was an Italian retrospective study of 135 pediatric patients with season and perennial AR and/or asthma (**Table 1**).[52] The investigators analyzed data related to health care costs 1 year before SLIT and during the 3 years during SLIT therapy. The outcomes measured included: number of exacerbations, clinic visits, absence from school, direct cost (medications, specialist visits, and SLIT), and indirect cost (costs associated lost time at school and parental lost time from work). Treatment with SLIT resulted in fewer exacerbations, medical visits, and lost days from school and work. Direct costs decreased 56%

Table 1
Studies comparing SLIT with SDT

Study	Comparators	Type	Perspective	Results
Berto et al,[52] 2005	1 y of SDT before SLIT; SLIT for 3 y	CEA	Health care system, society	Cost-savings with SLIT per health care system and society: Year before SLIT: mean annual health care costs/annual total costs per patient were €506 and €2672, respectively During SLIT: €224 (health care costs) and €629 (total cost) d
Berto et al,[57] 2006	Pollen SLIT for 3 y plus SDT as needed; SDT	CCA	Health care system, society	SCIT compared with SDT: Greater 6-y mean savings from payer and societal perspective More asthma cases avoided and patients improved
Bachert et al,[54] 2007	Grass SLIT for 3 y plus SDT as needed; SDT	CUA	Society	SLIT cost-effective cost per QALY; average 0.0287 QALYs per season compared with SDT
Beriot-Mathiot,[69] 2007	Grass SLIT for 3 y continuous or seasonal; SDT	CUA	Societal	Per ICER seasonal SLIT was cost-effective Continuous SLIT was cost-effective if sustained effect for ≥2 y after treatment
Canonica et al,[55] 2007	Grass SLIT for 3 y plus SDT as needed; SDT	CUA	Society	SLIT cost-effective per QALY: average 0.0167 QALYs per season compared with SDT
Berto et al,[58] 2008	Grass SLIT for 1 y; SDT for 1 y	CCA	3rd-party payer	Mean annual direct costs for SLIT greater than SDT €311.4 and €179.8, respectively
Nasser et al,[56] 2008	Grass SLIT for 3 y plus SDT as needed; SDT	CUA	Society	SLIT "very cost-effective" per QALY gained QALY gained at 9 y = 0.197; equivalent to an extra "72 d of perfect health" for patients treated with SLIT when compared with those receiving placebo
Ariano et al,[40] 2009	SLIT for 3 y plus SDT as needed; SDT	CCA	Health care system	Health care costs greater for SLIT plus SDT in Year 1, same in Years 2 and 3, and significantly lower in Years 4 and 5, compared with SDT
Ruggeri et al,[59] 2013	SLIT for 3 y plus SDT as needed; SDT	CEA	3rd-party payer, society	SLIT cost-effective per ICER; benefit of 0.127 QALYs in patients with medium AAdSS and 0.143 QALYs in patients with high AAdSS

Abbreviations: AAdSS, adjusted average symptom score; CCA, cost-consequence analysis; CUA, cost-utility analysis.
[a] Included in the Meadows et al, systematic review.[41]
[b] Included in the Hankin et al, systematic review.[58]
[c] Included in both systematic reviews.
From Cox L. Pharmacoeconomics of allergic diseases. In: Akdis CA, Agache I, editors. Global Atlas of Allergy. European Academy of Allergy and Clinical Immunology; 2014; with permission.

from €506 to €224 and indirect costs decreased 81% from €2166 to €406 during treatment with SLIT. Overall costs decreased 76% from €2672 pre-SLIT to €629 during SLIT treatment. The investigators only examined health care cost in patients with seasonal or perennial AR. It is presumed that the overall health care cost-savings would be even greater in patients with AR and asthma.

Several studies evaluated the health care economics of a randomized trial of SLIT grass-pollen tablets in adult patients with allergic rhinoconjunctvitis.[53] These studies considered the societal perspective over a 9-year horizon. In the Northern European cohort of this SLIT study, there was a significant improvement in QALY in the SLIT group (0.976 vs 0.947; $P<.001$), with annual treatment costs less than €2200.[54] Similarly in the Southern European cohort, SLIT was cost-effective at an annual cost in the range of €1500 to €1900.[55] For reference, to be considered cost-effective it was calculated that a drug must generate one QALY for less than €29,200. Finally, an analysis of the study data from the United Kingdom demonstrated that the cost of QALY gained was €6380, again suggesting that SLIT treatment provided pharmacoeconomic benefit.[56]

The Sublingual Immunotherapy Pollen Allergy Italy (SPAI) study evaluated the costs of using SLIT in association with standard therapy compared with standard treatment alone among 2200 adults with pollen-induced AR and asthma.[57] SLIT was associated with a 20.6% reduction in direct costs (-€626) and 43.7% reduction in indirect costs (-€1487). SLIT conferred a 32.8% reduction in direct and indirect costs.

The Sublingual Immunotherapy in Allergic Patients (SIMAP) study was a 1-year observational study of 102 Italian children and adults with grass-pollen- induced AR that evaluated the efficacy and safety of SLIT compared with SDT alone.[58] The mean annual treatment costs were higher in the SLIT versus SDT groups (€311 vs €180; $P<.0001$). The higher costs were caused by the costs of SLIT itself. The study also found that in both groups, patients with AR and asthma generated more costs than those with AR alone.

Ruggeri and colleagues[59] evaluated the cost-effectiveness of a five–grass pollen tablet in adults with grass pollen–induced AR. In this study, cost-effectiveness was stratified by low, medium, and high burden of disease based on average adjusted symptom score (AAdSS). Their analysis demonstrated that low AAdSS patients did not benefit from use of five–grass pollen SLIT, whereas patients with medium to high AAdSS did benefit. The five–grass pollen SLIT was found to cost €1024/QALY for patients with medium AAdSS and €1035/QALY for patients with high AAdSS. These numbers were lower than the critical threshold €30,000/QALY indicating that for patient with medium to high AAdSS, SLIT was a cost-effective treatment. In patients with low AAdSS, SLIT was not found to be cost-effective. To the contrary, the use of SLIT added to the cost of treatment without providing any significant clinical benefits, thus illustrating the importance of proper patient selection for AIT treatment.

Ronaldson and colleagues[60] performed a cost-utility analysis (CUA) in a model that follows two hypothetical cohorts of 1000 children with grass pollen allergic rhinoconjunctivitis, with or without asthma, who are treated with SLIT and symptomatic medications or SDT only. Their analysis demonstrated that the SLIT-treated group obtained an ICER of 0.10 QALYs per patient. The cost of SLIT treatment was €1202 higher than the SDT group. However, the ICER for the SLIT-treated group was €12,168/QALY, which fell lower than the threshold of €20,000 to €30,000/QALY that is used in the United Kingdom to deem a product cost-effective. This study again supports the cost-effectiveness of grass pollen AIT.

Hahn-Pederson and colleagues[61] evaluated the cost-effectiveness of an HDM SLIT tablet in the treatment of adults with HDM-induced allergic asthma. This was a CUA based on a phase III randomized controlled trial comparing the efficacy of ACARIZAX (ALK-Abello, Horsham, Denmark) with placebo. Both groups received conventional asthma pharmacotherapy. SLIT treatment resulted in an additional 0.66 QALY at an incremental cost of €2673. This equates to an ICER of €4041, which fell lower than the cost-effective threshold of €40,000. This study's results suggest that HDM SLIT is cost-effective in the treatment of adults with HDM-induced allergic asthma.

A German study compared the cost-effectiveness of HDM SLIT versus SDT alone in patients with moderate to severe HDM-induced AR.[62] The investigators performed a pharmacoeconomic analysis that examined a 9-year time horizon. They found that SLIT resulted in an additional QALY of 0.31 at an incremental cost of €2276. This resulted in an ICER of €7516 indicating that HDM SLIT in addition to pharmacotherapy is more cost-effective than pharmacotherapy alone.

PHARMACOECONOMICS OF SUBCUTANEOUS IMMUNOTHERAPY VERSUS SUBLINGUAL IMMUNOTHERAPY

Pokladnikova and colleagues[63] performed an economic evaluation of SCIT versus SLIT in adults with grass-induced rhinoconjunctivitis. Their analysis included the perspectives of third-party payers, patients, and society. After 3 years of treatment, SLIT and SCIT resulted in significant reductions in symptom scores and medication use. However, in the third year of study, SCIT demonstrated greater improvements in the visual analog scale and antihistamine use versus SLIT. From an economic perspective, SLIT proved to be less expensive. However, from a patient perspective SCIT was financially preferable to SLIT, particularly if the patient did not incur loss of income or travel expenses to receive SCIT. From the third-party payer perspective, the 3-year direct medical costs were €416 versus €482 for SLIT and SCIT groups, respectively. When both direct and indirect costs were considered, 3 years of treatment was €684 versus €1004 in the SLIT versus SCIT groups, respectively ($P<.001$). If patients in the SCIT group incurred no loss of income or productivity from receiving SCIT in a medically supervised setting then SCIT was overall financially preferable to SLIT.

A Danish study evaluated the budget impact of grass pollen–induced rhinoconjunctivitis comparing SQ-standardized grass AIT (Grazax; *Phleum pratense*, 75,000 SQ-T/2800 BAU, ALK) with SCIT (Alutard; *P pratense*, 100,000 SQ-U/mL, ALK).[64] The total direct and indirect costs associated with SLIT was €3789. This was €3460 less expensive than the company's SCIT product (Alutard). The authors suggested this cost-savings would allow for a health care system to treat an additional 600 patients with SLIT at no additional cost.

Westerhout and colleagues[65] evaluated the cost-effectiveness of grass pollen AIT (Oralair, Grazax, Anthony, France; Alutard SQ) in grass pollen–allergic rhinoconjunctivitis patients versus SDT alone. Patients were treated for 3 years and the assessment used a Markov model and a 9-year timeframe. The cost-utility ratio of Oralair versus SDT was €14,728 per QALY. When estimated incremental costs and incremental QALYs were considered, Oralair was determined to be the dominant strategy.

In 2014, Dranitsaris and Ellis[66] performed an indirect comparison of DBPC trials to evaluate the efficacy, safety, and cost between Oralair, Grazax, and grass pollen SCIT for the treatment of AR.[55] Twenty trials met their inclusion criteria.[66] Their analysis indicated that Oralair was less expensive than Grazax or SCIT. In the first year of treatment, Oralair use resulted in a cost savings of:

- $948 versus seasonal SCIT
- $1168 versus Grazax

- $2471 versus perennial SCIT

Most of the increased costs associated with SCIT were related to indirect costs caused by lost productivity and travel because of the requirement that SCIT be administered in a medically supervised setting. In the second and third years the pattern was similar with Oralair offering a cost savings of $868 versus perennial SCIT, $1883 versus seasonal SCIT, and $2344 versus Grazax. This model assumes that SCIT results in decreased productivity caused by lost hours from work for administration. If one were to make SCIT administration available, such that it required no lost work time (eg, an onsite medical clinic), then the total cost for perennial SCIT would be $1721 versus $1889.6 for Oralair. Thus, Oralair would be 9% more expensive than SCIT. This indicates that the cost differential between SLIT and SCIT could be reduced if administration of SCIT did not require lost time from work.

Verheggen and colleagues[67] using a Markov model and a 9-year time horizon evaluated the cost-effectiveness of Oralair (five-grass tablet) versus subcutaneous allergoid component for the treatment of grass pollen–induced allergic rhinoconjunctivitis. Oralair SLIT was associated with higher overall patient cost-savings of €458 per patient. Additionally, it was shown to be superior to SCIT in terms of clinical efficacy. SLIT resulted in an increased QALY of 0.036 and an ICER of €12,593 compared with allergoid SCIT. According to this study, there was 76% probability that the SLIT tablet was the most cost-effective treatment option.

Rheinhold and Bruggenjurgen[68] compared the cost-effectiveness of SCIT with Allergovit (Allergopharma, Germany) with Oralair SLIT using a Markov model with a timeframe of 9 years. Over the 9-year treatment period, the total per-person cost for SLIT was approximately 14% greater than for SCIT (€1159 for Allergovit vs €1322 for Oralair, respectively). In addition, SCIT treatment resulted in a per QALY gain of €11,000 compared with a €41,405 QALY gain for SLIT As a reference, cost-effective therapy is considered to be less than €40,000 to €50,000 per QALY gained. In this study, SCIT was more cost-effective than SLIT for treatment of grass pollen–induced rhinoconjunctivitis.

ALLERGEN IMMUNOTHERAPY PHARMACOECONOMICS IN SYSTEMATIC REVIEWS

In a review paper examining the efficacy of AIT for AR, Cox[27] summarized two systematic reviews that specifically examined AIT cost-effectiveness (**Table 2**). The most comprehensive review to date on AIT cost-efficacy was a systematic review and meta-analysis of studies that provided data on costs and clinical efficacy of SCIT and/or SLIT with SDT alone.[4] The systematic review was conducted by the National Institute for Health Research Health Technology Assessment (HTA) program.[4] The purpose of an HTA program is to produce high-quality research information on the effectiveness, costs, and broader impact of health technologies for those who use, manage, and provide care in the National Health Service. This HTA review used the electronic databases and trial registries (from inception up to April 2011).[4] They applied the standard systematic review methods for study selection, data extraction, and quality assessment of DBPC trials of SCIT or SLIT, SCIT compared with SLIT. Economic evaluations, meta-analysis, and indirect comparison meta-analysis were presented. The authors identified 14 economic evaluations and 2 reviews of economic evaluations (**Table 3**).[4] Four different types of cost-analyses were used in the 14 identified economic evaluation studies:

- 4 cost–consequences analyses
- 2 CEA

Table 2
Systematic reviews evaluating allergen immunotherapy health economics

Author, Year[a]	Economic Outcome Conclusion[b]	SCIT vs SDT[b]	SLIT Tablets vs SDT[b]	SLIT Drops vs SDT[b]	SCIT vs SLIT vs SDT[b]
Meadows et al,[4] 2013	14 Both SCIT and SLIT may be cost-effective from around 6 y	6 Cost-effective but varied in terms of payer perspective and timepoint	3 Cost-effective at ~ 6 y and various ICER	2 All favored SLIT	3 SCIT more cost-effective over time
Hankin & Cox,[29] 2014	23 Favored AIT over SDT	10 All favored SCIT	8 1 found higher costs with SLIT	1 Reduced costs by Year 4	4 All favored SLIT SLIT 48% cost-savings from healthcare system (HCS) perspective

[a] Included 3 studies that evaluated the actual total health care cost via claims analyses not included in the Meadows review.
[b] Number of studies evaluated.
From Cox L. The role of allergen immunotherapy in the management of allergic rhinitis. Am J Rhinol Allergy 2016;30(1):48-53; with permission.

Table 3
Studies comparing SCIT with SDT

Study	Comparators	Type	Perspective	Results
Schadlich & Brecht,[50] 2000	Pollen or HDM SCIT for 3 y plus SDT as needed; SDT	CEA	Society, health care system, 3rd-party payer	SCIT < SDT over 10 y Break-even point reached in the 7th y
Petersen et al,[44] 2005	Grass or HDM SCIT for 3–5 y plus SDT as needed; SDT	CEA	Society	Direct cost: SCIT > SDT If indirect costs of sick days included in the economic evaluation, SCIT costs < SDT
Ariano,[70] 2006	*Parietaria* SCIT for 3 y plus SDT as needed; SDT	CCA	Health care system, society	SCIT < SDT; 80% cost reduction found 3 y after stopping SCIT
Keiding & Jorgensen,[45] 2007	Grass SCIT for 3 y plus SDT as needed; SDT	CEA CUA	Health care system, society	SCIT cost-effectiveness per QALY; in the range of €10,000–€25,000 per QALY from perspective of the health care system
Omnes,[71] 2007	HDM or pollen SCIT 3–4 y plus SDT as needed; SDT	CEA	Society	Cost-effective per incremental cost of asthma cases avoided (ICER)
Bruggenjurgen et al,[47] 2008	SCIT for 3 y plus SDT as needed; SDT	CUA	3rd-party payer, society	Break-even point = 10 y After 15 y, annual cost savings of €140 per SCIT-treated patient
Hankin et al,[48] 2008	Costs 6 mo before and 6 mo after SCIT	CCA	Health care system	Weighted mean 6-mo savings/patient: $401
Hankin et al,[49] 2010	SCIT for 18 mo plus SDT as needed; SDT as needed for 18 mo	CCA	Health care system	SCIT 18-mo total health care costs 33% reduction compared with SDT
Hankin et al,[16] 2013	SCIT plus SDT as needed for 18 mo; SDT as needed for 18 mo	CCA	Health care system	SCIT 18-mo total health care costs compared with SDT: children = 42% reduction; adults = 30% reduction

Abbreviation: CCA, cost-consequence analysis.
From Cox L. Pharmacoeconomics of allergic diseases. In: Akdis CA, Agache I, editors. Global Atlas of Allergy. European Academy of Allergy and Clinical Immunology; 2014; with permission.

- 5 CUA
- 1 CEA and CUA
- 1 CEA and cost–benefit analyses
- 1 CEA and cost–consequences analyses

These cost-analyses differ in the way outcomes were measure or expressed, with CEAs, cost–benefit analyses, and CUAs typically reporting outcomes as the ICER. The ICER is calculated from QALY with the following formula:

$$ICER = \frac{\text{Cost of SCIT} - \text{Cost of ST}}{\text{QALYs for SCIT} - \text{QALYs for ST}}$$

The authors concluded that based on £20,000 to £30,000 per QALY, AIT became cost-effective in comparison with SDT alone 6 years of treatment initiation from the patient. From the National Health Services perspectives AIT was cost-effective after 7 years. Using the same threshold, SCIT was found to be cost-effective compared with SLIT after 5 years. The authors concluded that "… SCIT and SLIT may be cost-effective compared with SDT from around 6 years at a threshold of £20,000 to 30,000 per QALY."[4] Limited evidence indicated SCIT may more beneficial and less costly than SLIT. The authors did note that the studies used different outcome measures making it difficult to compare and combine results. They encouraged further research to "establish the comparative effectiveness of SCIT compared with SLIT and to provide more robust cost-effectiveness estimates."[4] All of the studies in this systematic review used single-allergen AIT.

Another systematic review of published studies that reported health economic outcomes associated with AIT conducted by Hankin and Cox[29] evaluated 23 studies that compared SLIT and/or SCIT with SDT (SCIT, 9; SLIT liquid drops, 2; SLIT tablets, 8; SCIT and SLIT, 4) and one directly comparing SLIT with SCIT (see **Table 1**). Only one early study comparing SCIT with SDT in adults with ragweed-allergic asthma failed to demonstrated significant cost-savings.[43] The review concluded that the remaining 23 comparative cost studies provided "compelling evidence for the cost savings of AIT (whether delivered subcutaneously or sublingually)." Four of the six studies comparing cost outcomes of SLIT with SCIT reported cost-savings favoring SLIT. All of the studies, except the three retrospective claims analyses studies of the Florida Medicaid reviewed previously in this paper, used single-allergen AIT.[16,48,49]

SUMMARY

The preponderance of the data suggests that AIT, with either SLIT or SCIT, is a cost-effective treatment option for patients with AR and/or asthma. One of this review's limitations is that most of the studies used one or two allergens. Additionally, most of the studies in this review were performed in European centers. Thus, the applicability to US patients may be limited. This is particularly relevant for the SCIT versus SLIT comparison in the United States because the typical US allergy-trained physician prescribes multiallergen AIT.[57] The cost of multiallergen SLIT using effective doses could be considerable.[58,59] SCIT in the United State is reimbursed by private and third-party payers with the definition of a dose being the volume administered (eg, 1 mL = dose). This reimbursement formula does not consider the number of allergens that are required to effectively treat the patients with AR. Thus, single-allergen SCIT is reimbursed the same multiallergen SCIT. In contrast, SLIT tablets only provide treatment of a single allergen and multiallergen allergic patients would have to take multiple tablets, which could be cost-prohibitive.[34,58] Clearly, in these patients, multiallergen SCIT would be less expensive than SLIT.

One of the arguments for SLIT over SCIT is that safe administration requires that SCIT is administered in a medically supervised setting, which is associated with indirect costs because of lost work time and reduced productivity. Most studies on SCIT cost-effectiveness assume that all patients will receive SCIT in a medical facility during usual business hours. Additionally, no study collected data directly from patients regarding the economic impact that SCIT had on them. However, in the United States, patients can receive SCIT outside of standard business hours and this would reduce the indirect costs of SCIT that is, "lost time from work." Another consideration is that many patients can continue their work electronically (eg, computer, smart phone) during the time they spend in medical clinic for SCIT treatment.

Overall, SLIT and SCIT are clinically efficacious and cost-effective treatment options for patients with AR and asthma. Whether SCIT is more cost-effective than SLIT or vice versa remains to be determined and requires more detailed pharmacoeconomic analysis that includes the direct and indirect costs of patients with AR, particularly multiallergen patients in the United States.

REFERENCES

1. Bousquet J, Khaltaev N, Cruz AA, et al. Allergic Rhinitis and its Impact on Asthma (ARIA) 2008 update (in collaboration with the World Health Organization, GA(2) LEN and AllerGen). Allergy 2008;63(Suppl 86):8–160.
2. Wheatley LM, Togias A. Clinical practice. Allergic rhinitis. N Engl J Med 2015;372:456–63.
3. Ozdoganoglu T, Songu M. The burden of allergic rhinitis and asthma. Ther Adv Respir Dis 2012;6:11–23.
4. Meadows A, Kaambwa B, Novielli N, et al. A systematic review and economic evaluation of subcutaneous and sublingual allergen immunotherapy in adults and children with seasonal allergic rhinitis. Health Technol Assess 2013;17:vi, xi-xiv, 1–322.
5. Wallace DV, Dykewicz MS, Bernstein DI, et al. The diagnosis and management of rhinitis: an updated practice parameter. J Allergy Clin Immunol 2008;122:S1–84.
6. Portnoy J, Miller JD, Williams PB, et al. Environmental assessment and exposure control of dust mites: a practice parameter. Ann Allergy Asthma Immunol 2013;111:465–507.
7. Phipatanakul W, Matsui E, Portnoy J, et al. Environmental assessment and exposure reduction of rodents: a practice parameter. Ann Allergy Asthma Immunol 2012;109:375–87.
8. Portnoy J, Chew GL, Phipatanakul W, et al. Environmental assessment and exposure reduction of cockroaches: a practice parameter. J Allergy Clin Immunol 2013;132:802–8.e1-25.
9. Portnoy J, Kennedy K, Sublett J, et al. Environmental assessment and exposure control: a practice parameter–furry animals. Ann Allergy Asthma Immunol 2012;108:223.e1-15.
10. Cox L, Nelson H, Lockey R, et al. Allergen immunotherapy: a practice parameter third update. J Allergy Clin Immunol 2011;127:S1–55.
11. Akdis M, Akdis CA. Mechanisms of allergen-specific immunotherapy: multiple suppressor factors at work in immune tolerance to allergens. J Allergy Clin Immunol 2014;133:621–31.

12. Bauchau V, Durham SR. Prevalence and rate of diagnosis of allergic rhinitis in Europe. Eur Respir J 2004;24:758–64.
13. Maurer M, Zuberbier T. Undertreatment of rhinitis symptoms in Europe: findings from a cross-sectional questionnaire survey. Allergy 2007;62:1057–63.
14. Sazonov V, Ambegaonkar BM, Bolge SC, et al. Frequency of diagnosis and treatment of allergic rhinitis among adults with asthma in Germany, France, and the UK: National Health and Wellness Survey. Curr Med Res Opin 2009; 25:1721–6.
15. Nolte H, Nepper-Christensen S, Backer V. Unawareness and undertreatment of asthma and allergic rhinitis in a general population. Respir Med 2006;100: 354–62.
16. Hankin CS, Cox L, Bronstone A, et al. Allergy immunotherapy: reduced health care costs in adults and children with allergic rhinitis. J Allergy Clin Immunol 2013;131:1084–91.
17. Marcellusi A, Viti R, Incorvaia C, et al. Direct and indirect costs associated with respiratory allergic diseases in Italy. A probabilistic cost of illness study. Recenti Prog Med 2015;106:517–27 [in Italian].
18. Minto H, Hogan AD. Allergic rhinitis is associated with otitis media with effusion: a birth cohort study. Pediatrics 2013;132:S29–30.
19. Peters AT, Spector S, Hsu J, et al. Diagnosis and management of rhinosinusitis: a practice parameter update. Ann Allergy Asthma Immunol 2014;113: 347–85.
20. Blaiss MS. Allergic rhinitis: direct and indirect costs. Allergy Asthma Proc 2010; 31:375–80.
21. Meltzer EO, Blaiss MS, Derebery MJ, et al. Burden of allergic rhinitis: results from the Pediatric Allergies in America survey. J Allergy Clin Immunol 2009;124: S43–70.
22. Long AA. Findings from a 1000-patient internet-based survey assessing the impact of morning symptoms on individuals with allergic rhinitis. Clin Ther 2007;29:342–51.
23. Blaiss MS. Pediatric allergic rhinitis: physical and mental complications. Allergy Asthma Proc 2008;29:1–6.
24. Sardana N, Craig TJ. Congestion and sleep impairment in allergic rhinitis. Asian Pac J Allergy Immunol 2011;29:297–306.
25. Meltzer EO, Nathan R, Derebery J, et al. Sleep, quality of life, and productivity impact of nasal symptoms in the United States: findings from the Burden of Rhinitis in America survey. Allergy Asthma Proc 2009;30:244–54.
26. Cox L. Allergy immunotherapy in reducing healthcare cost. Curr Opin Otolaryngol Head Neck Surg 2015;23:247–54.
27. Cox L. The role of allergen immunotherapy in the management of allergic rhinitis. Am J Rhinol Allergy 2016;30:48–53.
28. Kreiner-Moller E, Chawes BL, Caye-Thomasen P, et al. Allergic rhinitis is associated with otitis media with effusion: a birth cohort study. Clin Exp Allergy 2012;42: 1615–20.
29. Hankin CS, Cox L. Allergy immunotherapy: what is the evidence for cost saving? Curr Opin Allergy Clin Immunol 2014;14:363–70.
30. Schatz M. A survey of the burden of allergic rhinitis in the USA. Allergy 2007; 62(Suppl 85):9–16.
31. Cox L, Calderon MA. Allergen immunotherapy for atopic dermatitis: is there room for debate? J Allergy Clin Immunol Pract 2016;4:435–44.

32. Cox L, Williams B, Sicherer S, et al. Pearls and pitfalls of allergy diagnostic testing: report from the American College of Allergy, Asthma and Immunology/American Academy of Allergy, Asthma and Immunology Specific IgE Test Task Force. Ann Allergy Asthma Immunol 2008;101:580–92.

33. Allergies in America: a landmark survey of nasal allergy sufferers: adult. Available at: http://www.myallergiesinamerica.com./. Accessed October 4, 2008.

34. James LK, Shamji MH, Walker SM, et al. Long-term tolerance after allergen immunotherapy is accompanied by selective persistence of blocking antibodies. J Allergy Clin Immunol 2011;127:509–16.e1-5.

35. Marogna M, Tomassetti D, Bernasconi A, et al. Preventive effects of sublingual immunotherapy in childhood: an open randomized controlled study. Ann Allergy Asthma Immunol 2008;101:206–11.

36. Des Roches A, Paradis L, Menardo JL, et al. Immunotherapy with a standardized Dermatophagoides pteronyssinus extract. VI. Specific immunotherapy prevents the onset of new sensitizations in children. J Allergy Clin Immunol 1997;99:450–3.

37. Marogna M, Spadolini I, Massolo A, et al. Long-lasting effects of sublingual immunotherapy according to its duration: a 15-year prospective study. J Allergy Clin Immunol 2010;126:969–75.

38. Jacobsen L, Niggemann B, Dreborg S, et al. Specific immunotherapy has long-term preventive effect of seasonal and perennial asthma: 10-year follow-up on the PAT study. Allergy 2007;62:943–8.

39. Incorvaia C, Ariano R, Berto P, et al. Economic aspects of sublingual immunotherapy. Int J Immunopathol Pharmacol 2009;22:27–30.

40. Ariano R, Berto P, Incorvaia C, et al. Economic evaluation of sublingual immunotherapy vs. symptomatic treatment in allergic asthma. Ann Allergy Asthma Immunol 2009;103:254–9.

41. Alvarez-Cuesta E, Bousquet J, Canonica GW, et al. Standards for practical allergen-specific immunotherapy. Allergy 2006;61(Suppl 82):1–20.

42. Jutel M, Agache I, Bonini S, et al. International consensus on allergy immunotherapy. J Allergy Clin Immunol 2015;136(3):556–68.

43. Creticos PS, Reed CE, Norman PS, et al. Ragweed immunotherapy in adult asthma. N Engl J Med 1996;334:501–6.

44. Petersen KD, Gyrd-Hansen D, Dahl R. Health-economic analyses of subcutaneous specific immunotherapy for grass pollen and mite allergy. Allergol Immunopathol (Madr) 2005;33:296–302.

45. Keiding H, Jorgensen KP. A cost-effectiveness analysis of immunotherapy with SQ allergen extract for patients with seasonal allergic rhinoconjunctivitis in selected European countries. Curr Med Res Opin 2007;23:1113–20.

46. Frew AJ, Powell RJ, Corrigan CJ, et al. Efficacy and safety of specific immunotherapy with SQ allergen extract in treatment-resistant seasonal allergic rhinoconjunctivitis. J Allergy Clin Immunol 2006;117:319–25.

47. Bruggenjurgen B, Reinhold T, Brehler R, et al. Cost-effectiveness of specific subcutaneous immunotherapy in patients with allergic rhinitis and allergic asthma. Ann Allergy Asthma Immunol 2008;101:316–24.

48. Hankin CS, Cox L, Lang D, et al. Allergy immunotherapy among Medicaid-enrolled children with allergic rhinitis: patterns of care, resource use, and costs. J Allergy Clin Immunol 2008;121:227–32.

49. Hankin CS, Cox L, Lang D, et al. Allergen immunotherapy and health care cost benefits for children with allergic rhinitis: a large-scale, retrospective, matched cohort study. Ann Allergy Asthma Immunol 2010;104:79–85.

50. Schadlich PK, Brecht JG. Economic evaluation of specific immunotherapy versus symptomatic treatment of allergic rhinitis in Germany. Pharmacoeconomics 2000; 17:37–52.

51. Reinhold T, Ostermann J, Thum-Oltmer S, et al. Influence of subcutaneous specific immunotherapy on drug costs in children suffering from allergic asthma. Clin Transl Allergy 2013;3:30.

52. Berto P, Bassi M, Incorvaia C, et al. Cost effectiveness of sublingual immunotherapy in children with allergic rhinitis and asthma. Eur Ann Allergy Clin Immunol 2005;37:303–8.

53. Dahl R, Kapp A, Colombo G, et al. Efficacy and safety of sublingual immunotherapy with grass allergen tablets for seasonal allergic rhinoconjunctivitis. J Allergy Clin Immunol 2006;118:434–40.

54. Bachert C, Vestenbaek U, Christensen J, et al. Cost-effectiveness of grass allergen tablet (GRAZAX(R)) for the prevention of seasonal grass pollen induced rhinoconjunctivitis: a Northern European perspective. Clin Exp Allergy 2007;37: 772–9.

55. Canonica GW, Poulsen PB, Vestenbaek U. Cost-effectiveness of GRAZAX for prevention of grass pollen induced rhinoconjunctivitis in Southern Europe. Respir Med 2007;101:1885–94.

56. Nasser S, Vestenbaek U, Beriot-Mathiot A, et al. Cost-effectiveness of specific immunotherapy with Grazax in allergic rhinitis co-existing with asthma. Allergy 2008;63:1624–9.

57. Berto P, Passalacqua G, Crimi N, et al. Economic evaluation of sublingual immunotherapy vs symptomatic treatment in adults with pollen-induced respiratory allergy: the Sublingual Immunotherapy Pollen Allergy Italy (SPAI) study. Ann Allergy Asthma Immunol 2006;97:615–21.

58. Berto P, Frati F, Incorvaia C, et al. Comparison of costs of sublingual immunotherapy and drug treatment in grass-pollen induced allergy: results from the SI-MAP database study. Curr Med Res Opin 2008;24:261–6.

59. Ruggeri M, Oradei M, Frati F, et al. Economic evaluation of 5-grass pollen tablets versus placebo in the treatment of allergic rhinitis in adults. Clin Drug Investig 2013;33:343–9.

60. Ronaldson S, Taylor M, Bech PG, et al. Economic evaluation of SQ-standardized grass allergy immunotherapy tablet (Grazax((R))) in children. Clinicoecon Outcomes Res 2014;6:187–96.

61. Hahn-Pedersen J, Worm M, Green W, et al. Cost utility analysis of the SQ((R)) HDM SLIT-tablet in house dust mite allergic asthma patients in a German setting. Clinical and translational allergy 2016;6:35.

62. Green W, Kleine-Tebbe J, Klimek L, et al. Cost-effectiveness of SQ((R)) HDM SLIT-tablet in addition to pharmacotherapy for the treatment of house dust mite allergic rhinitis in Germany. Clinicoecon Outcomes Res 2017;9:77–84.

63. Pokladnikova J, Krcmova I, Vlcek J. Economic evaluation of sublingual vs subcutaneous allergen immunotherapy. Ann Allergy Asthma Immunol 2008;100: 482–9.

64. Ronborg SM, Svendsen UG, Micheelsen JS, et al. Budget impact analysis of two immunotherapy products for treatment of grass pollen-induced allergic rhinoconjunctivitis. Clinicoecon Outcomes Res 2012;4:253–60.

65. Westerhout KY, Verheggen BG, Schreder CH, et al. Cost effectiveness analysis of immunotherapy in patients with grass pollen allergic rhinoconjunctivitis in Germany. J Med Econ 2012;15:906–17.

66. Dranitsaris G, Ellis AK. Sublingual or subcutaneous immunotherapy for seasonal allergic rhinitis: an indirect analysis of efficacy, safety and cost. J Eval Clin Pract 2014;20:225–38.
67. Verheggen BG, Westerhout KY, Schreder CH, et al. Health economic comparison of SLIT allergen and SCIT allergoid immunotherapy in patients with seasonal grass-allergic rhinoconjunctivitis in Germany. Clin Transl Allergy 2015;5:1.
68. Reinhold T, Bruggenjurgen B. Cost-effectiveness of grass pollen SCIT compared with SLIT and symptomatic treatment. Allergo J Int 2017;26:7–15.
69. Beriot-Mathiot A, Vestenbaek U, Bo Poulsen P. Influence of time horizon and treatment patterns on cost-effectiveness measures: the case of allergen-specific immunotherapy with Grazax. Journal of medical economics 2007;10:215–28.
70. Ariano R, Berto P, Tracci D, et al. Pharmacoeconomics of allergen immunotherapy compared with symptomatic drug treatment in patients with allergic rhinitis and asthma. Allergy Asthma Proc 2006;27:159–63.
71. Omnes LF, Bousquet J, Scheinmann P, et al. Pharmacoeconomic assessment of specific immunotherapy versus current symptomatic treatment for allergic rhinitis and asthma in France. Eur Ann Allergy Clin Immunol 2007;39:148–56.

Evolution of Immune Responses in Food Immunotherapy

Johanna M. Smeekens, PhD*, Michael D. Kulis, PhD

KEYWORDS

• Food allergy • Immunotherapy • IgE • IgG4 • Th2 • Mast cells • Basophils

KEY POINTS

- Immunotherapy for food allergy transiently modifies the established allergic immune response.
- Changes in T-cell phenotypes following food allergy immunotherapy include decreased T helper 2–type cytokine production, expansion of regulatory T cells, and emergence of anergic allergen-specific T cells.
- Allergen-specific immunoglobulin G1 (IgG1), IgG2, IgG3, IgG4, IgA1, and IgA2 are increased with repeated antigen exposure during immunotherapy, whereas IgE initially increases but after several months of therapy is decreased from baseline levels.
- Clinical desensitization, as demonstrated by double-blind, placebo-controlled food challenges, following immunotherapy is associated with decreased degranulation responses of both mast cells and basophils.
- Although immunologic correlates to food allergen immunotherapy have been described, the field still lacks biomarkers that definitively can confirm a subject has achieved desensitization or sustained unresponsiveness.

INTRODUCTION
Epidemiology

Food allergy is a growing public health concern that affects an estimated 10% of adults[1] and 8% of children.[2,3] The prevalence of food allergy has increased over the past 2 decades.[4] The most common foods that cause allergic reactions are peanuts, tree nuts, shellfish, fish, soy, milk, egg, and wheat. Management of food allergy depends on strict avoidance of the eliciting food, because even trace amounts can

Disclosure Statement: The authors have nothing to disclose.
Funding: J.M. Smeekens is supported by an NIH T32 training grant (AI007062). M.D. Kulis is supported by NIH (1UM2 AI30836; 1R03AI140161-01; 2R01-AT004435-07AI) and DOD (W81XWH-16-1-0302).
UNC Department of Pediatrics, UNC Food Allergy Initiative, UNC Chapel Hill, 116 Manning Drive, Mary Ellen Jones Building, Room 3004, Chapel Hill, NC 27599, USA
* Corresponding author.
E-mail address: smeeken3@email.unc.edu

Immunol Allergy Clin N Am 40 (2020) 87–95
https://doi.org/10.1016/j.iac.2019.09.006
0889-8561/20/© 2019 Elsevier Inc. All rights reserved.
immunology.theclinics.com

lead to severe anaphylaxis.[5] The hypervigilance causes decreased quality of life in allergic individuals and their families and caretakers.[6] Unfortunately, accidental reactions occur quite frequently,[7] and the only way to treat them is with antihistamines and/ or epinephrine. In fact, an estimated 200,000 hospital emergency department visits are made each year as a result of food-induced anaphylaxis.[8]

Immunotherapy Approaches

Currently, there are no Food and Drug Administration–approved therapies to treat food allergies. However, several antigen-specific therapies are in clinical trials, including oral immunotherapy (OIT), epicutaneous immunotherapy (EPIT), and sublingual immunotherapy (SLIT). Phase 3 trials have been completed for an OIT drug formulated by Aimmune Therapeutics, AR101,[9] and an EPIT drug formulated by DBV Technologies, Viaskin.[10] The routes of administration and duration differ between therapies, but the overall design involves administering small but increasing doses of the food antigen over several months until a maintenance dose is achieved. The maintenance dose is continued indefinitely to reach and maintain a desensitized state, which is assessed by double-blind placebo-controlled food challenges. To date, immunotherapy trials have been conducted using peanut,[11–21] egg,[22–26] milk,[27–30] wheat,[31] and tree nuts.[32] In general, results from these clinical trials indicate that OIT is the most efficacious, as indicated by the amount of food protein ingested without dose-limiting symptoms. OIT also has the most side effects, including urticaria, wheezing, and upper respiratory and gastrointestinal symptoms, whereas EPIT and SLIT have few, mainly local side effects, but lower efficacy.[14,15,17,30] There appears to be a tradeoff between efficacy and adverse effects, and this may be related to the amount of antigen administered through the different routes. As shown in **Fig. 1**, OIT uses milligram-gram quantities (300–4000 mg); SLIT uses milligram quantities (2–5 mg), and EPIT uses microgram quantities (50–250 µg).

Immunobiology of Food Allergy

Food allergy is the result of an aberrant immunologic response involving mast cells, basophils, T cells, B cells, and immunoglobulin E (IgE).[33] Briefly, food antigens are taken up

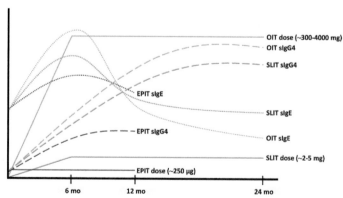

Fig. 1. Representative changes known to occur during allergen-specific OIT, SLIT, and EPIT. Relative allergen doses (*solid lines*) and the corresponding changes in allergen-specific IgE (sIgE; *dotted lines*) and IgG4 (sIgG4; *dashed lines*) in OIT (*blue*), SLIT (*green*), and EPIT (*red*) subjects.

by dendritic cells in the mucosa and presented to naïve T cells. T helper 2 (Th2) and T follicular helper cells then lead to B-cell production of antigen-specific IgE. IgE binds to FcεRI on basophils in circulation and mast cells in tissue, priming the immune system for an allergic reaction. Upon reexposure to the food, antigens are taken up and cross-link the FcεRI receptor on the surface of basophils and mast cells, which leads to degranulation and the release of mediators such as histamine.[5] The aim of this review is to give an overview of the immunologic changes that occur during immunotherapy. Specifically, the authors discuss T cells, B cells, and immunoglobulins, effector cells, and their evolution throughout OIT, SLIT, and EPIT.

T-CELL MODULATION

Gastrointestinal exposure through oral feeding usually results in immunologic tolerance to food antigens, a phenomenon termed oral tolerance.[34] When oral tolerance to food antigens fails, IgE-mediated food allergy may result. Oral tolerance is an antigen-specific state of immunologic unresponsiveness and can be induced by multiple mechanisms. Animal models have demonstrated that low-dose antigen exposure results in immune suppression by regulatory T cells (Tregs), whereas high-dose antigen exposure results in antigen-specific clonal deletion or T-cell anergy. Tolerance induction occurs in the mesenteric lymph nodes by tolerogenic CD103[+] dendritic cells that induce differentiation of naïve T cells into Tregs, leading to active suppression of the antigen-specific immune response.[35]

Once a food allergy is established, there is a clear Th2-skewed response to the allergen. Allergen-specific T cells are very rare in circulation; a tetramer study found 10 Ara h 1–specific T cells per million CD4[+] cells.[36] The T-cell response is dominated by the secretion of Th2 cytokines, including interleukin-4 (IL-4), IL-5, and IL-13. In addition, IL-9 has also been shown to be upregulated in response to food allergens in allergic individuals.[37] Allergic individuals also produce Th1 cytokines, including interferon-γ and tumor necrosis factor-α, along with IL-10 and IL-17, in response to the food allergen. Tregs and their cytokines are also present in allergic individuals. More recently, a new Th2 subset, referred to as Th2A cells (CD4[+] CD45RO[+]CRTh2[+]CD49D[+]CD27[−]CD161[+] cells), were identified that are present at higher quantities in allergic subjects compared with nonatopic subjects.[38] One aim of immunotherapy is to reverse the proallergic T-cell response, which may lead to tolerance.

Although there is no definitive T-cell signature in individuals who have undergone food allergen immunotherapy, overall trends are seen in this population. Generally, Th2 cytokines are decreased after immunotherapy, and Tregs are increased. For example, peanut OIT and SLIT lead to decreased IL-5 and IL-13 expression from restimulated peripheral blood mononuclear cells,[13,15,19,39] and a decreased number of Th2A cells have been shown with OIT.[38] Interestingly, a 10-fold difference in dose of peanut OIT (300 vs 3000 mg) did not result in meaningful differences in cytokine suppression.[39] OIT also leads to increased CD4[+]Foxp3[+] Tregs.[18,19] One study demonstrated that individuals who completed OIT and were classified as immune tolerant had decreased methylated sites on the Foxp3 locus of antigen-induced Tregs compared with nontolerant individuals,[18] indicating that Foxp3 methylation could be used as a biomarker to distinguish desensitization and sustained unresponsiveness. A previously unidentified subset of anergic CD4[+] T cells was identified in subjects who completed OIT.[40] Although no human data exist for T-cell changes during EPIT, a mouse study indicates that EPIT induces LAP[+] Tregs in the intestine, providing a potential mechanism underlying the efficacy of EPIT.[41]

B-CELL AND IMMUNOGLOBULIN CHANGES

B cells play a critical role in IgE production and maintaining IgE levels. B cells specific to any antigen are rare. Previous studies have used fluorescently labeled peanut allergens to show that there are very few peanut-specific B cells in the periphery of peanut-allergic individuals. One study showed that approximately 0.02% of B cells was Ara h 2 specific.[42] Another study showed that 0.0097% of B cells were Ara h 1 specific and 0.029% were Ara h 2 specific in peanut-allergic subjects; these quantities in both studies increased 3-fold during OIT.[43] In addition to changes in the number of B cells after immunotherapy, B-cell products, including IgE, IgG (IgG1, IgG2, IgG3 and IgG4) and IgA (IgA1 and IgA2), are also modulated in response to therapy.

Before immunotherapy, individuals generally have high levels of antigen-specific IgE and low levels of antigen-specific IgG and IgA. After immunotherapy is completed, antigen-specific IgG4 significantly increases, thereby increasing the ratio of IgG4 to IgE. These trends have been shown in immunotherapy to peanut, milk, and egg.[9,17,20,21,23,26,30,39,44,45] Importantly, even if antigen-specific IgE does not significantly decrease over the course of therapy, desensitization may still be induced.[15,19]

Immunoglobulin G and Immunoglobulin A Subclasses in Oral Immunotherapy and Sublingual Immunotherapy

Food immunotherapy involves chronic exposure to the antigen, which leads to increased serum antigen-specific IgG. These trends have been shown in OIT for peanut, milk, and egg. A previous study demonstrated that all peanut-specific IgG subtypes, including IgG1, IgG2, IgG3, and IgG4, increased after 1 year of OIT.[46] Importantly, the IgG fraction was shown to inhibit basophil activation by binding to the FcγRIIb receptor, indicating IgG may have protective effects as a result of OIT. Specifically, IgG4 accounts for most inhibition effects.[47] A more recent study found that IgG blocking effects are associated with sustained unresponsiveness in OIT subjects.[48] Many studies have shown increased IgG4 against whole antigen extract, purified allergens as well as specific epitopes in single antigen OIT.[21,43,49–51] In a multiallergen OIT study, IgG4 to all allergens increased after OIT.[52] These trends in IgG4 occur in OIT, SLIT, and EPIT and appear to be universal regardless of allergen (see Fig. 1). Interestingly, salivary IgG4 to α-lactalbumin, β-lactoglobulin, and casein has also been shown to increase during milk OIT in a published abstract.[53] These results indicate that IgG4 in the saliva and serum may be contributing to the protective effects seen during OIT.

Antigen-specific IgA in the serum also increases as a result of food immunotherapy. During a peanut OIT trial, Ara h 2–specific IgA increased.[43] Increases in IgA have also been shown during egg OIT, including IgA1 and IgA2 specific for egg white and allergen components.[54] Specifically, IgA and IgA2 to egg white significantly increased in individuals who achieved sustained unresponsiveness to egg, indicating that IgA may contribute to the protective effects. In addition to serum, IgA levels in the local mucosa have also been quantified during SLIT. Salivary peanut-specific IgA and secretory IgA were found to be increased during peanut SLIT, and these correlated with desensitization challenge outcomes.[55] All of these results indicate that IgA is another important factor in immunotherapy.

Immunoglobulin levels, specifically IgG4, vary significantly between therapies. In a direct comparison of peanut OIT and SLIT, peanut-specific IgG4 significantly increased after 12 months of therapy.[17] Although the quantity of IgG4 induced as a result of OIT was approximately 10-fold higher compared with SLIT, in the same trial, peanut-specific IgE was increased from baseline on SLIT, whereas it decreased for subjects on OIT. Other OIT and SLIT trials have demonstrated similar findings.[30] EPIT changes in IgG4 appear to be smaller in magnitude than SLIT, although no direct comparisons have been made between the therapies.

MAST CELL AND BASOPHIL ACTIVATION

The effector cells involved in anaphylaxis, namely mast cells and basophils, are also affected as a result of immunotherapy. Mast cells in the skin become less reactive during immunotherapy, as demonstrated by skin prick test (SPT) data.[21,23] In the same trial comparing peanut OIT and SLIT as described above, SPT wheal size decreased by about 3-fold in SLIT subjects, and by over 6-fold in OIT subjects after 12 months of therapy.[17] Mast cells in other mucosal surfaces, including the gastrointestinal tract, are more difficult to analyze; therefore, studies in humans have yet to be performed. As a result, animal models of desensitization have been developed to gain insight into underlying mechanisms. One study demonstrated that low-dose antigen exposure, below the threshold of an allergic reaction, leads to internalization of IgE on sensitized mast cells, thus preventing allergic reactions.[56] Another mechanism was discovered that indicates that actin rearrangement occurs during desensitization, which then inhibits calcium flux required for degranulation.[57]

Basophils are circulating effector cells that have similar properties to mast cells and can be readily studied. Basophil activation tests (BATs) are ex vivo assays that use whole blood to assess degranulation in response to allergens. Activation is typically monitored by CD63 or CD203c, which are quantified by flow cytometry. CD63 is present on granules and upon degranulation becomes fused with the cell membrane, whereas CD203c is constitutively expressed on the cell membrane and becomes upregulated upon activation. Both of these markers have been assessed during immunotherapy.[58] Researchers have theorized that BAT assays could be useful to monitor subjects on allergen immunotherapy. Notably, BAT assays have been shown to differentiate peanut-sensitized but tolerant individuals from peanut-sensitized and allergic individuals.[59] Therefore, once commercialized, BAT assays may be used to distinguish subjects who are desensitized from subjects who achieved sustained unresponsiveness during immunotherapy.

Similar to decreases in mast cell activation, basophil activation also decreases during immunotherapy. For subjects on OIT, basophils become hyporesponsive during the first few months. These results have been shown for peanut, milk, and egg.[23,30,60] During peanut SLIT, similar trends toward less reactive basophils have been shown.[15] BAT assays have yet to be reported for EPIT. Notably, decreases in basophil activation seem to be independent from immunoglobulin changes during the initial dose escalation and early buildup. Sustained basophil hyporesponsiveness has been associated with blocking effects of IgG.

FUTURE CONSIDERATIONS

Although the past decade has brought food allergy immunotherapy a wealth of clinical and immunologic knowledge, there is still much to be learned. The immunologic changes associated with food allergy immunotherapy are broadly applicable to many subjects, although biomarkers are lacking that (1) indicate who is a good candidate for OIT, SLIT, or EPIT and (2) can track subjects during immunotherapy to indicate when desensitization has occurred. Future studies may use omics-based approaches, along with systems biology to identify important, yet currently unknown, changes that occur while undergoing immunotherapy.[61,62]

SUMMARY

Food allergen immunotherapy definitively induces changes in T cells, B cells, and allergic effector cells. Many studies have demonstrated increases in allergen-specific IgG4 and subsequent decreases in allergen-specific IgE, with apparent underlying changes in T cells driving these responses. Ultimately, effector cells become less responsive to allergen encounters such that mast cell and basophil reactivity sharply decreases during long-term immunotherapy. Unfortunately, many of these immunologic changes are transient,[63] which leaves the field wondering whether immunotherapy can restore tolerance in food allergic patients.[64]

REFERENCES

1. Gupta RS, Warren CM, Smith BM, et al. Prevalence and severity of food allergies among US adults. JAMA Netw Open 2019;2(1):e185630.
2. Gupta RS, Springston EE, Warrier MR, et al. The prevalence, severity, and distribution of childhood food allergy in the United States. Pediatrics 2011;128(1): e9–17.
3. Gupta RS, Warren CM, Smith BM, et al. The public health impact of parent-reported childhood food allergies in the United States. Pediatrics 2018;142(6) [pii:e20181235].
4. Branum AM, Lukacs SL. Food allergy among U.S. children: trends in prevalence and hospitalizations. NCHS Data Brief 2008;(10):1–8.
5. Burks AW. Peanut allergy. Lancet 2008;371(9623):1538–46.
6. Avery NJ, King RM, Knight S, et al. Assessment of quality of life in children with peanut allergy. Pediatr Allergy Immunol 2003;14(5):378–82.
7. Fleischer DM, Perry TT, Atkins D, et al. Allergic reactions to foods in preschool-aged children in a prospective observational food allergy study. Pediatrics 2012;130(1):e25–32.
8. Clark S, Espinola JA, Rudders SA, et al. Frequency of US emergency department visits for food-related acute allergic reactions. J Allergy Clin Immunol 2011;127: 682–3.
9. PALISADE Group of Clinical Investigators, Vickery BP, Vereda A, Casale TB. AR101 oral immunotherapy for peanut allergy. N Engl J Med 2018;379(21): 1991–2001.
10. Fleischer DM, Greenhawt M, Sussman G, et al. Effect of epicutaneous immunotherapy vs placebo on reaction to peanut protein ingestion among children with peanut allergy: the PEPITES randomized clinical trial. JAMA 2019;321(10): 946–55.
11. Anagnostou K, Clark A, King Y, et al. Efficacy and safety of high-dose peanut oral immunotherapy with factors predicting outcome. Clin Exp Allergy 2011;41(9): 1273–81.
12. Bird JA, Feldman M, Arneson A, et al. Modified peanut oral immunotherapy protocol safely and effectively induces desensitization. J Allergy Clin Immunol Pract 2015;3(3):433–5.e1-3.
13. Blumchen K, Ulbricht H, Staden U, et al. Oral peanut immunotherapy in children with peanut anaphylaxis. J Allergy Clin Immunol 2010;126(1):83–91.e1.
14. Hofmann AM, Scurlock AM, Jones SM, et al. Safety of a peanut oral immunotherapy protocol in children with peanut allergy. J Allergy Clin Immunol 2009; 124(2):286–91, 291.e1-6.

15. Kim EH, Bird JA, Kulis M, et al. Sublingual immunotherapy for peanut allergy: clinical and immunologic evidence of desensitization. J Allergy Clin Immunol 2011; 127(3):640–6.e1.
16. MacGinnitie AJ, Rachid R, Gragg H, et al. Omalizumab facilitates rapid oral desensitization for peanut allergy. J Allergy Clin Immunol 2017;139(3):873–81.e8.
17. Narisety SD, Frischmeyer-Guerrerio PA, Keet CA, et al. A randomized, double-blind, placebo-controlled pilot study of sublingual versus oral immunotherapy for the treatment of peanut allergy. J Allergy Clin Immunol 2015;135(5): 1275–82.e1-6.
18. Syed A, Garcia MA, Lyu SC, et al. Peanut oral immunotherapy results in increased antigen-induced regulatory T-cell function and hypomethylation of forkhead box protein 3 (FOXP3). J Allergy Clin Immunol 2014;133(2):500–10.
19. Varshney P, Jones SM, Scurlock AM, et al. A randomized controlled study of peanut oral immunotherapy: clinical desensitization and modulation of the allergic response. J Allergy Clin Immunol 2011;127(3):654–60.
20. Vickery BP, Berglund JP, Burk CM, et al. Early oral immunotherapy in peanut-allergic preschool children is safe and highly effective. J Allergy Clin Immunol 2017;139(1):173–81.e8.
21. Vickery BP, Scurlock AM, Kulis M, et al. Sustained unresponsiveness to peanut in subjects who have completed peanut oral immunotherapy. J Allergy Clin Immunol 2014;133(2):468–75.
22. Buchanan AD, Green TD, Jones SM, et al. Egg oral immunotherapy in nonanaphylactic children with egg allergy. J Allergy Clin Immunol 2007;119(1):199–205.
23. Burks AW, Jones SM, Wood RA, et al. Oral immunotherapy for treatment of egg allergy in children. N Engl J Med 2012;367(3):233–43.
24. Jones SM, Burks AW, Keet C, et al, Consortium of Food Allergy Research (CoFAR). Long-term treatment with egg oral immunotherapy enhances sustained unresponsiveness that persists after cessation of therapy. J Allergy Clin Immunol 2016;137(4):1117–27.e10.
25. Lemon-Mule H, Sampson HA, Sicherer SH, et al. Immunologic changes in children with egg allergy ingesting extensively heated egg. J Allergy Clin Immunol 2008;122(5):977–83.e1.
26. Vickery BP, Pons L, Kulis M, et al. Individualized IgE-based dosing of egg oral immunotherapy and the development of tolerance. Ann Allergy Asthma Immunol 2010;105(6):444–50.
27. Kim JS, Nowak-Wegrzyn A, Sicherer SH, et al. Dietary baked milk accelerates the resolution of cow's milk allergy in children. J Allergy Clin Immunol 2011;128(1): 125–31.e2.
28. Nadeau KC, Schneider LC, Hoyte L, et al. Rapid oral desensitization in combination with omalizumab therapy in patients with cow's milk allergy. J Allergy Clin Immunol 2011;127(6):1622–4.
29. Skripak JM, Nash SD, Rowley H, et al. A randomized, double-blind, placebo-controlled study of milk oral immunotherapy for cow's milk allergy. J Allergy Clin Immunol 2008;122(6):1154–60.
30. Keet CA, Frischmeyer-Guerrerio PA, Thyagarajan A, et al. The safety and efficacy of sublingual and oral immunotherapy for milk allergy. J Allergy Clin Immunol 2012;129(2):448–55.e5.
31. Nowak-Wegrzyn A, Wood RA, Nadeau KC, et al. Multicenter, randomized, double-blind, placebo-controlled clinical trial of vital wheat gluten oral immunotherapy. J Allergy Clin Immunol 2019;143(2):651–61.e9.

32. Elizur A, Appel MY, Nachshon L, et al. Walnut oral immunotherapy for desensitisation of walnut and additional tree nut allergies (Nut CRACKER): a single-centre, prospective cohort study. Lancet Child Adolesc Health 2019;3(5):312–21.

33. Sicherer SH, Sampson HA. Food allergy: recent advances in pathophysiology and treatment. Annu Rev Med 2009;60:261–77.

34. Berin MC, Shreffler WG. Mechanisms underlying induction of tolerance to foods. Immunol Allergy Clin North Am 2016;36(1):87–102.

35. Tordesillas L, Berin MC. Mechanisms of oral tolerance. Clin Rev Allergy Immunol 2018;55(2):107–17.

36. DeLong JH, Simpson KH, Wambre E, et al. Ara h 1-reactive T cells in individuals with peanut allergy. J Allergy Clin Immunol 2011;127(5):1211–8.e3.

37. Brough HA, Cousins DJ, Munteanu A, et al. IL-9 is a key component of memory TH cell peanut-specific responses from children with peanut allergy. J Allergy Clin Immunol 2014;134(6):1329–38.e10.

38. Wambre E, Bajzik V, DeLong JH, et al. A phenotypically and functionally distinct human TH2 cell subpopulation is associated with allergic disorders. Sci Transl Med 2017;9(401) [pii:eaam9171].

39. Kulis M, Yue X, Guo R, et al. High and low dose oral immunotherapy similarly suppress pro-allergic cytokines and basophil activation in young children. Clin Exp Allergy 2019;49(2):180–9.

40. Ryan JF, Hovde R, Glanville J, et al. Successful immunotherapy induces previously unidentified allergen-specific CD4+ T-cell subsets. Proc Natl Acad Sci U S A 2016;113(9):E1286–95.

41. Tordesillas L, Mondoulet L, Blazquez AB, et al. Epicutaneous immunotherapy induces gastrointestinal LAP(+) regulatory T cells and prevents food-induced anaphylaxis. J Allergy Clin Immunol 2017;139(1):189–201.e4.

42. Hoh RA, Joshi SA, Liu Y, et al. Single B-cell deconvolution of peanut-specific antibody responses in allergic patients. J Allergy Clin Immunol 2016;137(1):157–67.

43. Patil SU, Ogunniyi AO, Calatroni A, et al. Peanut oral immunotherapy transiently expands circulating Ara h 2-specific B cells with a homologous repertoire in unrelated subjects. J Allergy Clin Immunol 2015;136(1):125–34.e12.

44. Bird JA, Spergel JM, Jones SM, et al, ARC001 Study Group. Efficacy and safety of AR101 in oral immunotherapy for peanut allergy: results of ARC001, a randomized, double-blind, placebo-controlled phase 2 clinical trial. J Allergy Clin Immunol Pract 2018;6(2):476–85.e3.

45. Jones SM, Sicherer SH, Burks AW, et al, Consortium of Food Allergy Research. Epicutaneous immunotherapy for the treatment of peanut allergy in children and young adults. J Allergy Clin Immunol 2017;139(4):1242–52.e9.

46. Burton OT, Logsdon SL, Zhou JS, et al. Oral immunotherapy induces IgG antibodies that act through FcgammaRIIb to suppress IgE-mediated hypersensitivity. J Allergy Clin Immunol 2014;134(6):1310–7.e6.

47. Santos AF, James LK, Bahnson HT, et al. IgG4 inhibits peanut-induced basophil and mast cell activation in peanut-tolerant children sensitized to peanut major allergens. J Allergy Clin Immunol 2015;135(5):1249–56.

48. Orgel K, Burk C, Smeekens J, et al. Blocking antibodies induced by peanut oral and sublingual immunotherapy suppress basophil activation and are associated with sustained unresponsiveness. Clin Exp Allergy 2019;49(4):461–70.

49. Burk CM, Kulis M, Leung N, et al. Utility of component analyses in subjects undergoing sublingual immunotherapy for peanut allergy. Clin Exp Allergy 2016;46(2):347–53.

50. Shreffler WG, Lencer DA, Bardina L, et al. IgE and IgG4 epitope mapping by microarray immunoassay reveals the diversity of immune response to the peanut allergen, Ara h 2. J Allergy Clin Immunol 2005;116(4):893–9.
51. Vickery BP, Lin J, Kulis M, et al. Peanut oral immunotherapy modifies IgE and IgG4 responses to major peanut allergens. J Allergy Clin Immunol 2013;131(1): 128–34.e1-3.
52. Andorf S, Purington N, Block WM, et al. Anti-IgE treatment with oral immunotherapy in multifood allergic participants: a double-blind, randomised, controlled trial. Lancet Gastroenterol Hepatol 2018;3(2):85–94.
53. Torabi B, Schneider O, Lejtenyi D, et al. Salivary IgG4 increases during milk oral immunotherapy. J Allergy Clin Immunol 2017;139(2):AB255.
54. Wright BL, Kulis M, Orgel KA, et al. Component-resolved analysis of IgA, IgE, and IgG4 during egg OIT identifies markers associated with sustained unresponsiveness. Allergy 2016;71(11):1552–60.
55. Kulis M, Saba K, Kim EH, et al. Increased peanut-specific IgA levels in saliva correlate with food challenge outcomes after peanut sublingual immunotherapy. J Allergy Clin Immunol 2012;129(4):1159–62.
56. Oka T, Rios EJ, Tsai M, et al. Rapid desensitization induces internalization of antigen-specific IgE on mouse mast cells. J Allergy Clin Immunol 2013;132(4): 922–32.e1-16.
57. Ang WX, Church AM, Kulis M, et al. Mast cell desensitization inhibits calcium flux and aberrantly remodels actin. J Clin Invest 2016;126(11):4103–18.
58. Thyagarajan A, Jones SM, Calatroni A, et al. Evidence of pathway-specific basophil anergy induced by peanut oral immunotherapy in peanut-allergic children. Clin Exp Allergy 2012;42(8):1197–205.
59. Santos AF, Douiri A, Becares N, et al. Basophil activation test discriminates between allergy and tolerance in peanut-sensitized children. J Allergy Clin Immunol 2014;134(3):645–52.
60. Jones SM, Pons L, Roberts JL, et al. Clinical efficacy and immune regulation with peanut oral immunotherapy. J Allergy Clin Immunol 2009;124(2):292–300, 300.e1-97.
61. Bunyavanich S, Schadt EE. Systems biology of asthma and allergic diseases: a multiscale approach. J Allergy Clin Immunol 2015;135(1):31–42.
62. Dhondalay GK, Rael E, Acharya S, et al. Food allergy and omics. J Allergy Clin Immunol 2018;141(1):20–9.
63. Gorelik M, Narisety SD, Guerrerio AL, et al. Suppression of the immunologic response to peanut during immunotherapy is often transient. J Allergy Clin Immunol 2015;135(5):1283–92.
64. Berin MC, Mayer L. Can we produce true tolerance in patients with food allergy? J Allergy Clin Immunol 2013;131(1):14–22.

Peanut Oral Immunotherapy
State of the Art

Mimi L.K. Tang, MBBS, PhD, FRACP, FRCPA[a,b,c,*],
Adriana C. Lozinsky, MSc, MD[a,1], Paxton Loke, MBBS, PhD, FRACP[a,b,1]

KEYWORDS

- Oral immunotherapy • Peanut • Desensitization • Sustained unresponsiveness
- Quality of life • Food challenge • Adjuvant

KEY POINTS

- Cumulative evidence shows that peanut oral immunotherapy (OIT) is effective at inducing desensitization through downregulation of effector pathways in the allergic reaction cascade; however, only a subset of patients achieve sustained unresponsiveness (remission), which requires redirection of the underlying allergic response toward tolerance.
- Desensitization refers to a temporary increase in reaction threshold and theoretically offers the patient protection from accidental exposure to small amounts of allergen; however, this incremental benefit is only maintained if the patient continues with regular (usually daily) treatment or allergen ingestion, and because the reaction threshold that is achieved can fluctuate over time, patients can and do react to their continuing treatment.
- A recent meta-analysis of peanut OIT randomized trials found that OIT is associated with a threefold greater risk of anaphylaxis and twofold greater risk of epinephrine use than allergen avoidance. Therefore, although peanut OIT can lead to the immunologic outcome of desensitization, this fails to reduce the number of allergic reactions or epinephrine use (for the treatment of allergic reactions) as intended, raising doubt as to whether OIT provides greater benefit over risk for patients.
- Improvement in patient quality of life may mitigate the risks associated with increased reactions; however, available low-level evidence indicates that OIT does not deliver an improved quality of life.
- Strategies to reduce adverse events associated with OIT and/or improve the ability for OIT to induce sustained unresponsiveness (which would remove the need for daily ongoing therapy) are required to improve the benefit-risk of peanut OIT.

[a] Allergy Immunology, Murdoch Children's Research Institute, Melbourne, Australia; [b] Department of Pediatrics, The University of Melbourne, Melbourne, Australia; [c] Department of Allergy and Immunology, The Royal Children's Hospital, Melbourne, Australia
[1] Present address: 50 Flemington Road, Parkville, Victoria 3052, Australia.
* Corresponding author. 50 Flemington Road, Parkville, Victoria 3052, Australia.
E-mail address: mimi.tang@rch.org.au

Immunol Allergy Clin N Am 40 (2020) 97–110
https://doi.org/10.1016/j.iac.2019.09.005
0889-8561/20/© 2019 Elsevier Inc. All rights reserved.
immunology.theclinics.com

INTRODUCTION

Oral immunotherapy (OIT) for the treatment of food allergy has generated intense research interest. OIT involves ingesting a daily dose of allergen, starting at a very low dose. Typically several increasing doses are administered on the first day (rush phase), followed by a buildup phase during which the last tolerated dose on rush day is continued daily with dose increases performed every 1 to 2 weeks until the maintenance dose is reached. Daily dosing at the top maintenance dose is then continued in the maintenance phase.[1] The measurable outcomes of OIT as a food allergy treatment are desensitization (DS) and sustained unresponsiveness.[2] DS is defined as an increase in the reaction eliciting threshold dose to the allergen while receiving active treatment.[2] This is a temporary state of protection that is only maintained while regular OIT dosing is continued (usually daily) and protection is lost rapidly (within 1–2 weeks) on discontinuation of regular allergen exposure.[3] Sustained unresponsiveness (SU) is a long-lasting state of nonreactivity to the food allergen that persists weeks or months after cessation of OIT.[2] It is currently considered that some level of intermittent allergen exposure is required to maintain SU although the amount or frequency of such exposure remains to be defined. DS is assessed by performing double-blind placebo-controlled food challenges (DBPCFC) before OIT and after maintenance dosing is achieved to demonstrate an increase in the reaction eliciting threshold for individual patients. SU is assessed by performing a DBPCFC at least 4 to 8 weeks after treatment has been discontinued (with continuing allergen elimination during this period). The optimal duration of allergen elimination before performing the SU challenge and the cumulative dose of allergen that should be tolerated in this SU challenge have not been standardized; however as the outcome of SU is intended to indicate an absence of the allergic response at the time of testing, the period of allergen elimination should be sufficient to exclude any residual DS effect and the cumulative dose of allergen tolerated should be at least equivalent to what would be used in a diagnostic food challenge where a negative challenge is considered to exclude presence of food allergy. Food OIT randomized trials have generally applied a period of 4 to 8 weeks allergen elimination before SU challenge as DS is expected to be lost in this time frame and the cumulative dose of peanut protein that is tolerated in the SU challenge should be at least 4 g peanut protein as in a diagnostic challenge.

Oral tolerance refers to the permanent resolution of allergy, a state of nonreactivity to allergen that does not require any ongoing allergen exposure. Tolerance is the ultimate aim of any food allergy treatment including OIT; however, such an outcome cannot currently be demonstrated within the context of food allergy clinical trials because permanence of an effect cannot be proven and accurate biomarkers with high sensitivity and specificity for detection of oral tolerance remain limited.[2] The absence of allergen-specific immunoglobulin E (sIgE) provides a reliable biomarker with high specificity for resolution of allergy yet has poor sensitivity as clinical allergy may resolve before allergen-specific IgE becomes negative. Improved biomarkers that can detect the resolution of allergy with high sensitivity in addition to being specific for absence of allergy are required. In the absence of additional biomarkers for tolerance acquisition, it has been suggested that demonstration of SU that persists years after discontinuation of treatment, so-called long-term SU, may offer a surrogate marker of oral tolerance.

PEANUT ORAL IMMUNOTHERAPY CLINICAL OUTCOMES

OIT has been evaluated in a broad range of food allergies, with peanut allergy drawing greatest interest. Most randomized controlled trials of peanut OIT have assessed for

DS with few evaluating SU. Cumulative evidence from meta-analyses indicates that OIT is effective at inducing DS in most treated subjects but is less effective at inducing SU with only a small subset of patients achieving SU even after 4 or 5 years of treatment. There is great heterogeneity in published peanut OIT randomized trials including differences in dose escalation schedules, maintenance doses, duration of treatment, cumulative allergen doses in study exit food challenge and duration of allergen elimination before assessment of SU.

Induction of Desensitization with Oral Immunotherapy

The first published trial of peanut OIT, an uncontrolled open-label study evaluating a variable maintenance dose of 300 to 1800 mg, reported a DS rate of 69% (27/39) by intention to treat (ITT) analysis, in which DS was defined as passing a 3.9 g peanut protein challenge.[4] The first double-blind placebo-controlled randomized trial[5] reported a DS rate of 84% (16/19) by ITT analysis in the OIT group (maintenance dose 4000 mg peanut protein) as compared with 0% (0/9) in the placebo group, where DS was defined as passing a 5-g peanut protein DBPCFC. Other published randomized controlled, open-label, and uncontrolled trials have reported DS rates ranging from 49% to 87%, with DS defined as tolerating 300 mg to 10 g peanut protein in the different studies (**Table 1**). A large phase 3 multicenter trial evaluating a proprietary peanut OIT (AR101; 300 mg peanut protein maintenance dose) was recently completed in 551 participants (age 4–55 years), with the primary analysis group limited to children aged 4 to 17 years (n = 496). Subjects were eligible to enroll in the trial if they had a reaction threshold at or below 100 mg peanut protein during DBPCFC at study entry; 67.2% in the active group (age 4–17 years) achieved DS to a dose of at least 600 mg (1043 mg cumulative) of peanut protein as compared with 4% in the placebo group at the exit DBPCFC.[17] No beneficial effect was observed in participants aged 18 to 55 years.[17] Peanut OIT has also been performed in the clinical setting (outside of clinical research) and a retrospective review of clinical cases reported that 81% of patients (211/262) were desensitized to a target maintenance dose of 3000 mg peanut protein and of those, nearly every patient passed a 6000 mg peanut protein DS challenge.[18] There was no control group and patient treatment was modified according to the judgment of the clinician, which may introduce potential biases.[18]

Induction of Sustained Unresponsiveness with Oral Immunotherapy

Few peanut OIT studies have examined for SU.[19–21] An uncontrolled study reported 2-week SU (SU assessed 2 weeks after treatment discontinuation/allergen elimination) in 13% (3/23) of children who received 500 mg peanut OIT for 2 months.[6] A second uncontrolled study (maintenance dose 4 g peanut protein for 5 years) reported 4-week SU (SU assessed at 4 weeks after treatment discontinuation/allergen elimination) in 31% (12/39) of children by ITT analysis.[9] However, as there was no entry peanut challenge and no control group, it is difficult to ascertain the benefit from OIT over and above natural resolution, which can occur in approximately 20% of children within 5 years.[22,23] An open-label controlled study of 4 g peanut protein OIT for 2 years in 43 subjects (5–45 years of age) reported 12-week SU in 30.4% (7/23) of the OIT group compared with 0% (0/20) of control subjects.[10] However only 3 (13%) of 23 passed a second food challenge after avoiding peanut for a further 3 months,[10] suggesting that SU was lost in more than 50% of initial treatment responders, within a short time frame. A study in preschool children aged up to 3 years (9–36 months) that compared peanut OIT at maintenance doses of 300 mg versus 3000 mg peanut protein over a median treatment period of 29 months and assessed for 4-week SU reported an SU rate of 78% in the 300-mg arm and 71% in the 3000-mg arm by ITT

Table 1
Published randomized controlled, open label and uncontrolled trials of Peanut OIT

Study	Design	Sample Size and Duration of OIT Treatment	Maintenance Dose (mg Peanut Protein)	Desensitization (ITT Analysis)	Sustained Unresponsiveness (ITT Analysis)
Jones et al,[4] 2009	Open label	39 36 mo	300–1800	3.9 g peanut protein OFC: 69% (27/39)	—
Blumchen et al,[6] 2010	Open label	23 8 wk	125	61% (14/23)	4 g peanut protein DBPCFC after 2 wk elimination: 13% (3/23)
Varshney et al,[5] 2011	Randomized, placebo-controlled	OIT n = 19; Placebo n = 9 48 wk	4000	5 g peanut protein DBPCFC: OIT 84% (16/19) vs Placebo 0% (0/9)	—
Anagnostou et al,[7] 2011	Open label	22 32 wk	800	6.6 g peanut protein OFC: 64% (14/22)	
Anagnostou et al,[8] 2014	Randomized controlled	OIT n = 49; Avoidance n = 50 26 wk	800	1.4 g peanut protein DBPCFC: OIT 49% (24/49) vs Avoidance 0% (0/50)	—
Vickery et al,[9] 2014	Open label	39 up to 5 y	1800–4000	—	5 g peanut protein DBPCFC after 4 wk elimination: 31% (12/39)
Syed et al,[10] 2014	Age-matched controlled	OIT n = 23; Avoidance n = 20 24 mo	4000	3.9 g peanut protein OFC: OIT 87% (20/23) vs Avoidance 0% (0/20)	3.9 g peanut protein OFC after 3 mo elimination: 30% (7/23); after 6 mo elimination: 13% (3/23)
Narisety et al,[11] 2015	Randomized OIT vs SLIT	OIT n = 11; SLIT n = 10 16–22 mo	OIT 2 g, SLIT 3.7 mg	10 g peanut protein OFC: 16 mo OIT 9% (1/11), 22 mo OIT + 6 mo SLIT 45% (5/11) vs 16 mo SLIT 0% (0/10), 22 mo SLIT + 6 mo OIT 50% (5/10)	10 g peanut protein OFC after 4 wk elimination: • 16 mo OIT 9% (1/11), • 22 mo OIT + 6 mo SLIT 27% (3/11) • 16 mo SLIT 0% (0/10), • 22 mo SLIT + 6 mo OIT 10% (1/10)

Study	Design	n	Maintenance dose (mg)	Outcome	Additional outcome
Vickery et al,[12] 2017	2 Doses of OIT	Low Dose n = 20; High Dose n = 17 up to 48 mo	300 (Low dose); 3000 (High dose)	5 g peanut protein DBPCFC: Low dose 85% (17/20) vs high dose 76% (13/17)	5 g peanut protein DBPCFC after 4 wk elimination: Low Dose 85% (17/20) vs High Dose 71% (12/17)
Kukkonen et al,[13] 2017	Randomized controlled	OIT n = 39; Avoidance n = 21; 8 mo	800	1.255 g peanut protein DBPCFC: OIT 67% (26/39) vs Avoidance 0% (0/21)	—
Bird et al,[14] 2018	Randomized, placebo-controlled	OIT n = 29; Placebo n = 26; Up to 36 wk	300	≥443 mg peanut protein DBPCFC: OIT 79% (23/29) vs Placebo 19% (5/26); 1043 mg peanut protein DBPCFC: OIT 62% (18/29) vs Placebo 0% (0/26)	—
PALISADE/Vickery et al,[17] 2018	Randomized, placebo-controlled	4–17 y old: OIT n = 372; Placebo n = 124; 12 mo	300	≥600 mg peanut protein DBPCFC: OIT 67.2% (250/372) vs Placebo 4% (5/124)	—
TAKE-AWAY/Reier-Nilsen, et al,[15] 2019	Randomized controlled	OIT n = 57; Avoidance n = 20; 24 mo	250–5000	7.5 g peanut protein OFC: OIT 61% (35/57)	—
Blumchen et al,[16] 2019	Randomized, placebo-controlled	OIT n = 31; Placebo n = 31; 16 mo	125–250	≥300 mg peanut protein OFC: OIT 74.2% (24/31) vs Placebo 16.1% (5/31)	—

Abbreviations: DBPCFC, double-blind placebo-controlled food challenge; ITT, intention to treat; OFC, oral food challenge; OIT, oral immunotherapy; SLIT, sublingual immunotherapy.

(*Modified from* Nurmatov U, Dhami S, Arasi S, et al. Allergen immunotherapy for IgE-mediated food allergy: a systematic review and meta-analysis. Allergy 2017;72(8):1133-1147.)

analysis.[12] However, in the absence of a "no-treatment" control group, these results must be interpreted with caution given that resolution of peanut allergy is most likely to occur in the first 5 years of life[22] and a recent study demonstrated that 22% of children outgrew their peanut allergy by age 4.[23]

SAFETY OF PEANUT ORAL IMMUNOTHERAPY

OIT as a standalone therapy is associated with a high rate of allergic reactions and consequently a high study withdrawal rate. Using data pooled from 3 peanut OIT studies (n = 104), Virkud and colleagues[24] reported that 80% of subjects receiving peanut OIT experienced adverse events (AEs), with 72% of these AEs occurring during buildup and 47% during maintenance. Forty-nine percent experienced gastrointestinal symptoms and up to 42% of participants experienced systemic reactions.[24] Twenty percent of participants receiving peanut OIT withdrew from these studies, with half withdrawing due to persistent gastrointestinal symptoms. Interestingly, higher overall AE rates were seen in participants with allergic rhinitis (2.9-fold) and larger peanut skin prick test (SPT) wheal size (1.4-fold for every 5-mm increase) but not baseline-specific peanut IgE.[24] The presence of asthma was associated with an increased AE rate (2.3-fold) only during the maintenance phase.[24] In the phase 3 multicenter peanut OIT trial of AR101 (PALISADE), more than 95% of participants age 4 to 17 years experienced AEs in both the active and placebo group.[17] Severe AEs were reported in 4.3% of the active group as compared with 0.8% of the placebo group and gastrointestinal AEs were reported in 85.8% of the active group compared with 69.4% of the placebo group.[17] Of concern, epinephrine was required for treatment of severe allergic reactions in 14.0% of those receiving active therapy as compared with 6.5% in the placebo group.[17] Furthermore, 21.5% of subjects receiving AR101 peanut OIT withdrew from the study compared with 8% from the placebo group; 11.6% of AR101 participants withdrew due to AEs and 6.5% due to gastrointestinal AEs, compared to 2.4% and 1.6% of the placebo group, respectively.[17] In a follow-up study of PALISADE, eligible AR101-treated participants continued on daily maintenance for another 6 months, and the rates of reaction did not reduce over time - the rate of AEs reported by AR101 treated subjects was 81.2% in the follow-on period and 88% in PALISADE.[25] A recent 2019 systematic review and meta-analysis of peanut OIT trials reported that peanut OIT increased the risk of anaphylaxis 3-fold and the use of epinephrine 2-fold as compared to no OIT/allergen avoidance.[26] Moreover, patients continuing on OIT must adopt lifestyle restrictions such as avoiding exercise and showering/bathing for at least 2 to 4 hours post-OIT dose, and the withholding of doses during infections, asthma exacerbations, and menstrual periods[26] which may limit the benefit to patients. The investigators concluded that the benefit from peanut OIT may not outweigh the risks and lifestyle impact associated with treatment.

Eosinophilic esophagitis (EoE) has been reported with OIT; however, it remains unclear whether OIT plays a direct causal role in development of EoE or if OIT instead unmasks preexisting EoE in food-allergic individuals (as a result of allergen exposure with OIT). A 2014 meta-analysis of EoE with OIT reported a prevalence of 2.7% (95% confidence interval 1.7%–4.0%),[27] which is not higher than the rate of EoE reported among food-allergic individuals (4.7%).[28] A review of all patients participating in peanut OIT clinical studies (including case reports, open-label, and randomized controlled trials) reported a rate of biopsy-confirmed EoE of 5.2%.[29] In a more recent meta-analysis that limited the analysis to randomized controlled trials, 3 cases of EoE were reported across 5 peanut OIT randomized controlled trials (n = 719), all of which occurred in patients receiving peanut OIT.[26] Furthermore, as baseline endoscopies are not routinely performed before starting OIT and endoscopy is also not performed routinely in patients with EoE-like symptoms during OIT, it is possible that allergen exposure during OIT reveals existing EoE that is asymptomatic while the patient is adhering to allergen avoidance. In a study in 21 adults, baseline endoscopies were performed before commencement of peanut OIT and 24% (5/21) were shown to have preexisting esophageal eosinophilia (>5 eosinophils per high-power field [eos/hpf]), whereas 14% (3/21) had greater than 15 eos/hpf associated with endoscopic changes.[30]

A critical yet unaddressed issue is the long-term safety of continuing DS with OIT. There is a lack of long-term follow-up data for peanut OIT. As the level of protection from DS is unstable and can be lost both in association with known cofactors (such as exercise, viral illness, asthma exacerbation, menstruation) and in the absence of any cofactors, patients continuing on OIT can react to their OIT dose despite having tolerated this same dose for many months.[24] It is therefore important to understand the long-term safety of being desensitized with OIT. Long-term and follow-up studies of DS with cow's milk OIT suggest that allergic reactions do not decrease over time. In a follow-up study conducted 5 years after children had been desensitized with cow's milk OIT, 50% of children were still experiencing reactions with more than 20% reporting at least a single episode of anaphylaxis in the preceding 12 months.[31] In another follow-up study conducted 7 years post-OIT, 64% of patients reported having 1 or more allergic reactions and 25% (33/132) required epinephrine for treatment of reactions.[32] Another concern is whether desensitized patients will adhere to continuing regular (daily) allergen dosing, which is necessary to maintain the DS state. Follow-up of 21 patients who were desensitized with peanut OIT or sublingual immunotherapy at 3 to 8 years after study completion revealed that only 57% (12/21) continued to ingest peanut with taste being the main reason for discontinuing regular peanut intake.[33]

Given the high rate of AEs associated with OIT that do not reduce substantially over time and the lifestyle restrictions placed on patients continuing on OIT/allergen ingestion, there is a need to develop alternate approaches that reduce the rate of AEs associated with OIT and/or increase the likelihood of achieving SUs.

IMPROVING TOLERABILITY AND EFFICACY OF PEANUT ORAL IMMUNOTHERAPY

There is a need for novel approaches that improve tolerability and efficacy of peanut OIT. The combined administration of OIT with adjuvant therapies has been investigated with the aim of improving safety or efficacy or both. The anti-IgE monoclonal antibody Omalizumab has been shown to reduce AEs and hence improve safety; however it has not been shown to improve the rate of SU.[34] Moreover, Omalizumab is expensive and must be used continually to avoid AEs associated with OIT.

Studies suggest that the use of immune response modifiers, such as probiotics or other Toll-like receptor (TLR) agonists alongside OIT may provide improved safety of OIT and effectiveness in inducing SU. A phase 2 proof of concept double-blind, placebo-controlled randomized trial evaluating *Lactobacillus rhamnosus* CGMCC 1.3724 in combination with peanut OIT (PPOIT) in 62 children with peanut allergy reported similar withdrawal rates in active and placebo-treated groups (9.7% in each group) with no study withdrawals due to AEs or gastrointestinal AEs and a high rate of 2-week to 6-week SU following 18 months of treatment.[35] ITT analysis showed that 74% of PPOIT-treated subjects achieved SU and 84% achieved DS to a cumulative dose of 4 g peanut protein.[35] Long-term follow-up of trial participants 4 years after completing treatment showed that PPOIT-treated subjects were significantly more likely to have continuing peanut intake than placebo participants (67% vs 4%; absolute difference 63%, 95% confidence interval 42–83; P = .001).[36] Furthermore, persistent SU (assessed by DBPCFC after 8 weeks of peanut elimination at 4 years posttreatment) was shown in 58.3% (7/12) of PPOIT-treated participants compared with 6.7% (1/15) of placebo participants (P = .012).[36] At 4 years posttreatment, PPOIT participants had significantly smaller peanut SPT and significantly higher peanut sIgG4:sIgE ratio in than placebo participants. These findings suggest that the addition of a live bacterial immune modifying adjuvant (*L rhamnosus* CGMCC 1.3724) alongside OIT can reduce AEs and increase effectiveness at inducing SU compared with OIT alone.[36] Further studies directly comparing PPOIT versus peanut OIT are required to confirm this.

TLR agonists such as TLR-9 CpG and TLR4 monophosphoryl lipid A and glucopyranosyl lipid A (MPL/GLA) have been shown in mouse models to reduce anaphylaxis[37] but efficacy at inducing SU has not been evaluated in clinical trials. Other adjuvants or adjunctive therapies such as the use of nanoparticles, peptide, and recombinant vaccine immunotherapy, interferon-gamma, leukotriene receptor antagonists, and ketotifen together either single or multifood OIT are currently being investigated, with studies either in pilot/preclinical and phase I trials.[37]

QUALITY OF LIFE FOR PEANUT ORAL IMMUNOTHERAPY

The benefit-risk profile of OIT may be enhanced if there is improvement in quality of life (QoL). Yet, few randomized controlled OIT trials have assessed patient QoL and there is currently no convincing evidence to suggest that OIT when compared with placebo improves QoL. A recent systematic review concluded that peanut OIT does not improve QoL (ie, no difference between groups) based on low-certainty evidence.[26] Open studies have suggested improved QoL while on OIT but do not report findings for a control group and QoL may improve as a result of participating in a study. On the other hand, QoL has been reported to deteriorate in some patients during OIT.[38] A summary of QoL outcome with peanut OIT is shown in **Table 2**. Thus far, the only study that demonstrated improved QoL after cessation of treatment was the PPOIT study evaluating the combination of *L rhamnosus* CGMCC 1.3724 with peanut OIT, and this improvement in QoL was shown to be related specifically to the acquisition of SU.[42] Further studies comparing QoL in desensitized patients (who experience frequent allergic reactions to their daily dose of allergen/OIT) and patients with SU (who are able to adopt ad libitum peanut intake) should be pursued to clarify the benefits offered by these different treatment outcomes.

SUMMARY AND FUTURE DIRECTIONS

Current peanut OIT approaches (where OIT is administered as a standalone therapy) are associated with frequent and severe AEs, and of greater concern result in higher rates of anaphylaxis, gastrointestinal AEs and epinephrine use than allergen avoidance.[17] Although OIT is effective at inducing desensitization, the ability to induce SU is limited. Desensitized patients must continue on regular (typically daily) dosing of allergen to maintain the desensitized state, yet they experience frequent allergic reactions to their daily allergen dose because the level of protection with desensitization is unstable and the underlying allergic response remains. In contrast, SU is considered to reflect redirection of the immune response away from allergy toward tolerance and is therefore expected to avoid allergic reactions following allergen ingestion. Novel approaches that improve the safety of OIT and increase the ability of OIT to induce SU

Table 2
A summary of QoL outcome with peanut OIT

Study	Design	Quality-of-Life Assessment	Findings
TAKE-AWAY/ Reier-Nilsen et al,[15] 2019	Open label, randomized: • 37/57 completed 2 y peanut OIT • 20 controls – observation/ peanut avoidance	At enrollment, end of updosing, and after 2 y of OIT. • Children: PedsQL v4.0 • Parents: PedsQL v4.0 parental proxy and FAQL-PB MCID $\geq$5.3	Mean change in QoL from enrollment to year 2: • Child self-report: 4.4 (0.5,8.3) • Parental proxy: 9.3 (4.3,14.3) • Two years of OIT improved child-QoL compared with controls as reported by parents, but not by the children. • These findings suggest that parents may overestimate improvement in child-QoL by OIT.
Blumchen et al,[16] 2019	Double-blind, randomized, placebo-controlled. 62 participants enrolled: • 31 OIT group • 31 placebo group	At enrollment and 4 wk after end of treatment/ final OFC: • Children/Teenagers: FAQLQ-CF/FAQLQ-TF • Parents: FAQLQ-PF MCID $\geq$0.5	• After final OFC, parents on the OIT group, but not on the placebo group reported MCID>0.5 within the domain "social and dietary limitation." • Comparing OIT and placebo groups, no significant difference was found in median change in HRQOL for all domains of the FA-QLQ-PF reported by parents after the treatment with OIT. • When compared HRQOL before and after OIT, children in the active group had the median improvement for the total score as well as for each domain of the FAQLQ-CF $\geq$0.5 of the MCID. • After final OFC, children on the OIT group, but not on the placebo group reported statistically significant improvement within the 2 domains: "risk of accidental exposure" and "emotional impact."

(continued on next page)

Table 2
(continued)

Study	Design	Quality-of-Life Assessment	Findings
Zhong et al,[39] 2018	Open trial No control group • 7/9 completed peanut OIT treatment	At enrollment, 2 wk after reaching maintenance dose and 4 wk after end of treatment: • Children/Teenagers: FAQLQ-CF/FAQLQ-TF • Parents: FAQLQ-PF	• The median baseline scores were 3.8, 4.1, and 7 out of a maximal possible 7 for PF, CF, and TF respectively. • 4 wk after end of treatment, FAQLQ-PF scores decreased by 0.5 (n = 5), FAQLQ-CF scores increased by 0.1 (n = 5) and FAQLQ-TF score decreased by 0.6 (n = 1). • There was no statistically significant improvement in QoL 4 wk after the end with peanut OIT.
STOP II Anagnostou et al,[8] 2014	Randomized, controlled, crossover trial. Phase I (26 wk) completed by: • 39/49 peanut OIT group • 46/50 controls –peanut avoidance Phase II (26 wk) controls allocated to receive active intervention	At enrollment and post –treatment. Performed only in the under 13-year-old participants: • Parents: FAQLQ-PF	• QoL scores were similar in active and control groups at baseline. • No comparative results between OIT and control group were reported at the end of the first phase of the study. • Both the active and control groups demonstrated a significant improvement (decrease) in Food Allergy QoL scores after OIT in the under-13-year-old participants: −1·61 and −1·41, respectively (both P<.001).
Factor et al,[40] 2012	Open trial No control group • 90/100 participants reached maintenance dose	At enrollment, and when achieving maintenance dose: • Children/Teenagers: FAQLQ-CF/FAQLQ-TF • Parents: FAQLQ-PF MCID ≥0.5	• A significant improvement in QoL was found in all survey domains, with the exception of the emotional impact domain on the adolescents' survey. • QoL significantly improved (P<.02) on all 30 questions when parents assessed their children 5–12 y old. • When children (8–12 y old) and teens assessed themselves, QoL improved (P<.05) on 22 of 24 questions and 12 of 18 questions, respectively.

(continued on next page)

Table 2 (continued)			
Study	**Design**	**Quality-of-Life Assessment**	**Findings**
Kamilaris et al,[41] 2012	Open label No control group • OIT: 16 children 9–36 mo old	At enrollment, completion of the buildup phase and 1 year of study maintenance	• Compared with baseline after participation in peanut OIT, parents report an increase in the areas of emotional, physical, and social well-being. • Issues relating to finding time to take the daily dose and remembering to take the daily dose were areas of stress reported by the parents. • Parents reported being less anxious about their child participating in activities in which they are not present and less anxious about their child becoming more independent in food selection.

Abbreviations: CF, child form; FAQLQ, food allergy quality of life questionnaire; HRQOL, health-related quality of life; MCID, minimal clinically important difference; OFC, oral food challenge; OIT, oral immunotherapy; PF, parent form; QoL, quality of life; TF, teenager form.

are required. Although a commercial peanut OIT treatment AR101 is currently being evaluated in a Biologics License Application by the US Food and Drug Administration[43] and may soon be available for clinical use, more studies are required to clarify the long-term safety of remaining desensitized in the real world.

REFERENCES

1. Wood RA. Food allergen immunotherapy: current status and prospects for the future. J Allergy Clin Immunol 2016;137(4):973–82.
2. Burks AW, Sampson HA, Plaut M, et al. Treatment for food allergy. J Allergy Clin Immunol 2018;141(1):1–9.
3. Loh W, Tang M. Adjuvant therapies in food immunotherapy. Immunol Allergy Clin North Am 2018;38(1):89–101.
4. Jones SM, Pons L, Roberts JL, et al. Clinical efficacy and immune regulation with peanut oral immunotherapy. J Allergy Clin Immunol 2009;124(2):292–300, 300.e1-97.
5. Varshney P, Jones SM, Scurlock AM, et al. A randomized controlled study of peanut oral immunotherapy: clinical desensitization and modulation of the allergic response. J Allergy Clin Immunol 2011;127(3):654–60.
6. Blumchen K, Ulbricht H, Staden U, et al. Oral peanut immunotherapy in children with peanut anaphylaxis. J Allergy Clin Immunol 2010;126(1):83–91.e1.
7. Anagnostou K, Clark A, King Y, et al. Efficacy and safety of high-dose peanut oral immunotherapy with factors predicting outcome. Clin Exp Allergy 2011;41(9): 1273–81.

8. Anagnostou K, Islam S, King Y, et al. Assessing the efficacy of oral immuno-therapy for the desensitisation of peanut allergy in children (STOP II): a phase 2 randomised controlled trial. Lancet 2014;383(9925):1297–304.

9. Vickery BP, Scurlock AM, Kulis M, et al. Sustained unresponsiveness to peanut in subjects who have completed peanut oral immunotherapy. J Allergy Clin Immunol 2014;133(2):468–75.

10. Syed A, Garcia MA, Lyu SC, et al. Peanut oral immunotherapy results in increased antigen-induced regulatory T-cell function and hypomethylation of forkhead box protein 3 (FOXP3). J Allergy Clin Immunol 2014;133(2):500–10.

11. Narisety SD, Frischmeyer-Guerrerio PA, Keet CA, et al. A randomized, double-blind, placebo-controlled pilot study of sublingual versus oral immunotherapy for the treatment of peanut allergy. J Allergy Clin Immunol 2015;135(5): 1275–82.e1-6.

12. Vickery BP, Berglund JP, Burk CM, et al. Early oral immunotherapy in peanut-allergic preschool children is safe and highly effective. J Allergy Clin Immunol 2017;139(1):173–81.e8.

13. Kukkonen AK, Uotila R, Malmberg LP, et al. Double-blind placebo-controlled challenge showed that peanut oral immunotherapy was effective for severe al-lergy without negative effects on airway inflammation. Acta Paediatr 2017; 106(2):274–81.

14. Bird JA, Spergel JM, Jones SM, et al. Efficacy and safety of AR101 in oral immu-notherapy for peanut allergy: results of ARC001, a randomized, double-blind, placebo-controlled phase 2 clinical trial. J Allergy Clin Immunol Pract 2018; 6(2):476–85.e3.

15. Reier-Nilsen T, Carlsen KCL, Michelsen MM, et al. Parent and child perception of quality of life in a randomized controlled peanut oral immunotherapy trial. Pediatr Allergy Immunol 2019;30(6):638–45.

16. Blumchen K, Trendelenburg V, Ahrens F, et al. Efficacy, safety, and quality of life in a multicenter, randomized, placebo-controlled trial of low-dose peanut oral immu-notherapy in children with peanut allergy. J Allergy Clin Immunol Pract 2019;7(2): 479–91.e10.

17. PALISADE Group of Clinical Investigators, Vickery BP, Vereda A, Casale TB, et al. AR101 oral immunotherapy for peanut allergy. N Engl J Med 2018;379(21): 1991–2001.

18. Wasserman RL, Hague AR, Pence DM, et al. Real-world experience with peanut oral immunotherapy: lessons learned from 270 patients. J Allergy Clin Immunol Pract 2019;7(2):418–26.e4.

19. Nurmatov U, Dhami S, Arasi S, et al. Allergen immunotherapy for IgE-mediated food allergy: a systematic review and meta-analysis. Allergy 2017;72(8): 1133–47.

20. Jones SM, Burks AW, Dupont C. State of the art on food allergen immuno-therapy: oral, sublingual, and epicutaneous. J Allergy Clin Immunol 2014; 133(2):318–23.

21. Tang ML, Martino DJ. Oral immunotherapy and tolerance induction in childhood. Pediatr Allergy Immunol 2013;24(6):512–20.

22. Ho MH, Wong WH, Heine RG, et al. Early clinical predictors of remission of pea-nut allergy in children. J Allergy Clin Immunol 2008;121(3):731–6.

23. Peters RL, Allen KJ, Dharmage SC, et al. Natural history of peanut allergy and predictors of resolution in the first 4 years of life: a population-based assessment. J Allergy Clin Immunol 2015;135(5):1257–66.e1-2.

24. Virkud YV, Burks AW, Steele PH, et al. Novel baseline predictors of adverse events during oral immunotherapy in children with peanut allergy. J Allergy Clin Immunol 2017;139(3):882–8.e5.

25. Carr TF, Shreffler WG, Griffin NM, et al. Longer-term safety and efficacy measures of AR101 oral immunotherapy for peanut allergy: results from a phase 3 follow-on study. J Allergy Clin Immunol 2019;143(2):AB256.

26. Chu DK, Wood RA, French S, et al. Oral immunotherapy for peanut allergy (PACE): a systematic review and meta-analysis of efficacy and safety. Lancet 2019;393(10187):2222–32.

27. Lucendo AJ, Arias A, Tenias JM. Relation between eosinophilic esophagitis and oral immunotherapy for food allergy: a systematic review with meta-analysis. Ann Allergy Asthma Immunol 2014;113(6):624–9.

28. Hill DA, Dudley JW, Spergel JM. The prevalence of eosinophilic esophagitis in pediatric patients with IgE-mediated food allergy. J Allergy Clin Immunol Pract 2017; 5(2):369–75.

29. Petroni D, Spergel JM. Eosinophilic esophagitis and symptoms possibly related to eosinophilic esophagitis in oral immunotherapy. Ann Allergy Asthma Immunol 2018;120(3):237–40.e4.

30. Wright BL, Fernandez-Becker NQ, Kambham N, et al. Baseline gastrointestinal eosinophilia is common in oral immunotherapy subjects with IgE-mediated peanut allergy. Front Immunol 2018;9:2624.

31. Keet CA, Seopaul S, Knorr S, et al. Long-term follow-up of oral immunotherapy for cow's milk allergy. J Allergy Clin Immunol 2013;132(3):737–9.e6.

32. Barbi E, Longo G, Berti I, et al. Adverse effects during specific oral tolerance induction: in home phase. Allergol Immunopathol (Madr) 2012;40(1):41–50.

33. Dantzer JA, Mudd KE, Wood RA. Long term follow-up of oral and sublingual immunotherapy for peanut allergy. J Allergy Clin Immunol 2019;143(2):AB247.

34. Hsiao KC, Tang MLK. Novel treatments for established food allergies. Curr Pediatr Rep 2016;4:178–85.

35. Tang ML, Ponsonby AL, Orsini F, et al. Administration of a probiotic with peanut oral immunotherapy: a randomized trial. J Allergy Clin Immunol 2015;135(3): 737–44.e8.

36. Hsiao KC, Ponsonby AL, Axelrad C, et al. Long-term clinical and immunological effects of probiotic and peanut oral immunotherapy after treatment cessation: 4-year follow-up of a randomised, double-blind, placebo-controlled trial. Lancet Child Adolesc Health 2017;1(2):97–105.

37. Virkud YV, Wang J, Shreffler WG. Enhancing the safety and efficacy of food allergy immunotherapy: a review of adjunctive therapies. Clin Rev Allergy Immunol 2018;55(2):172–89.

38. Rigbi NE, Goldberg MR, Levy MB, et al. Changes in patient quality of life during oral immunotherapy for food allergy. Allergy 2017;72(12):1883–90.

39. Zhong Y, Chew JL, Tan MM, et al. Efficacy and safety of oral immunotherapy for peanut allergy: a pilot study in Singaporean children. Asia Pac Allergy 2018; 9(1):e1.

40. Factor JM, Mendelson L, Lee J, et al. Effect of oral immunotherapy to peanut on food-specific quality of life. Ann Allergy Asthma Immunol 2012;109(5): 348–52.e2.

41. Kamilaris JS, Steele PH, Kulis MD, et al. Participation in peanut oral immunotherapy improves quality of life. J Allergy Clin Immunol 2012;129(2):AB29.

42. Dunn Galvin A, McMahon S, Ponsonby AL, et al, PPOIT study team. The longitudinal impact of probiotic and peanut oral immunotherapy on health-related quality of life. Allergy 2018;73(3):560–8.
43. Therapeutics A. U.S. FDA accepts BLA filing of aimmune therapeutics AR101 for peanut allergy. 2019. Available at: http://ir.aimmune.com/news-releases/news-release-details/us-fda-accepts-bla-filing-aimmune-therapeutics-ar101-peanut. Accessed May 17, 2019.

Safety of Food Oral Immunotherapy
What We Know, and What We Need to Learn

Sonia Vázquez-Cortés, MD[a], Paloma Jaqueti, MD[b],
Stefania Arasi, MD, PhD[c], Adrianna Machinena, MD[d],
Montserrat Alvaro-Lozano, MD, PhD[d],
Montserrat Fernández-Rivas, MD, PhD[e,*]

KEYWORDS

- Allergy • Food • Immunotherapy • Oral immunotherapy • Safety

KEY POINTS

- Compared with food avoidance, oral immunotherapy (OIT) for food allergy is associated with a higher incidence rate and risk of adverse reactions, including anaphylaxis.
- The lack of consistency in reporting adverse events in food OIT studies is the major limitation to establish precisely the safety profile, and therefore, an international consensus on safety reporting for OIT is needed.
- The analysis of large pooled clinical data sets and biological samples with integrated omics approaches is needed to identify risk factors and biomarkers associated with safety.
- The needs and opinions of patients/families on OIT should be taken into account for the management.
- It is absolutely necessary to stratify patients' risk of adverse reactions in order to manage them adequately with individualized care pathways.

INTRODUCTION

Food allergy (FA) has become a significant medical problem for which avoidance of the culprit foods and use of rescue medication in the event of an allergic reaction

[a] Allergy Department, Hospital Clinico San Carlos, IdISSC, ARADyAL, Prof. Martin Lagos s/n, Madrid 28040, Spain; [b] Allergy Department, Hospital Clinico San Carlos, IdISSC, Prof. Martin Lagos s/n, Madrid 28040, Spain; [c] Pediatric Allergology Unit, Department of Pediatric Medicine, Bambino Gesù Children's Research Hospital (IRCCS), Piazza S. Onofrio, Rome 00161, Italy; [d] Allergy and Clinical Immunology Department, Hospital Sant Joan de Deu, Secció d'Al-lergia i Immunologia Clínica, Passeig Sant Joan de Déu 2, Esplugues de Llobregat, Barcelona 08590, Spain; [e] Allergy Department, Hospital Clinico San Carlos, Medicine UCM, IdISSC, ARADyAL, Prof. Martin Lagos s/n, Madrid 28040, Spain
* Corresponding author.
E-mail address: mariamontserrat.fernandez@salud.madrid.org

Immunol Allergy Clin N Am 40 (2020) 111–133
https://doi.org/10.1016/j.iac.2019.09.013
0889-8561/20/© 2019 Elsevier Inc. All rights reserved.
immunology.theclinics.com

are recommended as the "standard of care."[1] In the last 2 decades, considerable research has been done on immunotherapy for FA with the aim of providing a therapy with a disease-modifying effect. Several routes of administration have been investigated, including subcutaneous, oral, sublingual, and epicutaneous ones. The largest body of evidence is on oral immunotherapy (OIT), which consists of the oral administration of progressively increasing doses of the food allergen until reaching a target dose (up-dosing phase) that is then taken regularly (maintenance phase).[2] Although the quality of studies performed is heterogeneous and the number of treated patients is limited, recent systematic reviews and metaanalysis[2,3] have shown that OIT is able to produce desensitization, in other words, to increase the threshold of reactivity to the food, provided the patient maintains the regular intake of the food allergen dose. In some individuals, this lack of reactivity to the food is maintained even after a period of cessation of exposure, a status known as sustained unresponsiveness (or remission).[4]

The evidence that OIT is able to induce desensitization has challenged the "standard of care" in FA, opening the gate to OIT in the management of (some) food allergic patients. However, OIT is associated with a significant number of adverse events, including adverse reactions (AR) directly related to the immunotherapy,[2,3] and this safety concern is at present the major barrier for OIT to become a therapeutic option in clinical practice.

In this article, the authors review the current evidence on safety of OIT (focusing on AR), address the limitations and gaps in the knowledge, and discuss some alternatives to fill the gaps in this quickly evolving area.

SAFETY OF FOOD ORAL IMMUNOTHERAPY: WHAT IS KNOWN

OIT has the inherent risk of producing AR that can go from mild oral symptoms to anaphylaxis. Frequency of reactions is higher during the up-dosing phase performed in the clinical setting. However, reactions may also appear at home to a dose previously tolerated in the clinic during the up-dosing, and even in the maintenance phase to doses tolerated previously for weeks or months. Patients and their families should be trained in the recognition and management of AR, including the early self-administration of epinephrine in anaphylaxis.[4] Reactions are the main reason for discontinuation. A few cases of severe, life-threatening anaphylaxis have been published,[5–8] but to the best of the authors' knowledge, no fatalities have been reported so far.

Evidence from Systematic Reviews and Metaanalysis

Safety aspects of OIT have been studied in 2 recent systematic reviews and metaanalyses. Nurmatov and colleagues[2] searched publications until March 31, 2016 on allergen immunotherapy for any FA administered through oral (OIT), sublingual (SLIT), epicutaneous, or subcutaneous (SCIT) routes. Thirty-one studies with 1259 participants were included: 25 randomized clinical trials (RCT) and 6 nonrandomized controlled clinical trials (CCT). OIT was studied in 18 RCTs and in 5 CCTs, and the FAs most commonly treated were milk, egg, and peanut in 16, 11, and 7 studies, respectively. The occurrence of local reactions (LR) (minor oropharyngeal/gastrointestinal [GI] reactions, perioral rash) and systemic reactions (SR) was analyzed. Because of heterogeneity in reporting adverse events, only 5 OIT trials (on milk 3, on egg 1, and on peanut 1) with a total number of 150 participants could be pooled in the metaanalysis of SR. In the metaanalysis of LR, 7 studies were pooled (3 on milk, 3 on egg, and 1 on milk and egg OIT) with 319 total participants. Despite this limited number of studies and patients treated, an increased risk of reactions was shown during OIT, both local (risk ratio [RR] of not experiencing a reaction in controls 2.12, 95% confidence interval [CI] 1.50–3.0) and systemic (RR of not experiencing a reaction in controls 1.16, 95% CI 1.03–1.30). Subgroup analysis showed an increased risk for SR in milk OIT, an increased risk for LR in milk and egg OIT, and that both conventional and rush protocols were associated with an increased risk of LR.

In the systematic review of Chu and colleagues,[3] published and unpublished RCTs comparing OIT for peanut allergy with placebo or avoidance were searched until December 6, 2018. Twelve studies (8 published between 2011 and 2018 and 4 unpublished) were included with 1041 participants, 767 from trials with proprietary formulations and 551 from a single phase 3 pivotal study.[9] The metaanalysis showed that peanut OIT increases anaphylaxis risk (RR 3.12, 95% CI 1.76–5.55), anaphylaxis frequency (incidence rate ratio 2.72, 95% CI 1.57–4.72), epinephrine use (RR 2.21, 95% CI 1.27–3.83), and serious adverse events (RR 1.92, 95% CI 1.0–3.66). When involvement of different organs/systems was analyzed, OIT increased the risk of having GI, mucocutaneous, and upper and lower respiratory reactions. These results were not modified by the OIT regimen (proprietary formulation or not, starting and target dose, treatment duration), or phase (buildup or maintenance), median participant age, and peanut threshold of reactivity in the entry oral food challenge.

Heterogeneity in Reporting Formats of Adverse Reactions in Oral Immunotherapy Studies

There is a high heterogeneity in the reporting formats of adverse events in OIT studies. It emerged already in the metaanalysis of Nurmatov[2] and reduced considerably the number of studies used in the quantitative synthesis. There is not yet a specific guideline on safety reporting of OIT in FA, and the proposed grading systems for SR in SCIT for nonfood allergens (reviewed in Ref.[9]) have not been applied in food OIT. Furthermore, there is considerable variability between systems used to grade SR in SCIT,[9] and food allergic reactions,[10] which, it is hoped, may be overcome with recent initiatives to harmonize this field.[11,12]

The authors have reviewed 52 studies for this article,[7–62] including 34 RCT, 10 CCT, and 8 real-life studies (RLS), dealing with peanut (n = 16), milk (n = 22), egg (n = 17), walnut (n = 1), sesame (n = 1), and wheat (n = 1) OIT (**Tables 1** and **2**).

In 64% of the studies reviewed, at least 80% of participants reached the target maintenance dose (mean 81.8%, range 21%–100%), and 0% to 36% (mean 11%) were withdrawn for AR. The frequency of patients with a certain AR is given in 84% of studies, whereas the total number of doses and the reaction rate per dose are provided in 40% and 45% of the studies, respectively. Only 40% report reactions separately per protocol phase, and there is scarce information on reactions in the long-term maintenance, because it is not covered within the time-frame of most RCT and CCT studies (**Tables 3** and **4**).

Severity grading of AR is done in 71% of articles reviewed (**Tables 5** and **6**) with different nonequivalent systems,[9,10] impairing comparisons across studies. Some trials present the frequency of severity graded reactions,[21,23,26,27,32,35,40,53,62] sometimes also depicted by phase.[7,17,26,27,31,37,48,52]

The authors have extracted the frequency of oropharyngeal, skin, GI, upper and lower respiratory reactions, and anaphylaxis (see **Tables 5** and **6**). Studies frequently provide the information in this line, per target organ/system involved, although some provide frequency of individual symptoms. Oral symptoms are sometimes excluded from the safety reporting, and upper and lower respiratory involvement may be presented in a single category (respiratory), with the consequent loss of information of the frequency of lower airway reactions, which are clinically relevant side effects.

Table 1
Characteristics of peanut, walnut, sesame, and wheat oral immunotherapy studies reviewed

Study	Country	Design	Participants N	Age Range (y)	Female (%)	Intervention Group OIT	N	Control Group Comparator	N
Varshney et al,[14] 2011	USA	RDBPCT	28	2–10	36	Peanut	19	Placebo	9
Anagnostou et al,[15] 2014	UK	Crossover RCT	99	7–16	29	Peanut	49	Avoidance[a]	50
Tang et al,[16] 2015	Australia	RDBPCT	62	1–10	40	Peanut + probiotic	31	Placebo	31
Narisety et al,[17] 2015	USA	RDBPCT	21	6–21	48	Peanut	10	Peanut SLIT[a]	11
Kukkonen et al,[7] 2017	Finland	CCT	60	6–18	42	Peanut	39	Avoidance	21
Vickery et al,[18] 2017	USA	RCT	37	9–36 mo	31	Peanut low and high dose	37	Avoidance (historical cohort)	154
Bird et al,[19] 2018	USA	RDBPCT	55	4–26	35	Peanut	29	Placebo	26
Fauquert et al,[20] 2018	France	RDBPCT	30	12–18	27	Peanut	21	Placebo	9
Nagakura et al,[21] 2018	Japan	CCT	34	5–18	26	Peanut	24	Avoidance	10
Vickery et al,[13] 2018	USA, Canada, Europe	RDBPCT	555	4–55	43	Peanut	416	Placebo	139
Nachshon et al,[22] 2018	Israel	RLS	145	≥4	38	Peanut	145		
Blumchen et al,[23] 2019	Germany	RDBPCT	62	3–17	39	Peanut	31	Placebo	31
Reier-Nilsen et al,[24] 2019	Norway	RCT	77	5–15	43	Peanut	57	Avoidance	20
Wasserman et al,[25] 2019	USA	RLS	270	4–18	40	Peanut	270		
Soller et al,[26] 2019	Canada	RLS	270	9–71 mo	41	Peanut	270		
MacGinnitie et al,[27] 2017	USA	RDBPCT	37	6–19	41	Peanut + omalizumab	29	Peanut OIT + placebo	8
Elizur et al,[28] 2019	Israel	CCT	73	4–20	30	Walnut	55	Avoidance	18
Nachshon et al,[29] 2019	Israel	CCT	75	≥4	36	Sesame	60	Avoidance	15
Nowak-Węgrzyn et al,[30] 2019	USA	crossover RDBPCT	46	4–30	22	Wheat low vs high dose	23	Placebo	23

Abbreviation: RDBPCT, randomized double-blind placebo-controlled trial.
[a] Start OIT after avoidance or SLIT.

Table 2
Characteristics of milk and egg oral immunotherapy studies reviewed

Study	Country	Design	Participants N	Participants Age Range (y)	Participants Female (%)	Intervention Group OIT	Intervention Group N	Control Group Comparator	Control Group N
Burks et al,[31] 2012	USA	RDBPCT	55	5–11		Egg	40	Placebo	15
Dello Iacono et al,[32] 2013	Italy	RCT	20	5–11	50	Egg	10	Avoidance	10
Fuentes-Aparicio et al,[33] 2013	Spain	RCT	72	4–15	25	Egg	40	Avoidance	32
Meglio et al,[34] 2013	Italy	RCT	20	≥4	40	Egg	10	Avoidance	10
Vazquez-Ortiz et al,[35] 2014	Spain	CCT	82	5–18	51	Egg	50	Avoidance	32
Caminiti et al,[36] 2015	Italy	RDBPCT	31	4–11	75	Egg	17	Placebo	14
Escudero et al,[37] 2015	Spain	RCT	61	5–17	37	Egg	30	Avoidance	31
Pérez-Rangel et al,[38] 2017	Spain	RCT	33	5–18	45	Egg	19	Avoidance[a]	14
Giavi et al,[39] 2016	Greece, Italy, Switzerland	RDBPCT	29	1–5.5	31	Egg	15	Placebo	14
Itoh-Nagato et al,[40] 2018	Japan	RCT	45	5–15	27	Egg	45	Avoidance[a]	22
Machinena et al,[41] 2019	Spain	RLS	43	>5	30	Egg	43		
Skripak et al,[42] 2008	USA	RDBPCT	20	6–17	40	Milk	13	Placebo	7
Longo et al,[43] 2008	Italy	RCT	60	5–17	35	Milk	30	Avoidance	30
Caminiti et al,[44] 2009	Italy	RDBPCT	13	5–10	38	Milk	10	Placebo	3
Pajno et al,[45] 2010	Italy	RSBPCT	30	4–10	43	Milk	15	Placebo	15
Martorell et al,[46] 2011	Spain	RCT	60	2–3	43	Milk	30	Avoidance	30
Salmivesi et al,[47] 2013	Finland	RDBPCT	28	6–14	57	Milk	18	Placebo	10
Vázquez-Ortiz et al,[48] 2013	Spain	RLS	81	5–18	38	Milk	81		

(continued on next page)

Table 2
(continued)

Study	Country	Design	N	Age Range (y)	Female (%)	OIT	N	Comparator	N
				Participants		**Intervention Group**		**Control Group**	
Lee et al,[49] 2013	Korea	RCT	31	7–12 mo	50	Milk	16	Avoidance	15
García-Ara et al,[50] 2013	Spain	CCT	55	4–14	37	Milk	36	Avoidance	19
Martínez-Botas et al,[51] 2015	Spain	CCT	32	4–7	32	Milk	25	Avoidance	7
Yanagida et al,[52] 2015	Japan	CCT	37	≥5	31	Milk	12	Avoidance[a]	25
Wood et al,[53] 2016	USA	RDBPCT	57	7–32	30	Milk + omalizumab	28	Milk OIT + placebo	29
Takahashi et al,[54] 2017	Japan	RCT	16	6–14		Milk + omalizumab	10	Avoidance	6
Mota et al,[55] 2018	Portugal	RLS	42	2–18	40	Milk	42		
Kauppila et al,[8] 2019	Finland	RLS	244	≥5	42	Milk	244		
De Schryver et al,[56] 2019	Canada	RCT	52	6–18	44	Milk	26	Avoidance[a]	26
Patriarca et al,[57] 1998	Italy	RCT[b]	20	5–13	50	Egg (n = 5), milk (n = 6)	11	Avoidance	9
Patriarca et al,[58] 2003	Italy	CCT[b]	75	3–55	58	Egg (n = 15) Milk (n = 29)	59	Avoidance	16
Patriarca et al,[59] 2007	Italy	CCT[b]	52	3–16	42	Egg (n = 17) Milk (n = 18)	42	Avoidance	10
Morisset et al,[60] 2007	France	RCT	150	1–8	35	Egg (n = 51) Milk (n = 28)	79	Avoidance	71
Staden et al,[61] 2007	Germany	RCT	45	0.6–12.9	36	Egg (n = 11) Milk (n = 14)	11	Avoidance	20
Arasi et al,[62] 2019	Italy	RLS	96	4–14	64	Egg (n = 14), milk (n = 20), plan for AR	34	Egg (n = 27) Milk (n = 35) No plan for AR	62

a Start OIT after avoidance.
b OIT for several foods reported together.

Table 3
Safety reporting in peanut, walnut, sesame, and wheat oral immunotherapy studies reviewed

Study	Differential Reporting During Phases	Report Total Doses Given	Report AR per Dose	Report Pt. per AR	% Pts Reached Maintenance Dose	% Pts Withdrawn for AR	Report Accidental Reactions in Controls
Peanut OIT							
Varshney et al,[14] 2011	Yes	No	No	Partially	84	16	No
Anagnostou et al,[15] 2014	No	Yes	Yes	Yes	84-91	5	No
Tang et al,[16] 2015	Yes	No	No	Yes	100	3.2	Yes
Narisety et al,[17] 2015	Yes	Yes	Yes	Yes	SLIT: 100 OIT: 91	SLIT 10; OIT 27 SLIT + OIT: 22.2	No
Kukkonen et al,[7] 2017	Yes	No	No	Yes	67 ITT; 83 PP	BU 10.3; M 12.9	No
Vickery et al,[18] 2017	Yes	No	Yes	Yes	86.5	8.1	No
Bird et al,[19] 2018	No	No	No	Yes	79	21	Yes
Fauquert et al,[20] 2018	No	No	Yes	Yes	81	9.5	Yes
Nagakura et al,[21] 2018	Yes	Yes	Yes	NM	92	NM	No
Vickery et al,[13] 2018	Yes	No	Yes	Yes	78	14	No
Nachshon et al,[22] 2018	Yes	No	No	Yes	78 (3000 mg) 92 (≥300 mg)	0.8	NA

(continued on next page)

Table 3
(continued)

Study	Differential Reporting During Phases	Report Total Doses Given	Report AR per Dose	Report Pt. per AR	% Pts Reached Maintenance Dose	% Pts Withdrawn for AR	Report Accidental Reactions in Controls
Blumchen et al,[23] 2019	Yes	Yes	Yes	Yes	74.2	6.5	Yes
Reier-Nilsen et al,[24] 2019	No	Yes	Yes	Yes	21.1 full dose 54.4 partial dose	26.7	No
Wasserman et al,[25] 2019	Yes	No	No	Yes	78	12.6	NA
Soller et al,[26] 2019	Yes	Yes	Unclear	Yes	90	Unclear (<10)	NA
MacGinnitie et al,[27] 2017	No	Yes	Yes	Yes	88.8	8.6	Yes
Walnut OIT							
Elizur et al,[28] 2019	Yes	Yes	Yes	Yes	89	5.4	Yes
Sesame OIT							
Nachshon et al,[29] 2019	No	Yes	Yes	Yes	88.4	NM	No
Wheat OIT							
Nowak-Węgrzyn et al,[30] 2019	Yes	Yes	Yes	Yes	82.6 low dose 57.1 high dose	10.9	Yes

Abbreviations: BU, build-up phase; ITT, intention to treat population; M, maintenance phase; NA, nonapplicable; NM, no mention; PP, per protocol population; Pts, participants.

Table 4
Safety reporting in egg and milk oral immunotherapy studies reviewed

Study	Differential Reporting During Phases	Report Total Doses Given	Report AR per Dose	Report Pt per AR	% Pts Reached Maintenance Dose	% Pts Withdrawn for AR	Report Accidental Reactions in Controls
Egg OIT							
Burks et al,[31] 2012	No	Yes	Yes	No	87.5	15	Yes
Dello Iacono et al,[32] 2013	No	No	No	No	0 (90 partial dose)	0	Yes
Fuentes-Aparicio et al,[33] 2013	No	No	No	Yes	92.5	7.5	No
Meglio et al,[34] 2013	No	No	No	No	80	10	No
Vazquez-Ortiz et al,[35] 2014	Yes	Yes	Yes	Yes	80	18	Yes
Caminiti et al,[36] 2015	Yes	No	No	Yes	94.1	5.9	No
Escudero et al,[37] 2015	Yes	Yes	Yes	Yes	93.3	6.7	No
Pérez-Rangel et al,[38] 2017	Yes	No	Yes	Yes	94	3	Yes
Giavi et al,[39] 2016	Unclear	Unclear	Unclear	No	100	0	Yes
Itoh-Nagato et al,[40] 2018	No	No	No	Yes	93.3	11.1	NM
Machinena et al,[41] 2019	Yes	Yes	Yes	Yes	76.7	16.3	NA
Milk OIT							
Skripak et al,[42] 2008	No	Yes	Yes	Yes	92.3	7.7	Yes
Longo et al,[43] 2008	Yes	No	No	No	36 (54–<150 mL)	10	Yes
Caminiti et al,[44] 2009	No	No	No	No	70 (10–<200 mL)	20	NM
Pajno et al,[45] 2010	No	No	No	Yes	76.9 (7.7–<200 mL)	15.4	No
Martorell et al,[46] 2011	No	Yes	Yes	Yes	90	3.3	Yes
Salmivesi et al,[47] 2013	No	No	No	Yes	88 (1 y); 85 (3 y)	11.1	Yes

(continued on next page)

Table 4
(continued)

Study	Differential Reporting During Phases	Report Total Doses Given	Report AR per Dose	Report Pt per AR	% Pts Reached Maintenance Dose	% Pts Withdrawn for AR	Report Accidental Reactions in Controls
Vázquez-Ortiz et al,[48] 2013	Yes	Yes	Yes	Yes	71.6 (20.9-<200 mL)	7.4	NA
Lee et al,[49] 2013	No	No	No	Yes	100	12.5	Yes
García-Ara et al,[50] 2013	Yes	No	No	Yes	92	5.5	Yes
Martínez-Botas et al,[51] 2015	No	Yes	Yes	Yes	100	0	NM
Yanagida et al,[52] 2015	No	Yes	Yes	No	58.3	0	No
Wood et al,[53] 2016	Yes	Yes	Yes	Yes	100 MOIT; 92.8 OIT	0 MOIT;14.3 OIT	NA
Takahashi et al,[54] 2017	Yes	Yes	AR per dose per Pt		100 MOIT	0	NM
Mota et al,[55] 2018	No	No	No	Yes	92.8	4.8	NA
Kauppila et al,[8] 2019	No	No	No	Yes	56	28	Yes
De Schryver et al,[56] 2019	Yes	No	No	Yes	73.2	26.8	Yes
Egg and milk OIT							
Patriarca et al,[57] 1998	No	No	No	Yes	CM 81.8; E 100	0	NM
Patriarca et al,[58] 2003	No	No	No	Yes	CM 65.5; E 83.3	CM 17; E 13.3	NM
Patriarca et al,[59] 2007	No	No	No	Yes	CM 66.7; E 83.3	CM 16.7; E 7.14	NM
Morisset et al,[60] 2007	No	No	No	No	CM 88.9; E 69.4	CM 11.1; E 14.3	NM
Staden et al,[61] 2007	No	No	No	Yes	64 (16 partial dose)	36	Yes
Arasi et al,[62] 2019	No	No	No	Yes	100	1	NA

Abbreviations: CM, milk; E, egg; MOIT, omalizumab and OIT.

Table 5
Symptoms and management of adverse reactions in the intervention group of peanut, walnut, sesame, and wheat oral immunotherapy studies reviewed

Study	Severity Grading	Skin	Oral	GI	Upper Respiratory	Lower Respiratory	Anaphylaxis	Epinephrine Use	Hospitalization ER, ICU
Peanut OIT									
Varshney et al,[14] 2011	No	NM	NM	NM	NM	NM	NM	10.5% Pt	No
Anagnostou et al,[15] 2014	No	13% Pt; 0.2% D	81% Pt; 6.3% D	Ab pain 57% Pt; 2.6% D	23% Pt; 0.4% D	23% Pt; 0.4% D	NM	2 = 1% Pt, 0.01% D	No
Tang et al,[16] 2015	No	41.2% Pt	0	11.7% Pt	0	44.2% Pt	9.7% Pt	9.7% Pt	No
Narisety et al,[17] 2015	Yes	2.8% D	24.2% D	9% D	6.9% D		9% Pt	36.3% Pt	No
Kukkonen et al,[7] 2017	Yes	Rash/eczema: BU 44%; M 18% Urticaria: BU 23% AE; M 24% AE	NM	Ab pain: BU 41%; M 18% Emesis: BU 10% AE; M 6% AE	NM	26% AE (BU) 21% AE (M)	0% AE (BU) 6% AE (M)	2.6% Pt	ER: BU: 4.6/10⁴ PtD M: 3/10⁴ PtD (28% Pt)
Vickery et al,[18] 2017a	Yes	Unclear >30 AE	Unclear	Unclear >57 AE	Unclear 20 AE	Unclear	Unclear	0.8% AE 6% Pt	No
Bird et al,[19] 2018	Yes	14% AE	10% AE	66% AE	48% AE		NM	3.4% Pt	1 SAE, 3.4% Pt
Fauquert et al,[20] 2018	Yes	81% AE	19% AE	76% AE	43% AE	57% AE	23.8% Pt 1/1000 D	9.5% Pt	No
Nagakura et al,[21] 2018	Yes	15.1% D	NM	28.6% D	15.1% D		NM	Hd 0% Hm 0.01% D	NM
Vickery et al,[13] 2018	Yes	66.9% AE	Pruritus 9.7% Pt	85.8% AE	81.2% AE		Unclear Systemic AR 14.2% Pt[b]	14% Pt	NM
Nachshon et al,[22] 2018	Yes	41% AE (BU)	NM	72% AE (BU)	41% AE (BU)	15% AE (BU)	Unclear	Hd 12.4% Pt Hm 14.5% FU 1.8%	No

(continued on next page)

Table 5
(continued)

Study	Severity Grading	Skin	Oral	GI	Upper Respiratory	Lower Respiratory	Anaphylaxis	Epinephrine Use	Hospitalization ER, ICU
Blumchen et al,[23] 2019	Yes	60% Pt	40% Pt	26.7% Pt	NM	43.3% Pt	0.02% SAE	2/2 (100%) SAE	OIT: H 9.7% Pt PB: ER 3.2%; H 12.9% Pt
Reier-Nilsen et al,[24] 2019	Yes	75.4% Pt 0.8% AE	86% Pt 5.9% AE	84.2% Pt 6% AE	64.9% Pt 0.3% AE		19.4% Pt 0.06% AE	10.5% Pt 0.03% AE	NM
Wasserman et al,[25] 2019	Yes	NM	NM	37.4% Pt	NM	NM	23% Pt[c]	23% Pt	No
Soller et al,[26] 2019	Yes	NM	NM	NM (1.1% EoE)	NM	NM	Unclear	4.1% Pt	1.11% Pt
MacGinnitie et al,[27] 2017	Yes	NM	NM	NM (8.1%Pt EoE)	NM	NM	Unclear	Unclear[d]	NM
Walnut OIT									
Elizur et al,[28] 2019	Yes	Hd: 38%Pt 1% D	Hd 9%Pt <1% D	Hd 47%Pt 2% D	Hd 53%Pt 2% D	Hd 15%Pt 1% D	NM	BU 20% Pt M 15% Pt FU 2% Pt	NM
Sesame OI									
Nachshon et al,[29] 2019	Yes	26.8% Pt 1.25% D	NM	53.5% Pt 2.5% D	42.5% Pt 2% D	9.4% Pt 0.4% D	NM	Hd: 0.5% D; 16.7% Pt Home 8.3% Pt 0.05% D	NM
Wheat OIT									
Nowak-Węgrzyn et al,[30] 2019	Yes	2.5% AE	2.2% AE	6.4% AE	7.3% AE	NM	NM	0.08% D	No

Abbreviations: Ab, abdominal; AE, adverse events; D, doses; ER, emergency room; FU, long-term follow-up; H, hospitalization; Hd, hospital dosing; Hm, home dosing; ICU, intensive care unit; PB, placebo; PtD, participant days.

[a] AEs presented in a figure; none of the multiple symptoms AE (n = 37) were considered anaphylaxis.
[b] Systemic allergic reactions in 14.2% Pt, mild 6.2% Pt, moderate 7.8% Pt, severe (considered anaphylaxis) 0.2% Pt.
[c] Epinephrine-treated reactions considered as anaphylaxis.
[d] Epinephrine needed in 14 reactions in 8 patients after 11 doses of omalizumab-OIT and 3 doses of OIT without omalizumab.

Table 6

Symptoms and management of adverse reactions in the intervention group of egg and milk oral immunotherapy studies reviewed

Study	Severity Grading	Skin	Oral	GI	Upper Respiratory	Lower Respiratory	Anaphylaxis	Epinephrine Use	Hospitalization ER, ICU
Egg OIT									
Burks et al,[31] 2012	Yes	4.4% D	15.4% D	5.5% D	7.8% D	No data	NM	No	No
Dello Iacono et al,[32] 2013	Yes	43.4% AE	39.6% AE	34% AE	32.1% AE	9.4% AE	NM	No	No
Fuentes-Aparicio et al,[33] 2013	No	16.7% AE	22.2% AE	58.3% AE	19.4% AE	25% AE	Unclear	12.5% Pt	No
Meglio et al,[34] 2013	Yes	30% Pt	50% Pt	50% Pt	0% Pt	30% Pt	No	NM	No
Vazquez-Ortiz et al,[35] 2014	Yes	20.5% AE	13.7% AE	37.2% AE	7.7% AE	18.8% AE	NM	26% Pt 0.1% D	NM
Caminiti et al,[36] 2015	Yes	5.9% Pt	0%	5.9% Pt	0%	0%	5.9% Pt	5.9% Pt	NM
Escudero et al, 2015[37]	Yes	B: 3.8% AE M: 9% AE 0.3% D	BU: 21.5% AE M: 53% AE 2.2% D	BU 82% AE M 44% AE 4% D	BU 11.4% AE M 24% AE 1.3% D	BU 6.3% AE 0.2% D	Unclear	3.3% Pt 0.04% D	No
Pérez-Rangel et al,[38] 2017	Yes	11% AE	19.4% AE	54.8% AE	7.7% AE	5.8% AE	1.3% AE	6.3% Pt	Unclear
Giavi et al,[39] 2016	Yes	Unclear	Unclear	Unclear	Unclear	Unclear	NM	No	No
Itoh-Nagato et al,[40] 2018	Yes	52.2% AE	NM	60% AE	52.2% AE	43.5% AE	2.2% AE	11.6% Pt	NM

(continued on next page)

Table 6
(continued)

Study	Severity Grading	Skin	Oral	GI	Upper Respiratory	Lower Respiratory	Anaphylaxis	Epinephrine Use	Hospitalization ER, ICU
Machinena et al,[41] 2019	Yes	NM	NM	NM	NM	NM	Unclear	13.9% Pt	No
Milk OIT									
Skripak et al,[42] 2008[a]	No	0.9% D	35.7% D	18.7% D	NM	8.1% D	1.2% D	0.2% D	No
Longo et al,[43] 2008	Yes	Hd 46.7% Pt Hm 23.3% Pt	Hd 100% Pt Hm 56.7% Pt	Hd 76.7% Pt Hm 46.7% Pt	Hd 60% Pt Hm 10% Pt	Hd 40% Pt Hm26.7% Pt	NM	Hd 13.3% Pt Hm 3.3% Pt	ER: 26.7% Pt
Caminiti et al,[44] 2009	No	10% Pt	20% Pt	30% Pt	30% Pt		30% Pt	20% Pt	No
Pajno et al,[45] 2010	No	7.7%Pt	15.4% Pt	38.5% Pt	30.8% Pt		23.1% Pt	15.4% Pt	No
Martorell et al,[46] 2011	Yes	67% Pt	NM	30% Pt	50% Pt		37% Pt	6.7% Pt	No
Salmivesi et al,[47] 2013	No	33.3%	44.4% Pt	50.5% Pt	11.1% Pt	19.2% Pt	0%	No	No
Vázquez-Ortiz et al,[48] 2013[b]	Yes	Unclear	Unclear	Unclear	Unclear	Unclear	8.7% AE 45.7% Pt	11.1% Pt 0.07%D	NM
Lee et al,[49] 2013	Yes	Unclear	Unclear	No	No	No	No	No	No
García-Ara et al,[50] 2013	No	Unclear	Unclear	Unclear	Unclear	Unclear	Unclear	3.3% Pt	No
Martínez-Botas et al,[51] 2015	Yes	17.4% AE	NM	33.3% AE	13.8% AE	48.7% AE	NM	NM	No
Yanagida et al,[52] 2015	Yes	Hd 3.6%D Hm 0.8%D	Hd 42.9% D Hm 13% D	Hd 5.3% D Hm 4.2% D	Hd 19.6% D Hm 4.3% D		NM	0% D	ER: 0.2% D
Wood et al,[53] 2016[c]	Yes	MOIT 0% D OIT BU 1.1 M 0.7%D	MOIT 0.6% D OIT BU 8.8% M 0.9% D	MOIT: 0% D OIT: BU 3%; M 0.4% D	MOIT: 0% D OIT: BU 2.5%; M 0.9% D		NM	No	No
Takahashi et al,[54] 2017	Yes	NM	NM	NM	NM	NM	NM	No	No

Study									
Mota et al,[55] 2018	Yes	40.5% Pt	9.5% Pt	11.9% Pt	9.5% Pt	11.9% Pt	4.8% Pt	4.8% Pt	No
Kauppila et al,[8] 2019[d]	No	HD 41% Pt LD 42% Pt	NM	HD 45% Pt LD 73% Pt	HD 40% Pt LD 69% Pt		Unclear	6.9%-14% Pt ICU 0.4% Pt	No
De Schryver et al,[56] 2019	Yes	NM	NM	NM	NM	NM	15.8% AE	0.6 AE per Pt ER: 3.8% Pt	No
Egg and milk OIT									
Patriarca et al,[57] 1998	No	CM 50% Pt HE 20% Pt	0%	CM16.7% Pt HE 20% Pt	0%	CM16.7% Pt HE 20% Pt	0%	No	No
Patriarca et al,[58] 2003	No	NM	NM	NM	NM	NM	NM	NM	No
Patriarca et al,[59] 2007	No	Unclear	Unclear	Unclear	Unclear	Unclear	Unclear	NM	No
Morisset et al,[60] 2007	No	Unclear	NM	Unclear	Unclear	Unclear	NM	NM	NM
Staden et al,[61] 2007	No	Unclear	NM	Unclear	Unclear		NM	NM	No
Arasi et al,[62] 2019	Yes	NM	NM	NM	NM	NM	NM (0%)[e]	NM	NM

Abbreviations: CM, cow's milk; HE, hen's egg; Hm, home dosing.

[a] LRs considered as oral, multiple systems reactions included under anaphylaxis.
[b] AE presented in a figure; multisystem reactions included under anaphylaxis.
[c] Median percent of doses.
[d] Data of BU phase presented, 1 life-threatening anaphylaxis requiring ICU treatment.
[e] Outcome presented is severe AE with medication plan.

Reporting per organ/system affected (and also per individual symptoms) does not provide the whole picture, because some of these organs can be affected simultaneously in a single reaction, and this information is sometimes lacking or it is unclear how it is captured (as SR or anaphylaxis?). To overcome this problem, some studies[18,48] include a category of "multiple symptoms" or "multisystem" for single reactions that involved multiple systems and report reactions per organ only when they are affected separately. Some studies indeed reported on SR and only considered a subset of them as anaphylaxis.[13] Wasserman and colleagues[25] reported on "epinephrine-treated reactions," which have been considered to be equivalent to anaphylaxis, according to their criteria to recommend epinephrine use.[63]

There is also an important variability in the reporting of medications needed to control the reactions, with some studies providing frequency of the different drugs used, and others only providing the frequency of epinephrine use (the latter collected in **Tables 5** and **6**).

Safety information on the placebo-treated groups shows that the placebo intervention entails more side effects[13,16,19,23,27,30,31] than the mere avoidance, but it is unclear how this should be taken into account in the interpretation of safety data. Furthermore, accidental reactions in controls are reported in 48% of trials (see **Tables 3** and **4**).

Anaphylaxis

Anaphylaxis and GI reactions are the 2 main reasons to discontinue OIT for AR. In the 52 articles reviewed, anaphylaxis was not mentioned in 19 (37%); in 12 (23%), the reporting was unclear, and 21 (40%) provided a frequency in different ways (percent of adverse events, percent of patients treated, per dose; see **Tables 5** and **6**). Anaphylaxis seems not to be adequately captured and likely there is additional anaphylaxis that fulfills the current diagnostic criteria[64] under reactions reported as "systemic," and "multiple symptoms" or multisystem reactions. Even the studies reporting on "epinephrine-treated reactions"[25] may underestimate anaphylaxis with some of the criteria for epinephrine use.[63]

Who are the patients at risk of developing anaphylaxis during OIT? Multiple factors may contribute to the occurrence and severity of AR and anaphylaxis during OIT; some are related to the protocol, others to the patient, and also cofactors may play a role (reviewed in Ref.[65]). In studies on milk and egg OIT,[35,48] it has been found that a high level of sensitization, low threshold of reactivity, higher severity of the reaction in the entry food challenge, and underlying asthma are associated with a higher frequency and severity of reactions. Some casein immunoglobulin E (IgE)-binding peptides detected baseline have been associated with a poorer safety profile.[51] Cofactors like exercise, intercurrent infections, tiredness, nonsteroidal anti-inflammatory drugs, and menses have been associated with anaphylaxis to doses tolerated previously.[65] Whether these cofactors contribute to the appearance and severity of the reaction or if they are merely coincidental is unclear. Other factors, like poor asthma or rhinitis control, dosing with an empty stomach, and irregular intake, have also been associated with a higher risk of reactions. Indeed, life-threatening reactions have been described in highly sensitized adolescents with uncontrolled asthma and suboptimal OIT compliance.[6,8]

In order to reduce the risk of AR, and especially, anaphylaxis, the effect of omalizumab has been studied.[27,53,54] Omalizumab seems to facilitate a rapid desensitization to peanut in highly sensitized patients[27] and improves the tolerance of milk OIT, with a significant reduction in the reaction rate per dose, in the number of reactions needing treatment, and in their severity, during both escalation and maintenance phases.[53,54] It is not yet known how long it should be maintained, and once discontinued, some patients experience AR with the maintenance dose previously tolerated.[66]

Gastrointestinal Reactions

GI reactions are frequently reported and are very often the reason for discontinuation, in both controlled trials and RLS (see **Tables 5** and **6**). Some of these GI symptoms correspond to immediate-onset IgE-mediated reactions that appear shortly after dosing. However, there are also some recurrent GI symptoms independent of dose timing with associated blood eosinophilia. They have been described in RLS and consist mainly of episodic vomiting more than 2 hours after dosing, less frequently in abdominal pain, and no dysphagia nor food impacttion.[25,28,29,67] They have been named OIT-induced GI and eosinophilic responses[67] and later, eosinophilic esophagitis-like OIT-related syndrome (ELORS).[25] Controlled studies do not make a difference in reporting between these time-dependent and independent GI reactions, and it is thus not possible to establish the actual incidence rate and risk separately.

ELORS symptoms appear early in the course of OIT,[25,67] but resolution of symptoms and decrease of eosinophilia with dose reductions[22,24,25,28,29,67] and short courses (1–4 weeks) of proton pump inhibitors (PPI) have been reported,[24,25] allowing most patients to reach maintenance dose. The authors are not aware of data of endoscopies performed in those withdrawn from therapy, nor in those who responded to dose adjustments or PPI and could resume OIT. Some of these patients do not respond to dose reduction, and in the few that have undergone endoscopy, eosinophilic esophagitis (EoE) was confirmed.[67]

New-onset EoE has been described during OIT studies. A metaanalysis[68] of 9 studies on peanut, milk, and egg OIT published until March 2014 estimated that 2.7% (95% CI 1.7–4.0) of patients newly developed EoE. This metaanalysis synthesized data of 708 participants treated and 17 EoE events and documented a significant publication bias in favor of studies reporting EoE. Interestingly, Chu and colleagues[3] only found 3 events of new EoE in 719 patients undergoing peanut OIT and could not establish the treatment effect.

Long-Term Safety

Long-term safety information comes mainly from RLS and shows that most patients are able to consume the food with no or mild reactions, but also that severe anaphylaxis may appear to doses previously tolerated. Because of heterogeneity in reporting, it is difficult to establish the incidence rate. Kukkonen and colleagues[7] reported an annual incidence rate of emergency room visits during a median follow-up of 30 months of 11% or 3/10,000 patient-days; Vickery and colleagues[18] reported 0.06% adverse events per person per dose in a 1- to 3-year maintenance, and Wasserman and colleagues[25] reported 9.9 epinephrine-treated reactions per 100 patient-years, all 3 being studies on peanut OIT. However, there are patients lost to follow-up who might have experienced AR, and mild AR might have not been reported by patients, or are not captured.[25] The frequency and severity of reactions seem to decrease with longer maintenance.[25,69] The analysis of circumstances surrounding these reactions points to the implication of some cofactors in around half of the events, and providing safety precautions to patients/families entails a significant reduction in AR.[62] Although cofactors may contribute to the appearance or severity of reactions, it is very likely that patients exercise (for instance) in many other occasions without having a reaction, but that type of information is not captured. Reactions during home maintenance are very worrying for patients and clinicians, and the identification of patients at risk is another unmet need. Interestingly, Kauppila and colleagues[8] found that high baseline milk-specific IgE and any GI or respiratory symptoms in the postbuildup phase were associated with milk anaphylaxis during maintenance.

SAFETY OF FOOD ORAL IMMUNOTHERAPY: WHAT ONE NEEDS TO LEARN

The lack of consistency in reporting adverse events in food OIT studies is the major limitation to establishing precisely the safety profile of this intervention, in the short and long terms. The authors still have open questions on when to start and end OIT, who are the best candidates with a good safety (and efficacy) profile that will most benefit from this intervention, and who are the higher-risk patients, in order to manage all of them adequately, with individualized care pathways.

Standardized Reporting of Safety

Because of the heterogeneity in reporting, it is not possible at present to estimate a rate per dose (or per 100 doses), a rate per patient, or exposure-adjusted rates, for adverse events in general, and for specific AR. In addition, besides reporting per organ/system involved, it is necessary to report on multisystem reactions and adequately identify anaphylaxis. Severity grading is also a parameter to include to provide a comprehensive view of AR, although a validated system accepted worldwide is not yet available.[9–12]

To overcome this problem, an international consensus on reporting structure for OIT studies is needed. It should involve multiple stakeholders, including clinicians, patients, and regulators, and the outcome could be an international guideline. Having a homogeneous reporting system will facilitate synthesis and metaanalysis of safety data, and identification of predictors of adverse events.

When to Start Oral Immunotherapy?

Most of the participants in OIT studies are children and adolescents, with adult patients included in some. There are no studies treating only adult patients, and a few studies[18,26,46,49] have exclusively treated infants and toddlers. For these reasons, in the European Academy of Allergy and Clinical Immunology guidelines on immunotherapy for FA,[4] no recommendation could be made on OIT for adult patients, and the recommendation for OIT to milk, egg, and peanut was for children "from around 4 to 5 years of age." This age recommendation was based on expert opinion, and not on scientific evidence. It is therefore important to establish whether OIT can be a potential treatment with an adequate safety and efficacy balance in adults, and in children less than 4 years of age, in order to know when to start OIT. In addition, it will be important to explore the interest, views, and compliance of adult patients, and parents of infants and toddlers submitted to OIT.

When To Stop Oral Immunotherapy?

In the frame of RCT, there are predefined criteria to discontinue therapy for safety reasons. In RLS, this is an individualized decision taken jointly by the allergy team with the patient and/or family. As previously reviewed, the main reasons to stop OIT are anaphylaxis and persistent, recurrent GI symptoms, although the frequency and severity of reactions that prompt discontinuation vary between studies. Severe anaphylaxis is a clear indication to stop OIT, but it could also be an indication to evaluate other therapeutic options, such as omalizumab.[66] There are patients experiencing anaphylaxis to a certain dose who have later completed the therapy[25] with dose adjustments, add-on medications to optimize control of atopic comorbidities (essentially asthma, and seasonal rhinitis), and intensive patient/family education.[62] The same applies to persistent/recurrent GI symptoms.[22,24,25] Information coming from RLS with a large series of patients and a higher flexibility in the management has shown that dose adjustments with or without antihistamine and PPI allowed most patients with ELORS to complete the therapy. These patients would have probably been discontinued in RCT, and therefore, carefully documented observations coming from clinical practice contribute to improve the understanding of the reactions and the clinical management of patients.

The analysis of pooled data sets (including RLS), and new observation and controlled studies, together with the patients/parents' opinions, would help answering this question.

What Are the Patients' Needs and Opinions on Oral Immunotherapy?

Patients in general, and especially parents of food allergic children, have a remarkable adherence to OIT despite repeated AR. According to Dunn-Galvin and Hourihane,[70] from a patient's point of view, "expected" severe AR with OIT are well accepted because they produce less anxiety than uncertain potential accidental reactions with avoidance. Parents who perceived a significantly higher likelihood of their child having a severe reaction and dying if food is ingested were the ones willing to participate in OIT studies. In addition, acceptance may also be driven by the close follow-up during OIT. Further investigation is needed on patients/parents' preferences and views of risks and benefits of OIT.

Stratification of Patients' Risk and Development of Care Pathways

Not all the patients undergoing OIT have a similar risk, and it is clearly stated in some publications that a few patients experienced the most AR.[35,42,48,51] The appearance of an AR and its severity results from a combination of multiple factors (related to the protocol, intrinsic to the patient, cofactors) that has interactions or additive effects that are still not understood.[65,71] Some factors and potential biomarkers have been identified in some milk and egg OIT studies, but further studies are needed to validate them and look for new ones. It could be done by combining and analyzing already existing data sets and biological samples from RCT, CCT, and RLS in collaborative research. In addition, the generation of an international registry of OIT (systemic) adverse events, and new observation and controlled trials applying a standardized safety reporting would help to stratify the patients' risk, and analyzing the effect of protocol factors, cofactors, and use of adjuvants on OIT safety.

In summary, the analysis of large pooled clinical data sets with comprehensive and homogeneous safety reporting, together with integrated omics approaches in biological samples of the same individuals, may uncovered endo-phenotypes and stratify patients' risk. This approach, combined with the patients/parents' needs and opinions on OIT, will allow the development of safe(r) personalized patient-tailored treatment algorithms, which are lacking at present. They will give OIT the right place as a treatment option in FA.

DISCLOSURE

The institution of S. Vázquez-Cortés, P. Jaqueti, and M. Fernández-Rivas has received grants from Aimmune. M. Fernández-Rivas has received consultancy fees from Aimmune and DBV and lecture fees from Aimmune Therapeutics, ALK-Abello, Allergy Therapeutics, Diater, HAL Allergy, and Thermo Fisher Scientific. M. Alvaro-Lozano has received consultancy fees from Sanofi Genentech. S. Arasi and A. Machinena do not have any conflicts of interest to disclose.

REFERENCES

1. Muraro A, Werfel T, Hoffmann-Sommergruber K, et al. EAACI food allergy and anaphylaxis guidelines: diagnosis and management of food allergy. Allergy 2014;69:1008–25.
2. Nurmatov U, Dhami S, Arasi S, et al. Allergen immunotherapy for IgE-mediated food allergy: a systematic review and meta-analysis. Allergy 2017;72:1133–47.
3. Chu DK, Wood RA, French S, et al. Oral immunotherapy for peanut allergy (PACE): a systematic review and meta-analysis of efficacy and safety. Lancet 2019;393:2222–32.
4. Pajno GB, Fernandez-Rivas M, Arasi S, et al. EAACI guidelines on allergen immunotherapy: IgE-mediated food allergy. Allergy 2018;73:799–815.
5. Nieto A, Fernandez-Silveira L, Mazon A, et al. Life-threatening asthma reaction caused by desensitization to milk. Allergy 2010;65:1342–3.
6. Vazquez-Ortiz M, Alvaro M, Piquer M, et al. Life-threatening anaphylaxis to egg and milk oral immunotherapy in asthmatic teenagers. Ann Allergy Asthma Immunol 2014;113:482–4.
7. Kukkonen AK, Uotila R, Malmberg LP, et al. Double-blind placebo-controlled challenge showed that peanut oral immunotherapy was effective for severe allergy without negative effects on airway inflammation. Acta Paediatr 2017;106:274–81.
8. Kauppila TK, Paassilta M, Kukkonen AK, et al. Outcome of oral immunotherapy for persistent cow's milk allergy from 11 years of experience in Finland. Pediatr Allergy Immunol 2019;30:356–62.
9. Vidal C, Rodríguez Del Río P, Gude F, et al. Comparison of international systemic adverse reactions due to allergen immunotherapy. J Allergy Clin Immunol Pract 2019;7:1298–305.
10. Eller E, Muraro A, Dahl R, et al. Assessing severity of anaphylaxis: a data-driven comparison of 23 instruments. Clin Transl Allergy 2018;8:29.
11. Cox LS, Sanchez-Borges M, Lockey RF. World Allergy Organization systemic allergic reaction grading system: is a modification needed? J Allergy Clin Immunol Pract 2017;5:58–62.
12. Muraro A, Fernandez-Rivas M, Beyer K, et al. The urgent need for a harmonized severity scoring system for acute allergic reactions. Allergy 2018;73:1792–800.
13. PALISADE Group of Clinical Investigators, Vickery BP, Vereda A, Casale TB, et al. AR101 oral immunotherapy for peanut allergy. N Engl J Med 2018;379:1991–2001.
14. Varshney P, Jones SM, Scurlock AM, et al. A randomized controlled study of peanut oral immunotherapy (OIT): clinical desensitization and modulation of the allergic response. J Allergy Clin Immunol 2011;127:654–60.
15. Anagnostou K, Islam S, King Y, et al. Assessing the efficacy of oral immunotherapy for the desensitisation of peanut allergy in children (STOP II): a phase 2 randomised controlled trial. J Allergy Clin Immunol 2014;135:737–44.e8.
16. Tang ML, Ponsonby AL, Orsini F, et al. Administration of a probiotic with peanut oral immunotherapy: a randomized trial. J Allergy Clin Immunol 2015;135:737–44.e8.
17. Narisety SD, Frischmeyer-Guerrerio PA, Keet CA, et al. A randomized, double-blind, placebo-controlled pilot study of sublingual versus oral immunotherapy for the treatment of peanut allergy. J Allergy Clin Immunol 2015;135:1275–82.e1-6.
18. Vickery BP, Berglund JP, Burk CM, et al. Early oral immunotherapy in peanut-allergic preschool children is safe and highly effective. J Allergy Clin Immunol 2017;139:173–81.e8.

19. Bird JA, Spergel JM, Jones SM, et al. Efficacy and safety of AR101 in oral immunotherapy for peanut allergy: results of ARC001, a randomized, double-blind, placebo-controlled phase 2 clinical trial. J Allergy Clin Immunol Pract 2018;6: 476–85.e3.
20. Fauquert JL, Michaud E, Pereira B, et al. Peanut gastrointestinal delivery oral immunotherapy in adolescents: results of the build-up phase of a randomized, double-blind, placebo-controlled trial (PITA study). Clin Exp Allergy 2018;48: 862–74.
21. Nagakura KI, Yanagida N, Sato S, et al. Low-dose oral immunotherapy for children with anaphylactic peanut allergy in Japan. Pediatr Allergy Immunol 2018; 29:512–8.
22. Nachshon L, Goldberg MR, Katz Y, et al. Long-term outcome of peanut oral immunotherapy–real-life experience. Pediatr Allergy Immunol 2018;29:519–26.
23. Blumchen K, Trendelenburg V, Ahrens F, et al. Efficacy, safety, and quality of life in a multicenter, randomized, placebo-controlled trial of low-dose peanut oral immunotherapy in children with peanut allergy. J Allergy Clin Immunol Pract 2019;7: 479–91.e10.
24. Reier-Nilsen T, Michelsen MM, Lødrup Carlsen KC, et al. Feasibility of desensitizing children highly allergic to peanut by high-dose oral immunotherapy. Allergy 2019;74:337–48.
25. Wasserman RL, Hague AR, Pence DM, et al. Real-world experience with peanut oral immunotherapy: lessons learned from 270 patients. J Allergy Clin Immunol Pract 2019;7:418–26.e4.
26. Soller L, Abrams EM, Carr S, et al. First real-world safety analysis of preschool peanut oral immunotherapy. J Allergy Clin Immunol Pract 2019 [pii:S2213-2198(19)30383-30386].
27. MacGinnitie AJ, Rachid R, Gragg H, et al. Omalizumab facilitates rapid oral desensitization for peanut allergy. J Allergy Clin Immunol 2017;139:873–81.e8.
28. Elizur A, Appel MY, Nachshon L, et al. Walnut oral immunotherapy for desensitisation of walnut and additional tree nut allergies (Nut CRACKER): a single-centre, prospective cohort study. Lancet Child Adolesc Health 2019;3:312–21.
29. Nachshon L, Goldberg MR, Levy MB, et al. Efficacy and safety of sesame oral immunotherapy–a real-world, single-center study. J Allergy Clin Immunol Pract 2019 [pii:S2213-2198(19)30488-X].
30. Nowak-Węgrzyn A, Wood RA, Nadeau KC, et al. Multicenter, randomized, double-blind, placebo-controlled clinical trial of vital wheat gluten oral immunotherapy. J Allergy Clin Immunol 2019;143:651–61.e9.
31. Burks AW, Jones SM, Wood RA, et al. Oral immunotherapy for treatment of egg allergy in children. N Engl J Med 2012;367:233–43.
32. Dello Iacono I, Tripodi S, Calvani M, et al. Specific oral tolerance induction with raw hen's egg in children with very severe egg allergy: a randomized controlled trial. Pediatr Allergy Immunol 2013;24:66–74.
33. Fuentes-Aparicio V, Alvarez-Perea A, Infante S, et al. Specific oral tolerance induction in paediatric patients with persistent egg allergy. Allergol Immunopathol (Madr) 2013;41:143–50.
34. Meglio P, Giampietro PG, Carello R, et al. Oral food desensitization in children with IgE-mediated hen's egg allergy: a new protocol with raw hen's egg. Pediatr Allergy Immunol 2013;24:75–83.
35. Vazquez-Ortiz M, Alvaro M, Piquer M, et al. Baseline specific IgE levels are useful to predict safety of oral immunotherapy in egg-allergic children. Clin Exp Allergy 2014;44:130–41.

36. Caminiti L, Pajno GB, Crisafulli G, et al. Oral immunotherapy for egg allergy: a double-blind placebo-controlled study, with post-desensitization follow-up. J Allergy Clin Immunol Pract 2015;3:532–9.

37. Escudero C, Rodríguez Del Río P, Sánchez-García S, et al. Early sustained unresponsiveness after short-course egg oral immunotherapy: a randomized controlled study in egg-allergic children. Clin Exp Allergy 2015;45:1833–43.

38. Pérez-Rangel I, Rodríguez Del Río P, Escudero C, et al. Efficacy and safety of high-dose rush oral immunotherapy in persistent egg allergic children: a randomized clinical trial. Ann Allergy Asthma Immunol 2017;118:356–64.e3.

39. Giavi S, Vissers YM, Muraro A, et al. Oral immunotherapy with low allergenic hydrolysed egg in egg allergic children. Allergy 2016;71:1575–84.

40. Itoh-Nagato N, Inoue Y, Nagao M, et al. Desensitization to a whole egg by rush oral immunotherapy improves the quality of life of guardians: a multicenter, randomized, parallel-group, delayed-start design study. Allergol Int 2018;67:209–16.

41. Machinena A, Lozano J, Piquer M, et al. Oral immunotherapy protocol for hen's egg allergic children: improving safety. Pediatr Allergy Immunol 2019. [Epub ahead of print].

42. Skripak JM, Nash SD, Rowley H, et al. A randomized, double-blind, placebo-controlled study of milk oral immunotherapy for cow's milk allergy. J Allergy Clin Immunol 2008;122:1154–60.

43. Longo G, Barbi E, Berti I, et al. Specific oral tolerance induction in children with very severe cow's milk-induced reactions. J Allergy Clin Immunol 2008;121:343–7.

44. Caminiti L, Passalacqua G, Barberi S, et al. A new protocol for specific oral tolerance induction in children with IgE-mediated cow's milk allergy. Allergy Asthma Proc 2009;30:443–8.

45. Pajno GB, Caminiti L, Ruggeri P, et al. Oral immunotherapy for cow's milk allergy with a weekly up-dosing regimen: a randomized single-blind controlled study. Ann Allergy Asthma Immunol 2010;105:376–81.

46. Martorell A, De la Hoz B, Ibáñez MD, et al. Oral desensitization as a useful treatment in 2-year-old children cow's milk allergy. Clin Exp Allergy 2011;41:1297–304.

47. Salmivesi S, Korppi M, Mäkelä MJ, et al. Milk oral immunotherapy is effective in school-aged children. Acta Paediatr 2013;102:172–6.

48. Vázquez-Ortiz M, Alvaro-Lozano M, Alsina L, et al. Safety and predictors of adverse events during oral immunotherapy for milk allergy: severity of reaction at oral challenge, specific IgE and prick test. Clin Exp Allergy 2013;43:92–102.

49. Lee JH, Kim WS, Kim H, et al. Increased cow's milk protein-specific IgG4 levels after oral desensitization in 7- to 12-month-old infants. Ann Allergy Asthma Immunol 2013;111:523–8.

50. García-Ara C, Pedrosa M, Belver MT, et al. Efficacy and safety of oral desensitization in children with cow's milk allergy according to their serum specific IgE level. Ann Allergy Asthma Immunol 2013;110:290–4.

51. Martínez-Botas J, Rodríguez-Álvarez M, Cerecedo I, et al. Identification of novel peptide biomarkers to predict safety and efficacy of cow's milk oral immunotherapy by peptide microarray. Clin Exp Allergy 2015;45:1071–84.

52. Yanagida N, Sato S, Asaumi T, et al. A single-center, case-control study of low-dose-induction oral immunotherapy with cow's milk. Int Arch Allergy Immunol 2015;168:131–7.

53. Wood RA, Kim JS, Lindblad R, et al. A randomized double-blind placebo-controlled study of omalizumab combined with oral immunotherapy for the treatment of cow's milk allergy. J Allergy Clin Immunol 2016;137:1103–10.e11.

54. Takahashi M, Soejima K, Taniuchi S, et al. Oral immunotherapy combined with omalizumab for high-risk cow's milk allergy: a randomized controlled trial. Sci Rep 2017;7:17453.
55. Mota I, Piedade S, Gaspar Â, et al. Cow's milk oral immunotherapy in real life: 8-year long-term follow-up study. Asia Pac Allergy 2018;8:e28.
56. De Schryver S, Mazer B, Clarke AE, et al. Adverse events in oral immunotherapy for the desensitization of cow's milk allergy in children: a randomized controlled trial. J Allergy Clin Immunol Pract 2019;7:1912–9.
57. Patriarca G, Schiavino D, Nucera E, et al. Food allergy in children: results of a standardized protocol for oral desensitization. Hepatogastroenterology 1998; 45:52–8.
58. Patriarca G, Nucera E, Roncallo C, et al. Oral desensitizing treatment in food allergy: clinical and immunological results. Aliment Pharmacol Ther 2003;17(3): 459–65.
59. Patriarca G, Nucera E, Pollastrini E, et al. Oral specific desensitization in food-allergic children. Dig Dis Sci 2007;52:1662–72.
60. Morisset M, Moneret-Vautrin DA, Guenard L, et al. Oral desensitization in children with milk and egg allergies obtains recovery in a significant proportion of cases. A randomized study in 60 children with cow's milk allergy and 90 children with egg allergy. Eur Ann Allergy Clin Immunol 2007;39:12–9.
61. Staden U, Rolinck-Werninghaus C, Brewe F, et al. Specific oral tolerance induction in food allergy in children: efficacy and clinical patterns of reaction. Allergy 2007;62:1261–9.
62. Arasi S, Caminiti L, Crisafulli G, et al. The safety of oral immunotherapy for food allergy during maintenance phase: effect of counselling on adverse reactions. World Allergy Organ J 2019;12:100010.
63. Wasserman RL, Factor JM, Baker JW, et al. Oral immunotherapy for peanut allergy: multipractice experience with epinephrine-treated reactions. J Allergy Clin Immunol Pract 2014;2:91–6.
64. Sampson HA, Muñoz-Furlong A, Campbell RL, et al. Second symposium on the definition and management of anaphylaxis: summary report. J Allergy Clin Immunol 2006;117:391–7.
65. Patel N, Vazquez-Ortiz M, Turner PJ. Risk factors for adverse reactions during OIT. Curr Treat Options Allergy 2019;6:164–74.
66. Martorell-Calatayud C, Michavila-Gomez A, Martorell Aragonés A, et al. Anti-IgE assisted desensitization to egg and cow's milk in patients refractory to conventional oral immunotherapy. Pediatr Allergy Immunol 2016;27:544–6.
67. Goldberg MR, Elizur A, Nachshon L, et al. Oral immunotherapy-induced gastrointestinal symptoms and peripheral blood eosinophil responses. J Allergy Clin Immunol 2017;139:1388–90.e4.
68. Lucendo AJ, Arias A, Tenias JM. Relation between eosinophilic esophagitis and oral immunotherapy for food allergy: a systematic review with meta-analysis. Ann Allergy Asthma Immunol 2014;113:624–9.
69. Jones SM, Burks AW, Keet C, et al. Long-term treatment with egg oral immunotherapy enhances sustained unresponsiveness that persists after cessation of therapy. J Allergy Clin Immunol 2016;137:1117–27.e10.
70. Dunn Galvin A, Hourihane JO. Psychosocial mediators of change and patient selection factors in oral immunotherapy trials. Clin Rev Allergy Immunol 2018;55: 217–36.
71. Turner PJ, Baumert JL, Beyer K, et al. Can we identify patients at risk of life-threatening allergic reactions to food? Allergy 2016;71:1241–55.

Sublingual and Patch Immunotherapy for Food Allergy

Jamie Waldron, MD*, Edwin H. Kim, MD, MS

KEYWORDS

- Peanut allergy • Sublingual immunotherapy • Epicutaneous immunotherapy
- Desensitization • Sustained unresponsiveness • Food allergy treatments

KEY POINTS

- Sublingual immunotherapy studies have demonstrated modest desensitization and excellent safety profile with longer studies indicating potential for sustained unresponsiveness.
- Epicutaneous immunotherapy studies have demonstrated modest desensitization in children younger than 11 years with excellent safety profile and adherence rates.
- Sublingual and epicutaneous immunotherapy methods could serve as alternative treatment options for peanut-allergic patients who are unable to tolerate oral immunotherapy.

INTRODUCTION

Food allergy is a significant public health problem in industrialized nations, but has also become an increasing problem globally.[1,2] An estimated 10.8% of adults[3] and 8.0% of children[4] in the United States have food allergies, and census data have indicated a tripling of prevalence over the past 10 to 15 years.[5] Although numerous foods are implicated in allergic disease, peanut allergy has been extensively studied, as it remains the most common food allergy, exhibits higher severity reaction on exposure, and only a fraction of people outgrow this allergy.[5]

Management of peanut allergy primarily focuses on avoidance measures with self-injectable epinephrine for treatment of accidental ingestions; there are no current Food and Drug Administration (FDA)-approved treatment options. Peanut allergy is also associated with poor quality of life for individuals diagnosed with peanut allergy and their caregivers, both of whom have expressed desire for treatment options for improvement in quality of life.[6,7] To meet this growing need, research has focused on multiple immunotherapy modalities for peanut food allergy, including oral (OIT), sublingual (SLIT), and epicutaneous (EPIT) immunotherapy.

University of North Carolina School of Medicine, 3004 Mary Ellen Jones Bldg, 116 Manning Dr, CB 8035, Chapel Hill, NC 27599, USA
* Corresponding author.
E-mail address: Jamie_Waldron@med.unc.edu

Immunol Allergy Clin N Am 40 (2020) 135–148
https://doi.org/10.1016/j.iac.2019.09.008
0889-8561/20/© 2019 Elsevier Inc. All rights reserved.
immunology.theclinics.com

Immunotherapy involves exposure to increasing doses of an allergen over time with the primary goal of providing clinical desensitization and possibly long-term tolerance. Desensitization is an increase in the threshold amount of food required to cause an allergic reaction that is dependent on regular exposure to the allergen, whereas tolerance is the nonresponsive state to an allergenic food that persists and is independent of routine exposure.[3] As specific clinical and immunologic indicators for tolerance have remained undefined, studies have primarily focused on the term sustained unresponsiveness (SU), defined as the phenomenon of persistence of desensitization for a defined time after discontinuation of immunotherapy (most studies have defined this as 4–8 weeks, although a specific time frame for SU remains undefined).[8,9] Clinical trials assessing food allergy immunotherapy have relied on double-blind, placebo-controlled food challenges (DBPCFC) to confirm reactivity at baseline and to assess treatment response while on therapy (desensitization) as well as after a prescribed amount of time off of therapy (SU). Food immunotherapy studies share common dosing phases of initial dose escalation, buildup dosing, and maintenance dosing; however, there remains significant variability in study protocol with regard to dosing, rate of dose escalation, and duration of therapy as food allergen immunotherapy methods remain under active investigation.

OIT has been extensively studied with current phase III trials being conducted in anticipation of FDA approval in the near future. OIT has shown promise for desensitization and potential for SU in a subset of patients, but is also associated with significant adverse side effects that may limit its use. Therefore, it is important to continue to pursue alternative therapeutic options for individuals that may not tolerate OIT or who wish to undergo therapy with a more acceptable side-effect profile. In this article, the authors have focused on advancements regarding investigational studies on SLIT and EPIT in peanut food allergy (**Table 1**).

SUBLINGUAL IMMUNOTHERAPY

SLIT was pursued as an alternative to OIT due to ease of administration, which involves holding a peanut protein solution sublingually for 2 minutes followed by swallowing of the solution. SLIT for food allergy includes phases that are similar to other forms of immunotherapy, including dose escalation and a maintenance phase. Maintenance doses have been determined by both the maximum amount of peanut protein in solution and the largest volume of liquid expected to be comfortably held in the sublingual space by a young child.[1] Investigations on SLIT also have been motivated by its safety profile, which is considered an advantage compared with alternative immunotherapy options. SLIT is thought to mediate its immune effects via oral Langerhans cells that take up antigen within the mouth and induce downstream immune modulation that results in antigen tolerance.[10] In addition, as SLIT is administered via a mucosal surface, it is possible that immunoglobulin IgA and secretory IgA involvement may help mitigate inflammatory response and play a role in downstream immune modulation.[11]

Early studies investigating immunotherapy for food allergies focused on cow's milk (CM) allergy. Keet and colleagues[12] were the first study to compare OIT and SLIT for food allergy in 2011. Thirty children (median age of 8 years) with CM allergy were randomized to SLIT or OIT; CM allergy was defined as documented CM allergy, CM-specific IgE (CM-sIgE) of greater than 0.35 kU/L, positive skin prick test (SPT) to CM, and positive baseline DBPCFC at study entry. All participants underwent initial dosing with SLIT with daily maintenance dose (DMD) of 3.7 mg for 8 weeks. Participants were then randomized in equal numbers into 1 of 3 groups: 2 OIT crossover

Table 1
Summary of key studies in peanut sublingual and epicutaneous immunotherapy

Food Immunotherapy Modality and Study	No. Subjects	Blinding	Maintenance Dosing	Treatment Duration	Comments
SLIT					
Kim et al,[1] 2011	18	Yes	2 mg	12 mo	First double-blind study of peanut SLIT
Fleischer et al,[13] 2013	40	Yes	1.4 vs 3.7 mg	12 mo	First multicenter study of peanut SLIT
Burks et al,[14] 2015	40	Yes	1.4 vs 3.7 mg	36 mo	First multicenter study of extended therapy peanut SLIT
Burk et al,[15] 2016	33	No	2 mg	12 mo	Immune markers to predict peanut SLIT response
Kim et al,[2] 2019	48	No	2 mg	36–60 mo	Efficacy of extended therapy peanut SLIT
OIT vs SLIT					
Narisety et al,[16] 2015	21	Yes	2000 mg (OIT) vs 3.7 mg (SLIT)	12–18 mo	First study comparing peanut OIT and SLIT
EPIT					
Jones et al,[21] 2016	96	Yes	20 vs 100 vs 250 vs 500 µg		Phase I multicenter study on safety of peanut EPIT
Jones et al,[8] 2016	74	Yes	100 vs 250 µg	12 mo	NIH-sponsored double-blind phase II study of peanut EPIT
Sampson et al,[22] 2017	221	Yes	50 vs 100 vs 250 µg	12 mo	Industry-sponsored double-blind phase IIb study of peanut EPIT
Fleischer et al,[6] 2019	356	Yes	250 µg	12 mo	Industry-sponsored double-blind phase III study of peanut EPIT

Abbreviations: EPIT, epicutaneous immunotherapy; NIH, National Institutes of Health; OIT, oral immunotherapy; SLIT, sublingual immunotherapy.

groups (DMD of 2000 mg in "OITA" vs 1000 mg in "OITB"), and continued SLIT, but at increased dose of 7 mg compared with entry SLIT dosing. Primary outcomes were safety, efficacy, and immunologic changes (CM-sIgE, IgG4, and basophil function) following 60 weeks of therapy. Efficacy was defined as proportion of subjects who would tolerate 10-fold or greater increase in milk protein during DBPCFC compared with baseline DBPCFC. Secondary end points included SU after 1 and 6 weeks after therapy cessation and adverse effects (AEs). Twenty-eight subjects completed 60 weeks of maintenance therapy; 2 subjects withdrew during dose escalation due to AEs (both participants were assigned to OIT, citing worsening eczema and concerns for eosinophilic esophagitis, respectively). DBPCFCs were performed at 12 and 60 weeks of maintenance therapy, with all participants having observed increase in median successfully consumed dose (SCD) compared with baseline; however, there was a significant increase in SCD with OIT therapy (79-fold and 64-fold for OITA and OITB, respectively) at 12 weeks and at 60 weeks (54-fold and 159-fold for OITA and OITB, respectively) when compared with SLIT treatment arm (7-fold and 40-fold at 12 and 60 weeks, respectively). For participants who successfully passed the 8000 mg DBPCFC at 60 weeks without rate-limiting symptoms, the assigned therapy was discontinued and the patient underwent 1-week DBPCFC and, if tolerated, underwent a second DBPCFC at 6 weeks after therapy was discontinued. One participant (10%) in SLIT, 8 (80%) of 10 in OITA, and 6 (60%) of 10 in OITB tolerated the 8000 mg and were eligible for DBPCFC off therapy; after 1 week, 2 subjects from OITB arm failed repeat DBPCFC. At 6 weeks after therapy, 4 subjects failed repeat DBPCFC (3 from OITA and 1 from OITB); 1 (10%) SLIT subject, 5 (50%) of 10 OITA subjects, and 3 (30%) of 10 OITB subjects had observed tolerance or SU at 6 weeks. Overall, CM-sIgE levels increased initially but decreased by study completion in OIT arms (there were no significant changes in CM-sIgEs in SLIT treatment arm), CM-sIgG$_4$ levels increased in all groups, SPT reactivity to CM decreased in all groups (no statistically significant difference among treatment arms), and basophil activity decreased in OIT arms (no significant change was observed in SLIT arm). With regard to safety, 29% of SLIT doses and 23% of OIT doses had associated symptoms; there were no significant differences in the rate of symptoms between treatment arms; however, there were more respiratory, gastrointestinal, and multisystem symptoms reported with OIT dosing compared with SLIT dosing. Two SLIT doses (due to aspiration of dosing) and 4 OIT doses (2 accidental ingestions, 1 maintenance, and 1 updosing) required epinephrine.

The first double-blind, placebo-controlled SLIT trial for peanut allergy was published by Kim and colleagues[1] in 2011. This study included 18 children aged 1 to 11 years old who were randomized to placebo (median age 4.7 years) versus active SLIT (median age 5.8 years); subjects in the active SLIT arm received a DMD of 2 mg for a total of 12 months. At the end of treatment, patients exhibited a 20-fold greater median SCD compared with those receiving placebo SLIT (1710 mg after peanut SLIT vs 85 mg after placebo); notably, this study did not include an entry DBPCFC and results reflect the direct comparison of end study DBPCFC between study arms. The investigators reported an initial increase followed by decrease to baseline levels in peanut-specific IgE (PN-sIgE) laboratory values, decreased basophil responsiveness to peanut, and increased PN-sIgG4, indicating diminished allergic response and potential for long-term immunologic change and tolerance. Regarding safety, the treatment group tolerated SLIT with few AEs; the primary AE was transient oropharyngeal symptoms reported in 9.3% doses in the treatment arm with 0.26% doses requiring antihistamines for symptomatic improvement; no epinephrine was required, supporting an overall favorable safety profile.

The first multicenter, randomized placebo-controlled trial for peanut SLIT was published by Fleischer and colleagues[13] in 2013. This study, conducted by the National Institutes of Health (NIH)-sponsored Consortium for Food Allergy Research (CoFAR), included an entry DBPCFC of up to 2000 mg peanut protein and then randomized 40 subjects (aged 12–37 years) to daily peanut SLIT (DMD of 1.386 mg) versus placebo, followed by a 5000 mg DBPCFC after 44 weeks. The primary measured outcome was percentage of responders, defined as a 10-fold increase in median SCD compared with baseline DBPCFC or consumption of a cumulative dose of 5000 mg peanut protein without dose-limiting symptoms. Seventy percent of subjects in the treatment arm were responders, that is, all met criteria of a 10-fold increase in median SCD compared with baseline oral food challenge (OFC). However, no participants were able to tolerate 5000 mg during the OFC. Participants were then unblinded and the placebo arm was crossed over to a "high-dose" active treatment group (DMD of 3.696 mg) for an additional 44 weeks, whereas the original treatment arm extended treatment on the same DMD (1.386 mg) for a total of 68 weeks for the second phase of this study. Seven (44%) high-dose crossover participants had observed a 10-fold increased SCD compared with baseline OFC. All initial responders remained responders at week 68. However, none of the week 44 nonresponders converted to responders with extended SLIT therapy. This suggests that SLIT therapy may benefit a limited subgroup of peanut-allergic subjects. In addition, no subject in the original treatment arm or crossover arm was able to tolerate a 5000 mg OFC, indicating a modest level of desensitization of unclear clinical significance. This study did uphold the safety profile of SLIT, with only 127 (1.1%) of 11,854 doses requiring treatment in phase I (125 doses required antihistamines, whereas 1 dose required albuterol, and 1 dose required both antihistamines and epinephrine) and 147 (2.9%) of 5030 doses requiring treatment in phase II (146 doses required antihistamine alone, whereas 1 dose required antihistamine and albuterol). Immunologic endpoints included a significant decrease in basophil reactivity after active SLIT compared with placebo, although there were no significant differences in PN-sIgE levels between treatment arms, suggesting that PN-sIgE at 12 months of therapy has poor predictive value for clinical outcomes with SLIT.

Building on the initial study by Fleischer and colleagues,[13] which suggested statistically significant but moderate desensitization after 44 weeks, Burks and colleagues[14] aimed to determine the potential for long-term desensitization with 3-year extended maintenance data from the original study. The previously enrolled 40 subjects were continued on "standard" peanut DMD SLIT (20 participants from the original "active" treatment arm with DMD of 1386 μg) and "high-dose" DMD SLIT (20 participants from the original "crossover" arm with DMD of 3696 μg). Participants underwent 5000 mg peanut protein DBPCFCs following 2 and 3 years of daily peanut SLIT, and an additional DBPCFC following an 8-week discontinuation of SLIT at study exit. By the study end, 4 (10%) of 37 SLIT-treated subjects (2 of 17 or 23.5% subjects from "high-dose" crossover SLIT arm and 2 of 20 or 10% subjects from "standard-dose" SLIT arm) were considered responders (by meeting criteria of 10-fold increase in median SCD compared with baseline DBPCFC) and all 4 achieved SU. This study continued to support the safety of SLIT with 98% of doses tolerated without adverse reaction when oropharyngeal symptoms were excluded; no symptoms were defined as severe or required epinephrine. Limitations of this study include an observed high dropout rate (>50%) despite overall perceived SLIT tolerance, thus making conclusions of long-term SLIT efficacy difficult to interpret due to small sample size. A slightly older population (median age of 14 years) was postulated as a potential reason for the high dropout rate, with 11 participants citing personal decision for study withdrawal, compared with previous studies, such as Kim and colleagues,[1] with younger participants (median age of 5.8 years) and no study withdrawals.

As previous publications indicated potential for response in a subgroup of peanut-allergic participants, a study by Burk and colleagues[15] in 2016 aimed to identify immune markers that could serve as predictors for clinical response to SLIT therapy.

Thirty-three subjects who were actively enrolled in SLIT trials had blood collected at study entry and exit; the study concluded with a 2500 mg DBPCFC of peanut protein after 12 months of SLIT therapy. Ten (30%) subjects passed the DBPCFC without symptoms and were considered desensitized; those who passed had significantly lower baseline levels of PN-sIgE, Ara h 2, and Ara h 3 subcomponent testing compared with subjects who did not pass exit OFC. The investigators suggested that PN-sIgE of greater than 81.3 kU/L and Ara h 2 sIgE of greater than 48.55 kU/L at baseline were able to discriminate and accurately predict a higher likelihood of failing the exit OFC, and thus were predictive of poor clinical response to SLIT therapy. However, this study was limited by small sample size and being a single-center trial.

Although various studies have been performed comparing specific immunotherapy methods with placebo, few studies have directly compared immunotherapy methods. Narisety and colleagues[16] published a randomized, double-blind, placebo-controlled study of SLIT versus OIT in 2015 to compare safety, efficacy, and mechanistic correlates of these 2 immunotherapy methods. This study consisted of an initial blinded monotherapy phase, followed by an unblinded combination therapy phase. The blinded phase consisted of 21 subjects (median age 11.1 years) with baseline OFCs who were randomized to active SLIT/placebo OIT (n = 10 at 3.7 mg SLIT DMD) or active OIT/placebo SLIT (n = 11 at 2000 mg OIT DMD) for 12 months of therapy; peanut desensitization was defined as 10-fold increase in SCD with 10,000 mg OFC compared with baseline OFC. During this blinding phase, 1 active SLIT (due to persistent gastrointestinal symptoms with dosing) and 4 active OIT subjects withdrew from study (1 due to diagnosis of eosinophilic esophagitis, 1 due to persistent gastrointestinal symptoms with dosing, 1 due to systemic reaction with dosing, and 1 due to noncompliance). Of those who completed the blinded phase to 12-month OFC, all participants achieved greater than 10-fold increase in SCD compared with baseline (9 of 9 participants in the SLIT arm and 7 of 7 participants in the OIT arm), although subjects in the OIT arm had significantly greater change in median SCD (21 mg at baseline vs 7246 mg after 12 months of therapy) compared with those in the SLIT arm (21 mg at baseline vs 496 mg after 12 months of therapy). One participant from the active OIT arm passed the 12-month OFC (as defined by tolerated cumulative ≥5000 mg OFC); he exhibited SU when rechallenged via OFC 4 weeks after discontinuing therapy. Participants in both treatment arms exhibited a decrease in SPT at 12 months, although the active OIT arm exhibited a greater change from baseline in SPT wheal diameter (12 mm vs 0 mm) compared with the active SLIT arm (9.3 mm vs 5.5 mm); PN-sIgE decreased in the active OIT arm at 12 months compared with baseline (169 kU/L vs 53 kU/L), whereas the active SLIT arm exhibited no significant difference compared with baseline (163 kU/L vs 273 kU/L) after 12 months of therapy. At 12 months, the study was unblinded and all participants who failed the 12-month OFC (as defined by development of dose-limiting symptoms during OFC preventing a cumulative ingestion of ≥5000 mg peanut protein) underwent an additional 6 months of active therapy combined with active alternative treatment to assess effect of dual therapy; 10,000 mg OFC was then performed at 18 months. Subjects who passed the 18-month OFC were then rechallenged via OFC 4 weeks after discontinuing all immunotherapy to assess SU. Five (71%) active SLIT/crossover OIT participants were able to pass exit OFC at 18 months, with only 1 demonstrating SU 4 weeks after discontinuing therapy (2 subjects withdrew during OIT buildup secondary to side effects). Four (67%) active OIT subjects passed exit OFC at 18 months with 3 exhibiting SU. Subjects achieving SU in either group were found to have lower PN-sIgE levels at baseline (median PN-sIgE of 79 kU/L) compared with those unable to achieve SU (median PN-sIgE of 257 kU/L), which is consistent with results from Burk and colleagues.[15] Another observation by the investigators included persistent safety profile for SLIT, as AEs were more commonly observed with OIT doses both during blinded monotherapy phase (43% OIT doses had AEs vs 9% of SLIT doses) and unblinded combined therapy (5.1% doses in active SLIT/crossover OIT vs 35.3% doses in active OIT/crossover SLIT). This study suggests that OIT appears to be more effective at achieving desensitization, but was also associated with significantly more adverse reactions and early study withdrawal.

More recently, Kim and colleagues[2] conducted a study on long-term SLIT with subjects receiving therapy up to 5 years. The investigators enrolled participants from a previous SLIT cohort and extended SLIT protocol (with DMD of 2 mg daily for up to 5 years); participants in the initial placebo cohort were crossed over into the active SLIT group. This study included 48 participants (median age 6.5 years) with history of clinical reaction to peanut and PN-sIgE of $\geq$7 kU/L at study entry. Subjects with SPT wheal less than 5 mm and PN-sIgE less than 15 kU/L who had completed at least 3 years of maintenance SLIT were allowed to complete therapy before 5 years (10 subjects met this criteria). Subjects completing maintenance SLIT (either after 5-year maintenance SLIT or by meeting criteria for early cessation) then underwent 5000 mg peanut protein DBPCFC. SU was also assessed by identical DBPCFC 2 to 4 weeks after cessation of SLIT therapy. Eleven (22.9%) subjects withdrew from the study before exit OFC, citing difficulty with compliance (n = 8), recurrent abdominal pain (n = 2), and other reasons (n = 1). Compliance in the 37 participants completing long-term SLIT was estimated at 95.5%. Thirty-two (87%) participants tolerated SCD of $\geq$750 mg during exit DBPCFC, whereas 12 (32%) of 37 tolerated the 5000 mg OFC with 10 of 12 demonstrating SU. Peanut SPT wheal, PN-sIgE, and basophil activation decreased significantly compared with baseline values. In addition, safety profile was upheld with 4.8% of doses having associated symptoms (most reported as transient oropharyngeal pruritus); antihistamine requirement was rare at 0.21% doses and no epinephrine was administered. This study suggests that extended peanut SLIT therapy provides clinically meaningful desensitization in most peanut-allergic children and can provide SUs in a subset of participants.

A significant advantage of SLIT has been its proven safety across studies. Study outcomes have shown modest desensitization, although there remains variability among therapeutic outcomes that warrant further investigation to support generalizability to peanut-allergic patients. In addition, many studies that report a modest desensitization response have also suggested that SLIT may have improved benefit in selected patient populations. Studies have used a wide range of dosing and treatment courses, although studies on longer maintenance courses have shown promise of improved clinical outcomes. Despite the safety and ease of administration, some trials had an unexpectedly high dropout rate, which is concerning for differences in overall treatment goals between investigators and participants. Further studies focused on clarifying treatment goals, dosing, and selection of appropriate patient population may aid in future applicability of SLIT for treatment of peanut food allergy.

EPICUTANEOUS IMMUNOTHERAPY

EPIT is another immunotherapy modality that has previously shown efficacy in other forms of allergic disease,[17,18] and has since been applied to food allergy.[8] This method is appealing due to its ease of administration. A patch with a peanut protein adsorbent film is applied to the skin for 24 hours during which there is passive absorption of peanut through skin pores where it is taken up by local dendritic cells. A new patch is applied in a few designated skin locations daily for maintenance dosing. Furthermore,

EPIT has the potential for a more robust safety profile compared with other immunotherapy methods, as murine studies have demonstrated a lack of systemic antigen absorption.[19] Prolonged epicutaneous delivery of antigen is thought to downregulate TH_2 immune response via enhanced T regulatory and TH_1 response[20]; antigen-driven activation of dermal dendritic cells that are trafficked to lymph nodes is thought to drive this immune modulation, mitigating systemic response to antigen exposure in murine models.[19]

Early phase I studies indicated safety and tolerability of EPIT by using Viaskin peanut product (DBV Technologies, Montrouge, France). Jones and colleagues[21] conducted the first phase I study, which was a randomized, double-blind, placebo-controlled multicenter study in which 100 subjects (median age 22 years) with peanut allergy were randomized to active EPIT (n = 80) versus placebo (n = 20). Subjects assigned to active EPIT were further randomized to 1 of 4 doses (0.02, 0.1, 0.25, and 0.5 mg). The primary outcomes were safety and tolerability of peanut EPIT as measured by presence and severity of treatment-emergent adverse events (TEAEs), treatment required, and adherence to therapy. Active treatment arms had no observed difference between rates of TEAEs, with 42 (52.5%) of 80 active EPIT subjects reporting TEAEs, 41.3% were mild severity and 11.3% were moderate severity; in comparison, 9 (45%) of 20 in the placebo group reported at least 1 TEAE with 30% mild severity and 15% moderate severity with no statistically significant difference in reported TEAEs in placebo and active EPIT groups. Most TEAEs were local reactions, including reports of patch-site erythema, pruritus, and edema. The study reported no severe adverse events or use of epinephrine and there was a high treatment adherence with 4 (4%) of 100 participants withdrawing from the study. OFC were not conducted in this study with peanut sensitization measured by PN-sIgE and SPT; there was no significant change in PN-sIgE or SPT in treatment groups during the study (specific levels were not reported).

Jones and colleagues in 2016[8] addressed the efficacy of EPIT in a phase II NIH-sponsored CoFAR, multicentered, double-blind, randomized, placebo-controlled study. Seventy-four participants (median age 8.2 years) with peanut food allergy (as defined by the following criteria: physician-diagnosed allergy or convincing clinical history with positive SPT or PN-sIgE >0.35 kU/L, and positive baseline OFC to cumulative dose of ≤1044 mg peanut protein) were randomized to receive 52 weeks of 1 of 3 treatments: placebo (n = 25), Viaskin 0.1 mg (VP100, n = 24), or Viaskin 0.25 mg (VP250, n = 25). The primary outcome was the percentage of responders at the end of study period, which was defined as passing a 5044-mg peanut protein DBPCFC or achieving a 10-fold or greater increase in median SCD from baseline. After 52 weeks, 3 (12%) of 25 placebo-treated participants, 11 (46%) of 24 VP100 participants, and 12 (48%) of 25 VP250 participants were considered responders (by achieving a 10-fold or greater increase in median SCD from baseline). However, only 1 participant (from the placebo group) passed the exit OFC (cumulative 5044 mg peanut protein). These findings indicate a modest but statistically significant treatment effect. Treatment success was higher among younger children (4–11 years) compared with older participants (>11 years), as older participants exhibited no statistically significant treatment effect. Significant immunologic differences were observed between treatment groups for peanut IgG4 levels and peanut IgG4/PN-sIgE ratios with participants in active treatment arms exhibiting increases in both when compared with those receiving placebo. No differences were observed for PN-sIgE levels or total IgE levels; a significant decrease in SPT wheal diameter compared with baseline was observed in the VP250 treatment arm only. Significant differences were observed with a decrease of basophil activation at a stimulant dose of 0.01 μg in treatment arms, but not at higher stimulant doses; this is consistent with a shift in threshold of reactivity to peanut rather than a loss of reactivity to peanut. There were 14.4% of placebo doses and 79.8% of VP100 and VP250 doses that resulted in reactions, predominantly mild local patch-site reactions. Although patch-site reactions were common and occurred with higher frequency in active treatment arms, most responded to oral antihistamines and/or topical corticosteroids (no reactions required epinephrine). The study had an overall high compliance at 97.1% for all groups, had high participant retention, indicating that EPIT was overall well tolerated.

Sampson and colleagues[22] conducted a larger multicentered industry-sponsored phase II trial in 2017 to identify the most effective dose and establish adverse event profile, efficacy, and acceptability of peanut EPIT. Study criteria were determined by eliciting dose, defined as the highest dose at which objective symptoms of an immediate hypersensitivity reaction develop. A total of 221 peanut-allergic patients who failed entry DBPCFC (as defined by eliciting dose of ≤300 mg peanut protein) were enrolled and randomized to 1 of 4 arms: 0.05-mg, 0.1-mg, 0.25-mg, or placebo Viaskin patch for 12 months. The primary efficacy end point was percentage of treatment responders, defined as a 10-fold increase in median SCD and/or tolerance of ≥1000 mg of peanut protein. A significant difference in response rates was observed at 12 months between the 0.25-mg patch arm (50%) and placebo groups (25%). No difference was seen between the placebo patch versus 0.1-mg patch, therefore the 0.5-mg patch was not analyzed. When response rate was stratified by age group, younger subjects (6–11 years) in the 0.25-mg patch group had significant response (53.6%) compared with their age bracket in the placebo group (19.4%), whereas the older subjects (>11 years) showed no difference in response between the 0.25-mg patch (46.4%) and placebo (32%). The percentage of patients with 1 or more AE was similar across all groups, although the rate of TEAEs related to investigational product was higher in treatment arms (94.6%–96.4%) compared with placebo (48.2%); most reported AEs were local skin reactions with no dose-related serious AEs observed. Immunologic changes included increase in peanut sIgG4 levels, decrease in median peanut SPT wheal diameter, and no change in overall PN-sIgE across all treatment arms when compared with placebo group.

Participants from the initial study phase were then recruited for a 2-year open-label extension trial to assess 36-month EPIT outcomes; volunteers were initially randomized to the 3 previously defined treatment arms, but then all were switched to 0.25-mg patch at the 6-month extension time period, as this was found to be the more efficacious dose. Eighty-nine (59.7%) participants were responders at 12-month extended treatment (24-month total study period), whereas 80 (64.5%) of 124 were responders at the 24-month extended treatment (36-month total study period). Although outcome data were collected through the 2-year extension phase, giving a total of 36-month data, comparison analyses were unable to be performed given the lack of placebo control group during the extension phase, thus warranting long-term DBPC trials for EPIT.

As previous studies on EPIT suggested an increased treatment benefit in younger populations and with 0.25-mg patch dosing, follow-up phase III trials were aimed at targeting this specific age range and dose. Fleischer and colleagues[6] published their phase III multicenter, randomized, double-blinded, placebo-controlled EPIT trial in 2019. A total of 356 peanut-allergic children aged 4 to 11 years (median age 7 years) who had objective reaction to an entry DBPCFC at dose of ≤300 mg peanut protein were recruited from 31 sites in 5 countries; subjects were randomized to receive daily 0.25-mg peanut patch (Viaskin) versus placebo patch for 12 months. The primary outcome was the percentage difference in responders between peanut patch and placebo patch based on eliciting dose determined by DBPCFC at baseline and month 12. Participants were considered responders based on results of baseline DBPCFC (if baseline eliciting dose was $\leq$10 mg, response was defined as eliciting dose of $\geq$300 mg; if baseline eliciting dose was 10–300 mg, response was defined as eliciting dose of $\geq$1000 mg). There was a statistically significant difference (P <.001) in responder rate with 35.3% responders in peanut-patch treatment arm versus 13.6% in placebo arm. However, the prespecified threshold of 15% or more on the lower bound of a 95% confidence interval around responder rate difference to determine positive trial result was not met (the 15% cutoff value was the accepted value as determined by discussion between the FDA and the investigators in the absence of guiding historical data; however, the investigators note there is no consensus regarding what threshold of sensitivity may confer clinically meaningful protection). As such, further hierarchical analyses of secondary and exploratory outcomes were not analyzed or reported. Most TEAEs were patch application site reactions, which occurred in 34.5% peanut patch and 11.9% of placebo patch. Skin reactions were more prominent during month 1, and were mostly grade 1 or 2. However, there were 10 (4.2%) reported serious TEAEs from the peanut-patch group and 6 (5.1%) from the placebo group; 3 participants in the peanut arm experienced 4 serious TEAEs that met criteria for anaphylaxis and were responsive to standard treatment with epinephrine, corticosteroids, and antihistamines. The all-cause rate of discontinuation was 10.5% and 9.3% in peanut-patch and placebo groups, respectively. Adherence was 98.5%.

Similar to SLIT therapy, EPIT studies have suggested a moderate desensitization response. Although treatment-related AEs were more prevalent with EPIT compared with SLIT, reactions were overall mild and readily treated with topical therapies. Despite these reported AEs, compliance with EPIT was commonly reported among studies, indicating a clear advantage over other immunotherapy methods (**Table 2**).

FUTURE CONSIDERATIONS/SUMMARY

As the impact of food allergy continues to be felt worldwide, there has been a shared desire among providers and patients for therapeutic options. Food allergy carries significant risk to health and safety for the food-allergic individual, but also increases burden on quality of life and health care utilization.[5] Food allergy not only impacts patients themselves, but entire family systems, and providers must recognize this to understand and address therapeutic goals. To help clarify these goals of therapy, Greenhawt and colleagues[7] interviewed caregivers of peanut-allergic children seeking enrollment in OIT or EPIT trials; a common theme among families was a desire for a protective buffer from accidental exposures. As most families viewed food allergy immunotherapy as an adjuvant to ongoing allergen avoidance, families expressed willingness to accept minimal or limited protection in exchange for minimal therapeutic risk.

As phase III trials of OIT are nearing completion with anticipated FDA approval, we are seeing the first generation of therapeutic options for food allergy come to fruition. OIT has been extensively studied, and appears to provide a greater degree of desensitization and increased tolerance of allergen in comparison with SLIT and EPIT. However, OIT also has a higher rate of AEs compared with other immunotherapies.

SLIT studies have demonstrated modest desensitization outcomes when compared with OIT, but exhibit advantageous improved safety profile with rare serious AEs. Across all SLIT studies, few doses of SLIT were associated with adverse side effects with most AEs involving transient oropharyngeal symptoms; even fewer doses

Table 2
Comparison of peanut immunotherapy methods

Study	Dosing			Safety			Efficacy	Proposed Mechanism of Action
	Initial Dose, mg	DMD, mg	Buildup Period, wk	Doses Causing Symptoms, %	Doses Requiring Epinephrine	Withdrawal Due to Symptoms	Median SCD	
OIT[23]								
Vickery et al,[23] 2018	3	300 mg	20	98.7%[a]	14%	11.6%	67.2%[b]	Activation of gut mucosal dendritic cells, which cause downstream immunomodulation with increased T regulatory response and suppression of Th2 response.
SLIT[1,12,14]								
Kim et al,[1] 2011	0.00025	2 mg	26	11.5%	0%	0%	1710 mg	Antigen is taken up by oral Langerhans cells to induce downstream immune modulation, resulting in antigen tolerance. IgA and secretory IgA may help mitigate inflammatory response and play a role in downstream immune modulation.
Fleischer et al,[13] 2013; Burks et al,[14] 2015	0.000066	1.386 mg	26	40.1%	0.01%	5%	371 mg	
Narisety et al,[16] 2015	0.000066	3.696 mg	18	9%	0%	10%	496 mg	

(continued on next page)

Table 2
(continued)

| Study | Dosing | | | Safety | | | Efficacy | Proposed Mechanism of Action |
	Initial Dose, mg	DMD, mg	Buildup Period, wk	Doses Causing Symptoms, %	Doses Requiring Epinephrine	Withdrawal Due to Symptoms	Median SCD	
EPIT[6,8,20]								
Sampson et al,[22] 2017	0.25 (3 h)	0.25 mg	3	96.4%	0.01%	0.6%	144 mg	Downregulation of TH_2 immune response via enhanced T regulatory and TH_1 response. Antigen-driven activation of dermal dendritic cells that are trafficked to lymph nodes is thought to drive immune modulation and mitigate systemic response to antigen exposure (as evidenced in murine models).
Jones et al,[8] 2016	0.25 (3 h)	0.25 mg	3	79.8%	0%	2%	144 mg	
Fleischer et al,[6] 2019	0.25 (3 h)	0.25 mg	2	59.7%	2.9%	1.7%	35.3%[b]	

Abbreviations: DBPCFC, double-blinded placebo-controlled food challenge; DMD, daily maintenance dose; EPIT, epicutaneous immunotherapy; Ig, immunoglobulin; OIT, oral immunotherapy; SCD, successfully consumed dose; SLIT, sublingual immunotherapy; SU, sustained unresponsiveness.
[a] Reported as % of participants that experienced an adverse event during intervention (active treatment).
[b] Responder rate or the percentage of participants that were considered responders.

required treatment and severe reactions requiring epinephrine were rare to absent. As current studies have used a variety of doses and duration of therapy, future studies would benefit from clarifying the optimal dose and duration of SLIT.

EPIT has also demonstrated modest desensitization in children, but proves advantageous with regard to high therapeutic adherence rates and excellent safety profile. Compared with SLIT, EPIT studies involved seemingly higher rate of AEs, although most of those reported were mild local skin site reactions that responded to topical therapies; the rate of serious AEs were rare among EPIT studies, suggesting a robust safety profile. As many current EPIT studies have focused on short-term outcomes, future investigation would benefit from long-term therapeutic outcomes.

As food allergy affects a heterogeneous group of individuals, therapeutic utility of food allergen immunotherapy will vary and a common threshold for therapeutic risk or clinical protection cannot be assumed for individuals desiring treatment. Although each immunotherapy method remains at different investigational stages, each method seems to have established a unique risk and benefit profile that is complementary to alternative immunotherapy options. With a shared goal of empowering food-allergic patients to meet each individual's specific treatment goals, it is important that we continue to pursue alternative immunotherapies, such as SLIT and EPIT, as a single therapeutic option with OIT may not prove feasible for all.

DISCLOSURE

The authors declare that they have no conflicting interests to disclose.

REFERENCES

1. Kim E, Bird JA, Kulis M, et al. Sublingual immunotherapy for peanut allergy: clinical and immunologic evidence of desensitization. J Allergy Clin Immunol 2011; 127:640–6.
2. Kim E, Yang L, Ye P, et al. Long-term sublingual immunotherapy for peanut allergy in children: clinical and immunologic evidence of desensitization. J Allergy Clin Immunol 2019;1–7.
3. Gupta RS, Warren CM, Smith BM, et al. Prevalence and severity of food allergies among US adults. JAMA Netw Open 2019;2(1):1–14.
4. Gupta RS, Springston EE, Warrier MR, et al. The prevalence, severity, and distribution of childhood food allergy in the United States. Pediatrics 2011;128(1): e9–17.
5. Cook QS, Kim EH. Update on peanut allergy: prevention and immunotherapy. Allergy Asthma Proc 2019;40:1–7.
6. Fleischer D, Greenhawt M, Sussman G, et al. Effect of epicutaneous immunotherapy vs placebo on reaction to peanut protein ingestion among children with peanut allergy: the pepites randomized clinical trial. JAMA 2019;321:946–55.
7. Greenhawt M, Marsh R, Gilbert H, et al. Understanding caregiver goals, benefits, and acceptable risks of peanut allergy therapies. Ann Allergy Asthma Immunol 2018;121:575–9.
8. Jones S, Sicherer S, Burks AW, et al. Epicutaneous immunotherapy for the treatment of peanut allergy in children and young adults. J Allergy Clin Immunol 2016; 139:1242–52.
9. Burks AW, Jones SM, Wood RA, et al. Oral immunotherapy for treatment of egg allergy in children. N Engl J Med 2012;367:233–43.

10. Allam JP, Peng WM, Appel T, et al. Toll-like receptor 4 ligation enforces tolerogenic properties of oral mucosal Langerhans cells. J Allergy Clin Immunol 2008;121(2):368–74.e1.
11. Kulis M, Saba K, Kim EH, et al. Increased peanut-specific IgA levels in saliva correlate with food challenge outcomes after peanut sublingual immunotherapy. J Allergy Clin Immunol 2012;129:1159–61.
12. Keet C, Frischmeyer-Guerrerio P, Thyagarajan A, et al. The safety and efficacy of sublingual and oral immunotherapy for milk allergy. J Allergy Clin Immunol 2011; 129:448–55.
13. Fleischer DM, Burks AW, Vickery BP, et al. Sublingual immunotherapy for peanut allergy: a randomized, double-blind, placebo-controlled multicenter trial. J Allergy Clin Immunol 2013;131:119–27.
14. Burks AW, Wood RA, Jones SM, et al. Sublingual immunotherapy for peanut allergy: long-term follow-up of a randomized multicenter trial. J Allergy Clin Immunol 2015;135:1240–8.
15. Burk CM, Kulis M, Leung N, et al. Utility of component analyses in subjects undergoing sublingual immunotherapy for peanut allergy. Clin Exp Allergy 2016;46: 347–53.
16. Narisety SD, Frischmeyer-Guerrerio PA, Keet CA, et al. A randomized, double-blind, placebo-controlled pilot study of sublingual versus oral immunotherapy for the treatment of peanut allergy. J Allergy Clin Immunol 2015;135:1275–82.
17. Senti G, Graf N, Haug S, et al. Epicutaneous allergen administration as a novel method of allergen-specific immunotherapy. J Allergy Clin Immunol 2009;124: 997–1002.
18. Senti G, von Moos S, Tay F, et al. Epicutaneous allergen-specific immunotherapy ameliorates grass pollen-induced rhinoconjunctivitis: a double-blind, placebo-controlled dose escalation study. J Allergy Clin Immunol 2012;129:128–35.
19. Dioszeghy V, Mondoulet L, Dhelft V, et al. Epicutaneous immunotherapy results in rapid allergen uptake by dendritic cells through intact skin and downregulates the allergen-specific response in sensitized mice. J Immunol 2011;186:5629–37.
20. Dioszeghy V, Mondoulet L, Dhelft V, et al. The regulatory T cells induction by epicutaneous immunotherapy is sustained and mediates long-term protection from eosinophilic disorders in peanut-sensitized mice. Clin Exp Allergy 2014;44: 867–81.
21. Jones SM, Agbotounou WK, Fleischer DM, et al. Safety of epicutaneous immunotherapy for the treatment of peanut allergy: a phase 1 study using the Viaskin patch. J Allergy Clin Immunol 2016;137:1258–60.e10.
22. Sampson H, Shreffler W, Yang WH, et al. Effect of varying doses of epicutaneous immunotherapy vs placebo on reaction to peanut protein exposure among patients with peanut sensitivity: a randomized clinical trial. JAMA 2017;318: 1798–809.
23. Vickery BP, Vereda A, Casale TB, et al. AR101 oral immunotherapy for peanut allergy. N Engl J Med 2018;379:1991–2001.

Food Allergy Immunotherapy with Adjuvants

Rory E. Nicolaides, MD[a,b], Christopher P. Parrish, MD[a,b],
J. Andrew Bird, MD[a,b],*

KEYWORDS

• Food allergy • OIT • SLIT • EPIT • Adjuvant therapy • Modified allergens

KEY POINTS

- Emerging forms of immunotherapy for food allergy (OIT, SLIT, and EPIT) have shown significant promise, but remain limited by concerns about efficacy, durability of effect, and/or safety.
- The next generation of treatments for food allergy will aim to improve the efficacy and/or safety of existing immunotherapy through immunomodulation.
- Future therapies will also aim to benefit patients suffering from multiple food allergies through effects that are not allergen-specific.

BACKGROUND/INTRODUCTION

Symptoms of food allergy typically develop in early childhood with approximately 8% of children believed to have a food allergy in the United States,[1] and recent

Disclosure Statement: Dr J.A. Bird reports personal fees from Food Allergy Research and Education, personal fees and non-financial support from American College of Allergy, Asthma and Immunology, grants from Nestle Health Sciences, personal fees from Nutricia North America, personal fees from Pharm-Olam International LTD, personal fees and other from Pfizer Pharmaceuticals, grants, personal fees and non-financial support from Aimmune Therapeutics, personal fees from Prota Therapeutics, personal fees from Allergy Therapeutics, Ltd, grants from NIH-NIAID, grants from Novartis, personal fees from AllerGenis, personal fees from Abbott Nutrition International, grants and personal fees from DBV Technologies, outside the submitted work. Dr C.P. Parrish reports personal fees from Aimmune Therapeutics, grants and non-financial support from DBV Technologies, grants from NIH-NIAID, grants form Novartis, grants from Regeneron, outside the submitted work.
[a] Department of Pediatrics, Division of Allergy and Immunology, University of Texas Southwestern Medical Center, 5323 Harry Hines Boulevard, Dallas, TX 75390-9063, USA;
[b] Department of Internal Medicine, Division of Allergy and Immunology, University of Texas Southwestern Medical Center, 5323 Harry Hines Boulevard, Dallas, TX 75390-9063, USA
* Corresponding author. Department of Pediatrics, Division of Allergy and Immunology, University of Texas Southwestern Medical Center, 5323 Harry Hines Boulevard, Dallas, TX 75390-9063.
E-mail address: Drew.Bird@utsouthwestern.edu

Immunol Allergy Clin N Am 40 (2020) 149–173
https://doi.org/10.1016/j.iac.2019.09.004
0889-8561/20/© 2019 Elsevier Inc. All rights reserved.

research suggests as many as 10.8% of US adults may have a food allergy.[2] At the present time there is no Food and Drug Administration (FDA)-approved therapy for treatment of food allergies and affected individuals must strictly avoid allergens in their diet while carrying auto-injectable epinephrine at all times. The burden of disease of food allergy is impacted by the continuous vigilance required to avoid ubiquitous food allergens and the potentially life-threatening nature of an anaphylactic reaction. The most commonly studied interventional therapies (oral immunotherapy [OIT], sublingual immunotherapy [SLIT], and epicutaneous immunotherapy [EPIT]) fall short in providing a completely satisfactory treatment for all patients. These approaches require daily exposure to allergen, and the pros and cons of each therapy have prevented allergists and patients alike from universal enthusiastic acceptance of one modality as superior to avoidance for all food allergic patients. This review briefly reviews the aforementioned therapies and expands on investigative therapies with potential future benefit.

OVERVIEW OF ORAL, SUBCUTANEOUS, EPICUTANEOUS, SUBCUTANEOUS IMMUNOTHERAPY

OIT is performed by gradually increasing the amount of allergen ingested over a period of time until a "maintenance dose" of allergen is attained. The initial doses of allergen are less than the triggering threshold. After an initial escalation day, participants return biweekly for dose escalation until the therapeutic dose is achieved. Peanut OIT has been studied more rigorously than OIT with other foods, and a recent phase 3, international, placebo-controlled trial using a standardized, manufactured peanut OIT product (AR101, Aimmune Therapeutics) showed that 67.2% of participants by intention to treat (85% of completers) met the primary endpoint, the ability to ingest 600 mg of peanut protein or more, without dose-limiting symptoms, after approximately 6 months of daily ingestion of 300 mg of peanut protein, whereas only 4% of placebo participants achieved this endpoint.[3]

Other methods of desensitization under investigation have been less successful in ensuring a consistent level of protection. SLIT involves placing a small amount of solubilized allergen under the tongue. Top SLIT doses are typically at least 1/100th those of maintenance OIT doses. The largest peanut SLIT trial to date enrolled 40 peanut-allergic adolescents and adults, evenly assigning patients to treatment and placebo.[4] A 10-fold or more increase in the reaction-triggering threshold was achieved by 70% of subjects assigned to treatment compared with 15% of placebo subjects. The median reactive dose increased from 3.5 mg to 496 mg after 44 weeks of therapy.

EPIT delivers allergen via an adhesive patch. Natural water loss from the skin displaces allergen from the patch and resident Langerhans cells (LC) selectively deliver antigen to local lymph nodes, initiating an immunologic response. EPIT patches contain 250 μg of peanut allergen, at least 1/100th that of typical SLIT doses and at least 1/1000th that of OIT doses. A recent phase 3 trial enrolled 356 participants and demonstrated a responder rate of 35.3% in peanut-patch–treated subjects versus 13.5% of placebo-treated subjects.[5]

Subcutaneous immunotherapy (SCIT) has been used for more than 100 years for treatment of environmental allergen sensitivities. SCIT for peanut allergy using intact allergen without modification or adjuvant has been studied in few subjects and abandoned as a therapeutic option because of frequent anaphylaxis and a high dropout rate.[6,7]

The balance between efficacy and safety is not perfectly met with any of the preceding therapeutic options. Although adverse effects (AEs) from peanut OIT are generally mild, they certainly exceed those of standard allergen avoidance or of patients receiving placebo, and use of auto-injectable epinephrine in treatment subjects significantly exceeds that of placebo-treated subjects.[8] Patients receiving SLIT and EPIT do not typically experience AEs on the same scale as patients receiving OIT; however, the safety benefit is met with a sacrifice in margin of efficacy for some patients, and at the present time serum biomarkers are not available to predict which patients will benefit most from which therapy. Each of the therapies, when effective, is believed to most often induce a transient state of benefit that diminishes with removal of the therapy or abstinence from the allergen for most allergic individuals. With these facts in mind, it is important to consider alternative approaches with adjuvants that would both augment the allergic response and protect the allergic individual from potential AEs.

IMMUNE MECHANISMS OF FOOD IMMUNOTHERAPY

Regardless of approach, the end-effect of immunotherapy is to increase the regulatory T-cell response and downregulate the manifestation of allergic symptoms associated with IgE cross-linking on mast cells and basophils. Allergen is initially taken up by dendritic cells and antigen-presenting cells (APCs). Dendritic cells migrate to local lymph nodes and induce production of allergen-specific regulatory T cells characterized by increased production of interleukin (IL)-10 and transforming growth factor (TGF)-beta.[9] TGF-beta suppresses mast cell reactivity, primarily through downregulation of FCεR1 on the cell surface of tissue mast cells and blood basophils. Concomitantly, Th1 production of interferon (IFN)-γ induces class-switch to immunoglobulin (Ig)E and increases specific IgG and IgA production. Allergen-specific IgG plays a crucial role by both binding and neutralizing allergen and through the induction of inhibitory signaling via FCγRIIB on mast cells and basophils. Prolonged exposure to allergen may lead to additional changes, including anergy and deletion of allergen-specific Th2 cells through repeated and frequent exposure to high doses of allergen, as has been demonstrated in patients receiving timothy grass pollen SCIT.[9] Additional changes specific to the type of therapy being used are outlined as follows.

OIT takes advantage of T regulatory cell (Treg) induction within gut-associated lymphoid tissue. In the initial stages of OIT, an increase in allergen-specific IgE is noted along with stimulation of resident Th2A cells and initial differentiation of naïve T cells into allergen-specific Th2 cells, increasing the proinflammatory response.[10] Repeated exposure to allergen leads to IgE endocytosis and actin rearrangement on mast cells and basophils, making these cells hyporesponsive. Over time, the Th2 cellular response decreases and allergen-specific IgG4 increases with a concomitant decrease in allergen-specific IgE. The Treg response strengthens with enhanced epigenetic modifications at the Foxp3 locus.

SLIT allows for allergen uptake through LCs in the sublingual ductal epithelial cells.[9] The safety of SLIT is associated with the relative paucity of mast cells and eosinophils in oral tissues.[11] Oral APCs exhibit a tolerogenic phenotype with LCs producing IL-10 and TGF-beta and expressing indoleamine 2,3-dioxygenase and macrophages producing IL-10, IL-12 and expressing retinaldehyde dehydrogenase 2 (RALDH-2). The default response of oral LCs, in the absence of allergen stimulation, is tolerance rather than inflammation. SLIT adjuvants take advantage of the default response and are primarily aimed at enhancing the induction of allergen-specific Th1 and/or Treg-cell responses via directed signaling to oral LCs and macrophages.

EPIT presents antigen to local LCs found in intact, noninflamed skin and allergen is undetectable in the peripheral circulation.[12] It has been theorized that EPIT may induce longer lasting protection than OIT or SLIT through the generation of gut-homing LAP + Foxp3- Tregs, which suppress mast cell activation via TGF-β–dependent mechanisms.[13] OIT also induces gut-homing Tregs; however, EPIT-induced Tregs have been shown to retain suppressive activities longer than those induced by OIT.[14]

LIMITATIONS OF FOOD IMMUNOTHERAPY

Immunotherapy for foods has shown promise but significant limitations in both efficacy and safety have prevented widespread clinical implementation. EPIT is limited mainly by its lower rate of efficacy.[5] Although rates of successful desensitization are generally much higher for SLIT and especially OIT, the effects are commonly lost after treatment cessation, as illustrated by low rates of sustained unresponsiveness.[15] In practical terms, this means that patients need to continue immunotherapy indefinitely to ensure ongoing protection. Significant modifications to lifestyle may be needed to accommodate dosing (eg, avoiding exercise for 2 hours after dosing, not dosing on an empty stomach) and this may create a substantial treatment burden over time. Furthermore, immunotherapy for foods is allergen-specific. Although studies of OIT with multiple foods have shown promise, the need to treat each individual food further increases the burden of treatment for the individual.

Safety concerns for food immunotherapy are related to allergic AEs. For EPIT and SLIT, AEs are generally limited and typically involve symptoms at the treatment site (skin and oral mucosa, respectively), whereas OIT presents more significant safety concerns. Systemic reactions, including anaphylaxis requiring epinephrine use, occur with OIT. A recent analysis estimated that peanut OIT implemented broadly would likely cause more anaphylaxis than it would prevent.[16] A systematic review and meta-analysis of peanut OIT safety and efficacy concluded with high certainty that current regimens increase allergic reactions and anaphylaxis when compared with placebo or avoidance.[8] Although no deaths have been attributed to OIT, a child in Japan was left ventilator dependent after a severe reaction during milk OIT (Motohiro Ebisawa, MD, PhD, personal correspondence, April 2018).

However, most reactions during OIT occur after intentional ingestion of an OIT dose, not on accidental ingestion. This arguably may lead to better preparedness and treatment of reactions when they do occur. Although exact rates of reactions due to accidental ingestion are not clear, they do commonly occur despite parental vigilance and label-reading.[17] Baumert and colleagues[18] estimated that an increase in peanut threshold of reactivity from ≤100 mg to 300 mg would reduce the risk of reaction due to peanut contamination of cookies, ice cream, doughnuts/snack cakes, and snack cake mixes by more than 95%. Although the phase 3 AR101 results did not report on rates of reactions due to accidental ingestion, at exit double-blind placebo-controlled food challenge (DBPCFC), 76.6% of subjects were able to tolerate a single dose of 300 mg,[3] indicating their threshold was higher than that identified by Baumert and colleagues[18] as clinically relevant for reduction of accidental reactions. This suggests that immunotherapy should drastically reduce rates of accidental reactions.

Gastrointestinal AEs from OIT are also frequent and are the most common cause of treatment discontinuation. Biopsy-proven eosinophilic esophagitis (EoE) has been documented in OIT subjects as well. A meta-analysis estimated the rate of EoE in those undergoing OIT at 2.7%.[19] A more recent analysis estimated the rate of EoE in subjects undergoing OIT at 5.1% based on confirmed cases, with up to 34.1% having symptoms possibly related to EoE.[20] However, asymptomatic mild gastrointestinal eosinophilia (involving the esophagus, gastric antrum, and/or duodenum) may be common at baseline in peanut-allergic adults before undergoing OIT.[21] Certain comorbidities (severe or uncontrolled asthma, severe atopic dermatitis, EoE) are generally considered contraindications to OIT, preventing treatment of many patients who potentially could benefit the most from therapy. Together these limitations in efficacy and safety illustrate an unmet need for alternative or adjunctive therapies to improve efficacy, safety, or both.

ORAL IMMUNOTHERAPY ADJUVANTS
Omalizumab

Omalizumab, a monoclonal antibody targeting the Fc portion of IgE antibodies, has been FDA-approved for allergic asthma and has shown promise in the treatment of food allergy as well, both as monotherapy and as an adjunct to OIT. Anti-IgE monotherapy with TNX-901 raised the threshold of reactivity for peanut,[22] whereas a phase II study with omalizumab was halted prematurely due to severe reactions during the entry oral food challenges (OFCs) (before drug administration) but the limited data before cessation suggested a similar effect.[23] Two studies showed an increase in threshold dose for various food allergens after omalizumab treatment.[24,25] Logically, these effects of omalizumab on food allergen thresholds should allow for more rapid escalation of OIT dosing and limit AEs such as urticaria and anaphylaxis. Thus, studies of omalizumab-facilitated OIT to date (**Table 1**) seem to confirm that omalizumab allows safer, more rapid desensitization but does not affect sustained unresponsiveness (SU) and additionally does not protect against EoE.

Milk
The first study of omalizumab as an adjunct to OIT was an open-label pilot study of 11 children with severe milk allergy.[26] After 9 weeks of pretreatment with omalizumab followed by 7 to 11 weeks of omalizumab-facilitated milk OIT, 9 of 10 passed a DBPCFC 8 weeks after omalizumab discontinuation and were able to incorporate >8 g/d (>240 mL milk) in their diet thereafter. Adverse reactions were mostly mild (1.8%), and epinephrine was used at a rate similar to previous OIT studies. In an open-label case series of 14 subjects with milk or egg allergy, all 5 milk-allergic subjects reached a maintenance dose of 6.6 g after 9 weeks of pretreatment with omalizumab[27]; however, 3 (60%) of 5 of the milk-allergic subjects relapsed with grade 3 or 4 anaphylaxis (Clark and Ewan grading[28])within 4 months of omalizumab cessation. The only randomized, placebo-controlled trial to date demonstrated marked improvements in safety outcomes (fewer adverse reactions, fewer reactions requiring treatment). There was no statistically significant benefit on rates of passing a 10-g desensitization OFC and SU rates were low for both groups.[29]

Peanut
In 2013, Schneider and colleagues[30] published the first open-label pilot study of omalizumab-facilitated peanut OIT in 13 highly allergic children. After 12 weeks of omalizumab pretreatment, 12 (92%) of 13 reached a maintenance dose of 2 g peanut protein after 8 weeks of OIT. Twelve weeks after omalizumab was discontinued, 85% passed a 4 g peanut protein DBPCFC and 92% tolerated an open 4-g challenge. Reactions were minimal (2% of doses) and mostly mild. MacGinnitie and colleagues[31] then demonstrated that omalizumab was superior to placebo in facilitating rapid peanut desensitization and 79% tolerating 2 g peanut protein 6 weeks after drug discontinuation. This number increased to a total of 31 (94%) of 33 subjects after treatment failures were offered open-label omalizumab. Despite the omalizumab arm receiving much higher doses of peanut protein, the overall rate of adverse reactions did not significantly differ. Yee and colleagues[32] subsequently reported on long-term

Table 1
Summary of food immunotherapy with adjuvants

Method of AIT + Adjuvants	Specific Adjuvants	Murine or Human	Reference	Condition or Disease	Study Design, Number of Participants, Age Range	Protocol; Duration and Dosing	Outcome and Other Significant Findings	Adverse Events
OIT	Omalizumab	Human	Nadeau et al,[26] 2011	Milk allergy	Phase I open label, 11 subjects, age 7–17 y (median 8 y)	Omalizumab monotherapy pretreatment × 9 wk → Omalizumab-facilitated OIT (rush to 1 g on day 1, weekly increase to 2 g) through wk 16 → OIT monotherapy through wk 24	Primary objective: 9 of 11 (82%) achieved 2000 mg/d dose within 7–11 wk of initial desensitization 9 passed DBPCFC (7250 mg) plus open challenge (4000 mg or 8000 mg), all 9 then tolerated >8000 mg/d (>240 mL)	1 dropout (abdominal pain, EoE ruled out) Reactions with 1.8% of doses (0.3% moderate, 0.1% severe)
		Human	Wood et al,[29] 2016	Milk allergy	DBPCRT, 57 subjects, age 7–32 y	Omalizumab (n = 28) or placebo (n = 29) → at mo 4 open-label milk OIT- 22–40 wk to reach maintenance (min 520 mg goal 3.8 g/d)→ Unblinded at mo 16 → Desensitization OFC and omalizumab discontinuation at mo 28 → Milk OIT discontinued at mo 30 (strict avoidance) → SU OFC at mo 32	SU: not assessed No benefit in efficacy (desensitization or SU) • Desensitization OFC (10 g) at wk 28 passed: 24/27 (88.9%) Omalizumab vs 20/28 (71.4%) placebo (P = .18) • SU OFC (10 g) at wk 32 passed: 13/27 (48.1%) Omalizumab vs 10/28 (35.7%) placebo (P = .42)	Significant improvement in safety in omalizumab group: • Doses per subject provoking symptoms (2.1% vs 16.1% P = .0005) • Dose-related reactions requiring treatment (0.0% vs 3.8%, P = .0008)
		Human	Martorell-Calatayud et al,[27] 2016	Milk or egg allergy	Open-label case series, 14 subjects (5 milk-allergic, 9 egg-allergic), age 3–13 y with prior failure of OIT	9 wk pretreatment with omalizumab → OIT to maintenance dose (6.6 g CM or 1.8 g EW) → omalizumab discontinued 2 mo after maintenance dose achieved	All patients (100%) achieved desensitization 8 of 14 (57.1%) continued maintenance OIT 6 of 14 (42.9%) patients relapsed with grade 3–4 anaphylaxis upon ingestion 2.5–4 mo after omalizumab discontinued (3 of 5 (60%) for CM; 3 of 9 (33%) for EW)	Only 4 (28%) developed mild reactions during induction phase of OIT

| Human | Schneider et al,[30] 2013 | Peanut allergy | Open-label, 13 subjects, median age 10 y, failed entry DBPCFC at 100 mg dose or lower, and median peanut-specific IgE level of 229 kUA/L | 12-wk omalizumab pretreatment → Day 1 OIT to max 250 mg peanut protein (cumulative dose 490 mg) → ~8 wk peanut OIT up-dosing to maintenance (2 g peanut protein) → Omalizumab discontinued, maintenance OIT continued for 12 wk → 4 g peanut protein DBPCFC | OIT day 1:
• 13 of 13 (100%) ingested max cumulative 490 mg peanut protein (7 without symptoms, 6 with minimal symptoms)
After 8 wk OIT (20 wk omalizumab):
• 12 of 13 (92%) reached 2 g peanut protein maintenance dose 12 wk after omalizumab discontinued (with OIT continued): 11 of 13 (85%) tolerated 4 g peanut protein DBPCFC | 2.0% of doses associated with reactions (1.8% of doses with mild symptoms, 0.2% of doses with moderate symptoms, 0.06% with severe symptoms)
1 subject withdrew due to persistent nausea/vomiting after reaching 1250 mg dose No reactions to omalizumab |

(continued on next page)

Table 1
(continued)

Method of AIT + Adjuvants	Specific Adjuvants	Murine or Human	Reference	Condition or Disease	Study Design, Number of Participants, Age Range	Protocol; Duration and Dosing	Outcome and Other Significant Findings	Adverse Events
		Human	MacGinnitie et al,[31] 2017	Peanut allergy	DBPCRCT, 37 subjects, median age 10 y	Omalizumab (n = 29) vs placebo (n = 8) 12 wk pretreatment → Day 1 OIT to 250 mg peanut protein (CTD 490 mg) → Peanut OIT weekly up-dosing to 2 g → After week 19 study drug discontinued → 4 g OFC 12 wk later → 4 g or 2 g daily maintenance Treatment failures (unable to tolerate 250 mg peanut protein after 8 wk desensitization) → open-label omalizumab and peanut OIT	12 of 13 (92%) tolerated open 4 g peanut protein challenge SU: not assessed OIT day 1: • Omalizumab: 23 of 29 (79%) tolerated max 250 mg dose (490 mg CTD) • Placebo: 1 of 8 (13%) tolerated max 250 mg dose (490 mg CTD) Tolerance of 2 g peanut dose 6 wk after study drug withdrawal (primary endpoint): • Omalizumab: 23 of 29 (79%) • Placebo: 1 of 8 (13%) Treatment failures: • Omalizumab 2 of 27 (7.4%) • Placebo 6 of 8 (75%) • All tolerated 2 g while on open-label omalizumab In total 31 of 33 (94%) of subjects who received omalizumab and peanut OIT tolerated 2 g peanut	2 of 33 (6%) who received both omalizumab (blinded or open-label) and peanut OIT had symptoms suggestive of EoE (1 [3%] biopsy-proven) 1 of 8 (13%) of placebo patients had biopsy-proven EoE while on OIT 6 of 22 (27%) who passed 4 g open challenge had allergic reactions to 4 g maintenance dose (4 [18%] required epinephrine) but tolerated decreased dose of 2 g thereafter No statistically significant difference in rate of reactions in omalizumab (7.8% of doses) vs placebo (16.8% of doses) arms (P = .15) despite omalizumab group

Model	Reference	Allergy	Study design/subjects	Protocol/dosing	Efficacy results	Adverse effects/safety
					6 wk after omalizumab stopped 4 g open challenge 12 wk after omalizumab stopped: • Omalizumab: 22 of 27 (81%) passed • Placebo: 1 of 8 (13%) passed SU: not assessed	receiving much higher doses
Human	Yee et al,[32] 2019	Peanut allergy	LTFU of the 13 subjects from Scheider et al 2013 study	LTFU visits every ~6 mo up to 72 mo Allowed to change peanut dose formulations; optional spacing of dosing from daily to every-other-day to twice weekly to weekly Dose adjusted if symptoms occurred (ranged from 500 mg to 3500 mg)	7 of 13 (54%) continued peanut OIT through mo 72 QoL improved from baseline in all subjects SU: not assessed	6 of 13 (46%) discontinued due to adverse reactions Higher peanut IgE and Ara h2 IgE associated with discontinuation 1 of 13 (7.7%) developed EoE
Human	Bégin et al,[34] 2014	Multiple food allergy	Open label, 25 subjects, median age 7 y Up to 5 foods (mean 3.6 foods): peanut (all), milk, egg, tree nuts, wheat, sesame.	8-wk omalizumab pretreatment → rapid desensitization Omalizumab discontinued at week 16 Maintenance OIT dose 4 g/food daily	OIT day 1: • 19 of 25 (76%) reached max first day dose (250 mg protein per food) with minimal or no symptoms All patents reached dose of 1 g/food by 3 mo of OIT 88% reached max dose 4 g/food by 9 mo of OIT SU: not assessed	5.3% of home doses triggered reactions 94% of reactions were mild Reaction rates dropped by 70% after 6 mo of therapy 1 severe reaction after reaching 4 g/food maintenance, treated with epinephrine
Human	Andorf et al,[35] 2017	Multiple food allergy	Observational LTFU of Bégin 2014 with additional subjects without peanut allergy (total 34)	Same as Bégin 2014 except maintenance dose of 2 g to 4 g (high dose) vs 300 mg (low dose) LTFU visits every 6–12 mo	All passed 2 g OFC to each of their food allergens at the end of LTFU Choice of low vs high maintenance dose: • All 6 almond subject and all 8 pecan chose low dose	No change in maintenance dose due to safety concerns Reactions occurred with 3.5% of maintenance doses (95.6% mild)

(continued on next page)

Table 1
(continued)

Method of AIT + Adjuvants	Specific Adjuvants	Murine or Human	Reference	Condition or Disease	Study Design, Number of Participants, Age Range	Protocol; Duration and Dosing	Outcome and Other Significant Findings	Adverse Events
		Human	Andorf et al,[78] 2018	Multiple food allergy	DBPCRCT, 48 subjects, median age 8 y (2–5 foods, mean 3.3 foods)	Followed median 53 mo (32–62 mo) 8-wk pretreatment omalizumab (n = 36) vs placebo (n = 12) → rapid desensitization Study drug discontinued at week 16 Exit DBPCFC at week 36	• 73% of egg and 80% of milk chose high dose Week 30 2 g protein/food DBPCFC: 30 of 36 (83%) omalizumab passed 4 of 12 (33%) placebo	No severe adverse events Lower rates of AEs in omalizumab group
		Human	Andorf et al,[36] 2019	Multiple food allergy	RCT, 70 subjects (age 5–22 y), multiple food allergies (confirmed by DBPCFC)	16 wk of open-label omalizumab (weeks 0–16) 22 wk of multifood OIT (weeks 8–30) If 1 g/food maintenance dose reached by week 28–29, then randomized 1:1:1 to 1 g, 300 mg, or 0 mg for 6 wk (weeks 30–36) DBPCFC at wk 36	10 dropouts (5 failed desensitization) 34 of 40 (85%) on active treatment (1 g or 300 mg) vs 11 of 20 (55%) on 0 g tolerated 2 g of each food allergen Highest failure rates with cashew and peanut Threshold of reactivity increased even for 9 failures (CTD increased from 15 mg to 750 mg) 6-wk SU (0 g arm): 55% passed 2 g DBPCFC	No clinically significant difference in rates of AEs among groups BUT higher 4 doses of epinephrine given in 1 g arm vs 1 in 0 g arm and 0 in 300 mg arm
	Probiotics	Human	Tang et al,[43] 2015	Peanut allergy	DBPCRT, 62 subjects, 1–10 y	Peanut OIT (peanut flour, 50% peanut protein) combined with probiotic *Lactobacillus rhamnosus* CGMCC (1.3724 at a fixed dose of 2×10^{10} CFU) (PPOIT), or placebo OIT without	Possible SU achieved in 82.1% with PPOIT & 3.6% with placebo (P<.001) Desensitization with DBPCFC (cumulative dose 4 g peanut protein) achieved in 89.7% receiving PPOIT and 7.1% receiving placebo ($P \leq 001$)	PPOIT was well tolerated with no participants withdrawing because of AE. Number needed to treat of 9 to produce clinical benefit in 7 children

	Type	Reference	Allergy	Study design	Intervention/dosing	Outcome	Adverse events
	Human	Hsiao et al,[79] 2017	Peanut allergy	4-y follow-up on previously reported cohort	probiotic, once daily for 18 mo	58% of PPOIT vs 7% of placebo subjects demonstrated 8-wk SU ($P<.012$)	
Dupilumab	Human	NCT03682770; recruiting	Peanut allergy	Phase 2, Multicenter, DBPCRT; 156 subjects; 6–17 y	dupilumab + AR101 (peanut OIT) or placebo; every 2 wk	Desensitization with DBPCFC at wk 28	
FAHF	Murine	Srivastava et al,[48] 2017	Peanut and tree nut allergy	Placebo-controlled RCT, 3 groups: sham treatment (water), OIT alone, OIT + 3-wk prior and 3-wk BF2 cotreatment (dose 12 mg/d)	Mice were sensitized with, then underwent, 1 d peanut (PN), walnut (WN), and cashew (CSH) rush OIT plus 3 wk of maintenance dosing of 6.25 mg PN/WN/CSH cocktail; OFC at 1, 2, 5, 6 wk after therapy	1-wk after OFC: BF2 treatment significantly enhanced OIT desensitization (37.5% OIT mice reacted vs 18% BF2+OIT mice, $P<.01$). BF2+OIT produced more sustained protection than OIT alone at 5–6 wk after OFC with all 3 foods (100% sham, 91% OIT only, 23% BF2+OIT mice reacted with median score lower vs sham $P<.05$). BF2+OIT prevented OIT increase of antigen specific IgE, and pro-tolerogenic IFN-γ/IL4 and IL10/IL4 ratios ($P<.05$–.01 vs OIT alone), associated with more persistent protection	BF2 reduced rush OIT build-up dose phase AE: 43% of OIT- only mice had moderate to severe reactions vs 12% of BF2+OIT with mild reactions and lower median symptom scores ($P<.001$)
	Human	Wang et al,[49] 2015	Peanut, tree nut, sesame, fish, and/or shellfish allergy	DBPCRT; 68 subjects; 12–45 y	FAHF-2 tablets 15 g/d or placebo, with DBPCFC to a max 5 g protein after 6 mo	By ITT, placebo group had higher eliciting and cumulative dose ($P = .05$) at final DBPCFC; no difference in requiring epinephrine to treat reactions ($P = .55$); no significant difference in immunologic parameters (allergen-specific IgE, IgG4, cytokine production, or BAT)	Total 387 AE, none severe, no difference in the number reported per subject between groups. GI complaints most common. Notably, 44% subject has poor drug adherence for at least 1/3 of study period

(continued on next page)

Table 1
(continued)

Method of AIT + Specific Adjuvants	Murine or Human	Reference	Condition or Disease	Study Design, Number of Participants, Age Range	Protocol; Duration and Dosing	Outcome and Other Significant Findings	Adverse Events
E-B-FAHF-2 + Omalizumab	Human	NCT02879006; recruiting	Milk, egg, peanut, almond, cashew, hazelnut, walnut, sesame, and/or wheat allergy	DBPCRT, phase 2; 34 subjects, 6–40 y	All subjects = multiallergen OIT + omalizumab × 4 mo (2 mo pre-OIT + 2 mo build-up phase). Then randomized to E-B-FAHF-2 or placebo, OIT therapy (1 gm each food allergen) × 2 years, with post OFC	Primary outcome: SUs evaluated by the absence of dose-limiting symptoms to a cumulative dose of 4444 protein; secondary outcome of desensitizing to 4444 mg and/or 7444 mg or higher	
Interferon-gamma	Human	Noh & Lee,[54] 2009	Egg, milk, or wheat allergy	Case control; 25 subjects (IFN-γ + OIT n = 10, OIT alone n = 5, IFN-γ alone n = 5, no treatment n = 5), children	SC IFN-γ given 10–20 min before each dose of OIT, then OFC done at therapy completion and 3 mo post; duration was dependent on food	10 subjects who received IFN-γ + OIT achieved SU. No subjects achieved SU or desensitization with OIT alone, IFN-γ alone, or no treatment. IFN-γ + OIT associated with increased food-specific IgE, but reduced SPT wheal	All OIT participants failed to complete OIT protocol and withdrew because of frequent and severe reactions
	Human	Noh & Jang,[55] 2014	Milk, egg, wheat, soy	Case control; 25 subjects (IFN-γ + dual OIT[a] n = 10, IFN-γ + classic OIT[b] n = 5, OIT alone n = 5, no treatment n = 5), children	SC IFN-γ (3×10^6 IU/m^2) given 10–20 min before doses of OIT per protocol; duration was dependent on food. No assessment of SU	Desensitization achieved in 10/10 and 5/5 subjects who received dual OIT and classic OIT, respectively. No subjects desensitized who received OIT alone or no treatment	

(continued on next page)

SLIT CpG-nanoparticles	Murine	Srivastava et al,[60] 2016	Peanut allergy	Total 90 mice in 7 groups (n = 10–22/group) 4 weekly gavages with either CpG/PN-NPs, individual vehicle components (5 groups), or no treatment; then 5 monthly peanut OFCs	Mice treated with CpG/PN-NPs, compared with none of the vehicle components or control mice, were significantly protected from anaphylaxis in all OFCs (lower median symptom scores $P<.01$ vs .001 vs sham, higher post-challenge body temperatures $P<.05–.001$ for CpG/PN-NPs vs sham treatment, lower 30 min post-OCF blood histamine levels $P<.05–.001$ between the treatment and vehicle control groups), and had decreased spIgE/IgG1 (observed at all challenges except the first challenge at week 14, $P<.05–.001$), and increase in peanut-specific IgG2a (TH1-associated immunoglobulin) levels ($P<.05–.01$) at all 5 OFCs
	Murine	Kulis et al,[59] 2013	Peanut allergy	Prophylactic model (a) and therapeutic model (b) a. 0.5 mg peanut protein ± 30 ug of 3 types of CpG molecules (ODNs) on days 1, 8, and 22 via intraperitoneal (i.p.) injection; day 36, 1 mg protein i.p. injection challenge. b. 3 groups, placebo, peanut alone, or peanut plus type A, B, or C CpG. IT on days 36, 39, 43, 46, 50, and 53; i.p. challenge on day 63	a. Type B ODNs inhibited anaphylaxis in the sensitization protocol (lower symptom scores $P<.01$, body temperature $P<.001$, and mouse mast cell protease 1 release $P<.05$ vs sham) compared with sham treatment. b. Co-administration of type B ODN + peanut protein reduced anaphylactic reactions $P<.01$, increased IFN-γ $P<.001$ and peanut-IgG2a $P<.01–.001$, without a significant decrease in peanut IgE or IL-4 responses

Table 1
(continued)

Method of AIT + Adjuvants / Specific Adjuvants	Murine or Human	Reference	Condition or Disease	Study Design, Number of Participants, Age Range	Protocol; Duration and Dosing	Outcome and Other Significant Findings	Adverse Events
	Murine	Zhu et al,[58] 2007	Peanut allergy	Prevention model (a) and therapeutic model (b); 5 mice per group	a. Sensitization 3 times with oral peanut ± IMO; 1 mg peanut challenge day 28 b. Sensitization and days 0 & 14, starting on day 21 treated 4 times every 4 d with oral IMO; challenge day 34	a. Combination of IMO/peanut vs peanut only decreased IgE, IL-5, IL-13, and increased IgG2a and IFN-γ levels (all $P<.05$) b. IM vs PBS-treated treated mice showed decreased IgE, IL-5, and IL-13 levels, and increased IgG2a and IFN-γ levels in the serum, intestines, and spleen cells (all $P<.05$)	
SCIT / LAMP-vax DNA	Human	NCT03755713, recruiting	Peanut allergy	Phase 1, Randomized, Placebo-Controlled, 3 cohorts with 10 subjects each, ages 12–17 y	ID administration of ASP0892 (ARA-LAMP-vax) in 3 cohorts: ASP8062 low-dose, high-dose, placebo	Evaluate safety, tolerability and immune responses	
	Human	NCT02851277, recruitment completed	Peanut allergy	Phase 1, randomized, placebo-controlled, 30 subjects, 18–55 y	ID administration: ASP8062 low dose, high dose, placebo. IM administration: high dose and placebo; once every 2 wk for 4 doses	Evaluate safety, tolerability and immune responses	
HAL-MPE1	Human	Bindslev-Jensen et al,[67] 2017	Peanut allergy	DBPCRT, treatment group with HAL-MPE1 (11 subjects) or placebo (6 subjects)	Randomized to receive 15–20 weekly incremental doses of subcutaneous HAL-MPE1or placebo	After HAL-MPE1, there were more frequent but generally mild (redness and no wheal sizes exceeding 5 cm) local reactions, and no late systemic reactions	

Human	NCT02991885	Peanut allergy	DBPCRT, 42 participants, 5–50 y	Weekly subcutaneous HAL-MPE1or placebo Day 42– SC treatment with 200 µL of the different test preparations (PE or MPE ± Al(OH)3) or PBS ± Al(OH)3, 2 ×/wk for 6 wk. Challenges: 12 mg PE IG day 91, IP 0.1 mg PE days 98 and 112	Assessing safety, tolerability and immunologic effects	
Murine	Van der Kleij et al,[66] 2019	Peanut allergy	n = 6 sensitized mice per group		HAL-MPE1 reduces allergenicity while still retaining immunogenicity of peanut extract (did not affect peanut-specific human T-cell proliferation in vitro ($P = .23$), induced IgG responses cross-reactive with native PE, reduced IgE binding to Ara h 2 and Ara h 6, and reduced basophil activation ($P<.01$) and mediator release)	
Human	NCT02382718	Fish allergy	DBPCRT, 45 participants, 18–65 y	SC injections of mCyp c 1 (or placebo) in an up-dosing phase (build up from 6ng– 60 µg over 10 injections in an 8 week period), followed by maintenance phase (60 µg once at 2 wk, then 4 monthly injections ×4 mo)	Assessing efficacy and safety	
PVX-108	Prickett et al,[72] 2019 AAAAI abstract, ACTRN1 261700069233 6	Peanut allergy	DBPCRT, 66 subjects (Stage 1: 48 subjects, stage 2: 18 subjects), 18–65 y	8 cohorts received either ID PVX108 or placebo in increasing doses; final cohort–6 IDs of 150 nmol × 16 wk	Serum from peanut-allergic demonstrated a lack of basophil reactivity to PVX108 vs peanut extract	No participants experienced any serious AE, only mild to moderate and mostly related to injection site reactions
CpG-nano-particles	Pali-Scholl et al,[73] 2013 Murine	Peanut allergy	Murine model	SC injection of protamine nanoparticles complexed with Ara h 2	Favorable increase in Ara h 2-specific IgG2a without detectable Ara h 2-specific IgE	

(continued on next page)

Table 1
(continued)

Method of AIT + Adjuvants	Specific Adjuvants	Murine or Human	Reference	Condition or Disease	Study Design, Number of Participants, Age Range	Protocol; Duration and Dosing	Outcome and Other Significant Findings	Adverse Events
Mucosal		Human	Wood et al,[75] 2013	Peanut allergy	Controls: 5 healthy adults, Subjects: 10 peanut-allergic adults, ages 18–50 y	Rectal administration of EMPT-123. Controls: 4 weekly escalating doses to max study dose 3063 µg. Subjects: 10 weekly escalating doses from 10 µg to 3063 µg, then 3 biweekly doses of 3063 µg	Significant reduction in SPT titration (10.0 within-subject change; $P = .02$) and basophil activation; no significant changes for total IgE, peanut IgE, or peanut IgG4	50% of participants unable to complete the dosing regimen (2 mild & 1 moderate reaction) and 20% experiencing severe allergic reactions (anaphylaxis)

Abbreviations: AE, adverse event; AIT, allergen-specific immunotherapy; ARA-LAMP-vax, a multivalent peanut (Ara h1, h2, h3) LAMP-DNA plasmid vaccine; BAT, basophil activation test; DBPCFC, double-blind placebo-controlled food challenge; DBPCRT, double-blind placebo-controlled randomized trial; EoE, eosinophilic esophagitis; HAL-MPE1, aluminum hydroxide adsorbed modified peanut extract; ID, intradermal; Ig, immunoglobulin; IM, intramuscular; IMO, immune modulatory oligonucleotide; ITT, intention to treat; LAMP-vax, lysosomal associated membrane protein vaccine; LTFU, long-term follow-up; ODNs, oligodeoxynucleotide molecules; OFC, oral food challenge; OIT, oral immunotherapy; PPOIT, peanut OIT combined with probiotic; RCT, randomized control trial; SC, subcutaneous; SCIT, subcutaneous immunotherapy; SLIT, sublingual immunotherapy; SPT, skin prick test; SU, sustained unresponsiveness.
[a] Dual OIT: a dose of interferon-gamma with OIT in the morning and a dose of OIT alone in the evening.
[b] Classic OIT: single daily dose of interferon-gamma with OIT.

follow-up from the pilot study by Schneider and colleagues[30] that 6 (46%) of 13 subjects discontinued OIT due to adverse reactions, indicating that omalizumab did not alter the need for nor increase the tolerability of long-term ongoing therapy.

Multifood oral immunotherapy

Thirty percent of children with food allergy react to multiple foods.[33] As such, the ability to simultaneously treat all of an individual's food allergies is highly desirable. Although the benefits of immunotherapy are allergen-specific, omalizumab's effects are not. Thus, omalizumab has potential to be used to treat children with multiple food allergies. Bégin and colleagues[34] treated 25 subjects with omalizumab (8 weeks pretreatment and 8 additional weeks during OIT) and multifood OIT for up to 5 allergens. Nineteen (76%) of 25 tolerated the maximum day 1 initial dose escalation, all patients reached a maintenance dose of 1 g/food by 3 months of OIT, and reactions occurred with 5.3% of doses and were mostly mild. Long-term follow-up of these subjects plus 9 additional (34 total) revealed that all subjects passed 2 g OFC to each food after a median of 53 months.[35]

Another study by Andorf and colleagues[36] examined the durability of 30 weeks of omalizumab-facilitated multifood desensitization by comparing various maintenance doses of each food beginning 14 weeks after omalizumab discontinuation. Thirty-four (85%) of 40 randomized to continued active OIT (1 g or 300 mg) passed a DBPCFC after 6 weeks on the assigned dose, versus 20 (55%) among those who discontinued OIT. Durability of effect varied by food. Threshold of reactivity was increased even among those who failed the challenge. SU was not examined. A large upcoming multicenter phase 3 trial aims to provide deeper insight into omalizumab as monotherapy and as an adjunct to multifood OIT and whether subjects can maintain dietary consumption of the foods after omalizumab cessation over longer follow-up (NCT03881696).

Probiotics and Oral Immunotherapy

The increase in both prevalence and severity of food allergy has occurred simultaneously with global changes in environment and lifestyle. Some of these factors have been associated with gut microbiome dysbiosis and proposed to correlate with the development of food allergy, leading to recent investigations into the role of probiotics on immune tolerance mechanisms in food allergy.[37–40] Early studies demonstrated that cow's milk formula containing the probiotic *Lactobacillus rhamnosus* GG accelerated immune tolerance acquisition in cow's milk–allergic children, confirmed on 3-year follow-up.[41,42] The efficacy of probiotics as an adjuvant for OIT has been recently studied in an Australian cohort of peanut-allergic children. Subjects were randomized to receive 18 months of either peanut OIT combined with probiotic (PPOIT) or placebo OIT without probiotic.[43] Desensitization was achieved in 89.7% receiving PPOIT and 7.1% receiving placebo, and possible SU in 82.1% with PPOIT and 3.6% with placebo. Four-year follow-up showed that 58% of PPOIT compared with 7% of placebo subjects demonstrated 8-week SU,[44] suggesting long-lasting clinical benefit of this combined therapy. An additional benefit to PPOIT is that it was well tolerated with no participants withdrawing because of adverse events, in contrast to reported rates of OIT withdrawal ranging from 10% to 30%. Subjects participating in the trial did not all undergo entry food challenges to verify allergic status, and the length of time abstaining from therapy to measure SU varied among participants, with some abstaining for only 2 weeks before the SU challenge. Future studies into the efficacy of PPOIT will better elucidate its potential superiority to OIT without a probiotic supplement.

Dupilumab and Oral Immunotherapy

Dupilumab is a monoclonal antibody that targets the IL-4-receptor-alpha, effectively inhibiting both IL-4 and IL-13. It is currently being studied in combination with AR101 for peanut allergy (NCT03682770).[45] It is already FDA-approved for moderate to severe asthma and eczema, and investigation is ongoing for its use in eosinophilic esophagitis (NCT02379052).[46] Although the ultimate benefit of dupilumab for facilitating OIT and improving the safety of OIT remains to be seen, the potential of dupilumab to improve control of severe comorbidities may theoretically expand the use of OIT to subjects in whom OIT otherwise may be contraindicated.

Food Allergy Herbal Formula and Oral Immunotherapy

It has been suggested that Chinese herbal medicines can be of value in treating a myriad of diseases, including allergies. Initial murine model studies demonstrated that treatment with FAHF-2 (food allergy herbal formula 2) eliminated anaphylaxis and downregulated Th2 responses in peanut-allergic mice.[47] More recent studies by this group using B-FAHF-2 (BF2) with peanut and tree nut OIT in sensitized mice demonstrated an advantage to adjuvant therapy.[48] Benefits included reduced frequency of and less severe adverse reactions during OIT build-up, enhanced OIT desensitization, more sustained protection, and pro-tolerogenic cytokine profile. The only human study to date was disappointing, with no clinical benefit and none of the expected immunomodulatory effects versus placebo, possibly due in part to poor adherence.[49] Ongoing areas of investigation include a DBPCRT using multiallergen OIT with omalizumab, followed by OIT with B-FAHF-2 for 2 years (NCT02879006).[50]

Interferon-γ

The role of IFN-γ in food allergy has been explored in murine models as well as in patients with cow's milk allergy, both demonstrating allergy resolution.[51–53] Its role in combination with OIT has been investigated in 2 case control studies. The first involved 25 children with egg, milk, or wheat allergy.[54] All 10 subjects who received IFN-γ with OIT achieved SU at 3 months, in contrast to no subjects achieving SU or desensitization with either treatment independently. Of note, all patients who received OIT alone failed to complete the OIT protocol and withdrew because of frequent and severe reactions. A later case control study of a similar pediatric cohort examined the use of IFN-γ with either classic or dual OIT.[55] Classic OIT involved a single daily dose of IFN-γ with OIT, compared with dual OIT with a dose of IFN-γ with OIT in the morning followed by a dose of OIT alone in the evening. All patients who received dual OIT and classic OIT achieved desensitization, compared with no patients who received OIT alone or no treatment. Although studies are limited, this suggests the addition of IFN-γ improved OIT tolerability and achieving desensitization.

SUBLINGUAL IMMUNOTHERAPY ADJUVANTS
Sublingual Immunotherapy cytosine-phosphate-guanine (CpG)-Nanoparticles

Although there has been great interest in adjuvant therapies using probiotics and other whole-cell bacteria, it has also been suggested that microbial macromolecules expressing toll-like receptor (TLR) ligands may provide similar adjuvant activity to activate the host immune system. CpG oligodeoxynucleotides (ODNs) are TLR9 ligands that induce Th1[56] and Treg[57] immunity, as demonstrated by the differentiation of T cells stimulated by CpG-activated dendritic cells into Tregs that suppress effector T-cell responses. Two studies demonstrated a reduction in peanut-induced anaphylaxis in hypersensitive mice when treated with orally administered or injected peanut combined with CpG both prophylactically and therapeutically.[58,59] In a mouse model of peanut immunotherapy, OIT with CpG-coated poly(lactic-co-glycolic-acid) nanoparticles containing peanut extract (CpG/PN-NPs) improved allergic disease in peanut-sensitive mice.[60] Only the mice treated with CpG/PN-NPs were significantly protected from anaphylaxis in all OFCs, developed a sustained and significant decrease in both peanut-specific IgE and IgG1 (TH2-associated immunoglobulin), as well as an increase in peanut-specific IgG2a (TH1-associated immunoglobulin). Overall, CpG/PN-NPs peanut OIT in a mouse model was found to be well tolerated, induced persistent protection from anaphylaxis, and conferred beneficial regulation of peanut-specific immune responses with favorable alteration in cytokine profiles. Further studies are needed to elucidate whether the same CpG sequences are immunostimulatory in mice and humans.

SUBCUTANEOUS IMMUNOTHERAPY
Lysosomal Associated Membrane Protein-vax DNA

DNA vaccines have been studied in a variety of diseases. Of particular interest in allergy is the use of LAMP (lysosomal associated membrane protein) technology to treat pollen allergies, and in novel therapeutic approaches in peanut allergy. This approach involves inserting DNA encoding the allergen in a plasmid containing the coding sequence for LAMP, such that when APCs take up the plasmid it induces synthesis of an allergen-LAMP fusion protein hypothesized to elicit Th1 responses.[61] Studies by Su and colleagues[62] using this approach with Japanese red cedar allergy in murine models showed it was not only effective in eliciting Th1-type immune responses, but also has a favorable safety profile and produces active immunologic effects.[63] Current investigations include phase I, randomized controlled studies evaluating the safety, tolerability and immune responses in peanut-allergic adolescents (NCT03755713[64]) and adults (NCT02851277[65]) receiving varying doses of intradermal or intramuscular injections of ASP0892 (ARA-LAMP-vax), a multivalent peanut (Ara h1, h2, h3) LAMP-DNA plasmid vaccine.

Subcutaneous Immunotherapy (Modified Allergen) (Aluminum Hydroxide Adsorbed Modified Peanut Extract)

The need for the development of a modified peanut extract to facilitate the clinical application SCIT for peanut allergy was recognized after early attempts with peanut extract resulted in many severe systemic reactions.[6] Subsequent studies demonstrated that aluminum hydroxide adsorbed modified peanut extract (HAL-MPE1) reduces allergenicity while still retaining immunogenicity of peanut extract (PE).[66] In their in vivo mouse model, immunotherapy with Ara h 2 and 6 chemically modified (MPE) was capable of reducing allergic responses while maintaining immunologic potency. This data suggest greater safety in the preparation of MPE compared with PE potentially enabling higher and clinically effective dosing and supports further development of MPEs for SCIT. Human trials have examined the use of incremental escalating doses weekly with either HAL-MPE1 or placebo in peanut-allergic subjects.[67] Although early and late local reactions were more frequently observed after HAL-MPE1 compared with placebo, they were generally of mild intensity with no late systemic reactions exceeding grade I. The investigators suggested that this incidence and intensity of early and late local and systemic reactions supported the safety and tolerability of treatment with HAL-MPE1, and that 4 to 5 months of weekly dose escalations effectively induced immunologic changes. A similar but larger study with

42 participants ages 5 to 50 years is ongoing (NCT02991885).[68] This approach is also being investigated beyond peanut allergy using a novel biotechnological product, the recombinant hypoallergenic parvalbumin mCyp c 1, for SCIT in the treatment of fish allergy. This molecule has proven to be safe, hypoallergenic and immunogenic in a phase I/IIa study,[69] and is now being investigated in a multinational phase IIb study (NCT02382718).[70]

Peptide-Based Vaccines (PVX-108)

Furthering the concept of using modified allergens is an approach using synthetic peptides representing T-cell epitope sequences of the major peanut allergens Ara h 1 and Ara h 2. This is theorized to target allergen-specific T cells without causing IgE-mediated inflammatory cell activation.[71] A novel therapeutic product, PVX108, for intradermal immunotherapy demonstrated a favorable safety profile in a phase 1 trial (ACTRN12617000692336).[72] No participants experienced any serious adverse events, and immunologic assays confirmed lack of basophil reactivity to PVX108 in contrast to peanut extract. A phase 2 clinical trial is planned in children.

Subcutaneous Immunotherapy + CpG

Another approach for allergen-specific immunotherapy is to use protamines, arginine-rich proteins that spontaneously assemble into nanoparticles with CpG-ODNs, which drive the immune response toward Th1. A murine model using subcutaneous administration of protamine nanoparticles complexed with Ara h 2 observed a favorable increase in Ara h 2-specific IgG2a without detectable Ara h 2-specific IgE.[73] Findings suggest that protamine-based nanoparticles with CpG-ODN counteract the allergen induced Th2-dominated immune response and may be considered a novel allergen immunotherapy delivery system.

MUCOSAL IMMUNOTHERAPY

The use of heat-killed (HK) bacterial adjuvants is another variation on recombinant proteins in immunotherapy to reduce clinical reactivity wile maintain tolerogenic immune responses. The safety and potential efficacy of this approach at inducing long-term downregulation of peanut hypersensitivity was observed in a murine model of rectally administered HK *Escherichia coli* producing engineered (mutated) Ara h1, 2, and 3 (HKE-MP123).[74] Despite these promising preclinical studies, a later phase 1 study conducted to assess the safety of this vaccine had rather unexpected results as rectal administration of EMP-123 resulted in frequent adverse reactions, with 50% of participants unable to complete the dosing regimen and 20% experiencing severe allergic reactions.[75] Thus, although it was hypothesized that rectal administration would capitalize on the rich immunologic colonic environment to enhance tolerance development and allow safe administration of larger antigen doses, it is unknown whether the highly absorptive nature of the colonic mucosa potentially enhanced the observed risk of AEs. The investigators suggest that a more conservative approach using slower escalation and daily dosing may have minimized these reactions.

FUTURE AREAS OF INVESTIGATION
Ibrutinib

Ibrutinib is a Bruton tyrosine kinase (BTK) inhibitor that has been hypothesized to be useful in preventing allergic reactions, as BTK is a key component of not only B-cell receptor signaling but also plays a role in activation of mast cells and basophils via FcεRI signaling. A pilot study in 2 patients with chronic lymphocytic leukemia demonstrated that ibrutinib completely eliminated skin test reactivity and IgE-mediated basophil activation test (BAT) responses to aeroallergens within 1 week of starting treatment.[76] This same group expanded on this work in a study of peanut and tree nut allergic patients who were given a standard FDA-approved dose of 420 mg of ibrutinib daily for 1 week.[77] Skin prick test analysis after 2 doses showed a sustained significant decrease in wheal and flare in all subjects for all allergens tested (average reduction 76.6% for wheal and 86.0% for flare, both $P<.0001$), as well as suppression of IgE-mediated BAT responses ($P = .0002$ at days 2 and 4, $P<.0001$ on day 7); however, serum-specific IgE to foods were unchanged at follow-up and responses were not sustained. After cessation of ibrutinib treatment, approximately 80% of SPT areas returned to within 80% of baseline diameter within 1 week, and IgE-mediated BAT responses recovered within days. Ibrutinib was considered safe and well tolerated with no serious adverse reaction; however, the study was limited by a small sample size (n = 6). Further investigation is necessary to evaluate potential use in preventing allergic reactions.

SUMMARY

Although there are currently no FDA-approved therapies for treatment of life-threatening food allergies, it is expected that the treatment landscape will change dramatically in the coming years. It is likely that physicians will have a choice of allergen-specific therapies in the near future; however, the treatment options most likely to appear on the market will not be tolerable for all food allergic patients, will not provide significant benefit for all patients, will not be sustainable long-term for all patients, and will not address the needs of patients with multiple food allergies. In an effort to improve safety and efficacy the next generation of investigative therapeutics will focus on targeted immune modulation and a decreased risk of anaphylaxis with therapy. Broader consideration will also be given to multifood allergic patients as non–allergen-specific therapies target prevention of anaphylaxis irrespective of the allergen. The treatment landscape for food allergy is changing quickly, and refined approaches to therapy will provide more comprehensive benefit to the most severely affected food allergic patients.

REFERENCES

1. Gupta RS, Warren CM, Smith BM, et al. The public health impact of parent-reported childhood food allergies in the United States. Pediatrics 2018;142(6) [pii:e20181235].
2. Gupta RS, Warren CM, Smith BM, et al. Prevalence and severity of food allergies among US adults. JAMA Netw Open 2019;2(1):e185630.
3. Investigators PGoC, Vickery BP, Vereda A, et al. AR101 oral immunotherapy for peanut allergy. N Engl J Med 2018;379(21):1991–2001.
4. Fleischer DM, Burks AW, Vickery BP, et al. Sublingual immunotherapy for peanut allergy: a randomized, double-blind, placebo-controlled multicenter trial. J Allergy Clin Immunol 2013;131(1):119–27.e1-7.
5. Fleischer DM, Greenhawt M, Sussman G, et al. Effect of epicutaneous immunotherapy vs placebo on reaction to peanut protein ingestion among children with peanut allergy: the PEPITES Randomized Clinical Trial. JAMA 2019; 321(10):946–55.
6. Nelson HS, Lahr J, Rule R, et al. Treatment of anaphylactic sensitivity to peanuts by immunotherapy with injections of aqueous peanut extract. J Allergy Clin Immunol 1997;99(6 Pt 1):744–51.

7. Oppenheimer JJ, Nelson HS, Bock SA, et al. Treatment of peanut allergy with rush immunotherapy. J Allergy Clin Immunol 1992;90(2):256–62.
8. Chu DK, Wood RA, French S, et al. Oral immunotherapy for peanut allergy (PACE): a systematic review and meta-analysis of efficacy and safety. Lancet 2019;393(10187):2222–32.
9. Feuille E, Nowak-Wegrzyn A. Allergen-specific immunotherapies for food allergy. Allergy Asthma Immunol Res 2018;10(3):189–206.
10. Kulis MD, Patil SU, Wambre E, et al. Immune mechanisms of oral immunotherapy. J Allergy Clin Immunol 2018;141(2):491–8.
11. Moingeon P, Lombardi V, Baron-Bodo V, et al. Enhancing allergen-presentation platforms for sublingual immunotherapy. J Allergy Clin Immunol Pract 2017;5(1):23–31.
12. Bird JA, Sanchez-Borges M, Ansotegui IJ, et al. Skin as an immune organ and clinical applications of skin-based immunotherapy. World Allergy Organ J 2018;11(1):38.
13. Tordesillas L, Mondoulet L, Blazquez AB, et al. Epicutaneous immunotherapy induces gastrointestinal LAP(+) regulatory T cells and prevents food-induced anaphylaxis. J Allergy Clin Immunol 2017;139(1):189–201.e4.
14. Dioszeghy V, Mondoulet L, Puteaux E, et al. Differences in phenotype, homing properties and suppressive activities of regulatory T cells induced by epicutaneous, oral or sublingual immunotherapy in mice sensitized to peanut. Cell Mol Immunol 2017;14(9):770–82.
15. Gernez Y, Nowak-Wegrzyn A. Immunotherapy for food allergy: are we there yet? J Allergy Clin Immunol Pract 2017;5(2):250–72.
16. Shaker MS. An economic analysis of a peanut oral immunotherapy study in children. J Allergy Clin Immunol Pract 2017;5(6):1707–16.
17. De Schryver S, Clarke A, La Vieille S, et al. Food-induced anaphylaxis to a known food allergen in children often occurs despite adult supervision. Pediatr Allergy Immunol 2017;28(7):715–7.
18. Baumert JL, Taylor SL, Koppelman SJ. Quantitative assessment of the safety benefits associated with increasing clinical peanut thresholds through immunotherapy. J Allergy Clin Immunol Pract 2018;6(2):457–65.e4.
19. Lucendo AJ, Arias A, Tenias JM. Relation between eosinophilic esophagitis and oral immunotherapy for food allergy: a systematic review with meta-analysis. Ann Allergy Asthma Immunol 2014;113(6):624–9.
20. Petroni D, Spergel JM. Eosinophilic esophagitis and symptoms possibly related to eosinophilic esophagitis in oral immunotherapy. Ann Allergy Asthma Immunol 2018;120(3):237–40.e4.
21. Wright BL, Fernandez-Becker NQ, Kambham N, et al. Baseline gastrointestinal eosinophilia is common in oral immunotherapy subjects with IgE-mediated peanut allergy. Front Immunol 2018;9:2624.
22. Leung DY, Sampson HA, Yunginger JW, et al. Effect of anti-IgE therapy in patients with peanut allergy. N Engl J Med 2003;348(11):986–93.
23. Sampson HA, Leung DY, Burks AW, et al. A phase II, randomized, double-blind, parallel-group, placebo-controlled oral food challenge trial of Xolair (omalizumab) in peanut allergy. J Allergy Clin Immunol 2011;127(5):1309–10.e1.
24. Savage JH, Courneya JP, Sterba PM, et al. Kinetics of mast cell, basophil, and oral food challenge responses in omalizumab-treated adults with peanut allergy. J Allergy Clin Immunol 2012;130(5):1123–9.e2.
25. Fiocchi A, Artesani MC, Riccardi C, et al. Impact of omalizumab on food allergy in patients treated for asthma: a real-life study. J Allergy Clin Immunol Pract 2019; 7(6):1901–9.e5.

26. Nadeau KC, Schneider LC, Hoyte L, et al. Rapid oral desensitization in combination with omalizumab therapy in patients with cow's milk allergy. J Allergy Clin Immunol 2011;127(6):1622–4.
27. Martorell-Calatayud C, Michavila-Gomez A, Martorell-Aragones A, et al. Anti-IgE-assisted desensitization to egg and cow's milk in patients refractory to conventional oral immunotherapy. Pediatr Allergy Immunol 2016;27(5):544–6.
28. Clark AT, Ewan PW. Food allergy in childhood. Arch Dis Child 2003;88(1):79–81.
29. Wood RA, Kim JS, Lindblad R, et al. A randomized, double-blind, placebo-controlled study of omalizumab combined with oral immunotherapy for the treatment of cow's milk allergy. J Allergy Clin Immunol 2016;137(4):1103–10.e11.
30. Schneider LC, Rachid R, LeBovidge J, et al. A pilot study of omalizumab to facilitate rapid oral desensitization in high-risk peanut-allergic patients. J Allergy Clin Immunol 2013;132(6):1368–74.
31. MacGinnitie AJ, Rachid R, Gragg H, et al. Omalizumab facilitates rapid oral desensitization for peanut allergy. J Allergy Clin Immunol 2017;139(3):873–81.e8.
32. Yee CSK, Albuhairi S, Noh E, et al. Long-term outcome of peanut oral immunotherapy facilitated initially by omalizumab. J Allergy Clin Immunol Pract 2019; 7(2):451–61.e7.
33. Gupta RS, Springston EE, Warrier MR, et al. The prevalence, severity, and distribution of childhood food allergy in the United States. Pediatrics 2011;128(1):e9–17.
34. Bégin P, Dominguez T, Wilson SP, et al. Phase 1 results of safety and tolerability in a rush oral immunotherapy protocol to multiple foods using Omalizumab. Allergy Asthma Clin Immunol 2014;10(1):7.
35. Andorf S, Manohar M, Dominguez T, et al. Observational long-term follow-up study of rapid food oral immunotherapy with omalizumab. Allergy Asthma Clin Immunol 2017;13:51.
36. Andorf S, Purington N, Kumar D, et al. A phase 2 randomized controlled multisite study using omalizumab-facilitated rapid desensitization to test continued vs discontinued dosing in multifood allergic individuals. EClinicalMedicine 2019;7: 27–38.
37. Plunkett CH, Nagler CR. The influence of the microbiome on allergic sensitization to food. J Immunol 2017;198(2):581–9.
38. Zhao W, Ho HE, Bunyavanich S. The gut microbiome in food allergy. Ann Allergy Asthma Immunol 2019;122(3):276–82.
39. Pascal M, Perez-Gordo M, Caballero T, et al. Microbiome and allergic diseases. Front Immunol 2018;9:1584.
40. Berni Canani R, Paparo L, Nocerino R, et al. Gut microbiome as target for innovative strategies against food allergy. Front Immunol 2019;10:191.
41. Berni Canani R, Nocerino R, Terrin G, et al. Formula selection for management of children with cow's milk allergy influences the rate of acquisition of tolerance: a prospective multicenter study. J Pediatr 2013;163(3):771–7.e1.
42. Berni Canani R, Di Costanzo M, Bedogni G, et al. Extensively hydrolyzed casein formula containing Lactobacillus rhamnosus GG reduces the occurrence of other allergic manifestations in children with cow's milk allergy: 3-year randomized controlled trial. J Allergy Clin Immunol 2017;139(6):1906–13.e4.
43. Tang ML, Ponsonby AL, Orsini F, et al. Administration of a probiotic with peanut oral immunotherapy: a randomized trial. J Allergy Clin Immunol 2015;135(3):737–44.e8.
44. Hsiao K-C, Ponsonby A-L, Axelrad C, et al. Long-term clinical and immunological effects of probiotic and peanut oral immunotherapy after treatment cessation: 4-year follow-up of a randomised, double-blind, placebo-controlled trial. Lancet Child Adolesc Health 2017;1(2):97–105.

45. Campbell RL, Bashore CJ, Lee S, et al. Predictors of repeat epinephrine administration for Emergency Department patients with anaphylaxis. J Allergy Clin Immunol Pract 2015;3(4):576–84.
46. Bock SA, Muñoz-Furlong A, Sampson HA. Fatalities due to anaphylactic reactions to foods. J Allergy Clin Immunol 2001;107(1):191–3.
47. Srivastava KD, Kattan JD, Zou ZM, et al. The Chinese herbal medicine formula FAHF-2 completely blocks anaphylactic reactions in a murine model of peanut allergy. J Allergy Clin Immunol 2005;115(1):171–8.
48. Srivastava KD, Song Y, Yang N, et al. B-FAHF-2 plus oral immunotherapy (OIT) is safer and more effective than OIT alone in a murine model of concurrent peanut/tree nut allergy. Clin Exp Allergy 2017;47(8):1038–49.
49. Wang J, Jones SM, Pongracic JA, et al. Safety, clinical, and immunologic efficacy of a Chinese herbal medicine (Food Allergy Herbal Formula-2) for food allergy. J Allergy Clin Immunol 2015;136(4):962–70.e1.
50. Ogawa Y, Grant JA. Mediators of anaphylaxis. Immunol Allergy Clin North Am 2007;27(2):249–60.
51. Lee HO, Miller SD, Hurst SD, et al. Interferon gamma induction during oral tolerance reduces T-cell migration to sites of inflammation. Gastroenterology 2000;119(1):129–38.
52. Suomalainen H, Soppi E, Laine S, et al. Immunologic disturbances in cow's milk allergy, 2: evidence for defective interferon-gamma generation. Pediatr Allergy Immunol 1993;4(4):203–7.
53. Kweon MN, Fujihashi K, VanCott JL, et al. Lack of orally induced systemic unresponsiveness in IFN-gamma knockout mice. J Immunol 1998;160(4):1687–93.
54. Noh G, Lee SS. A pilot study of interferon-gamma-induced specific oral tolerance induction (ISOTI) for immunoglobulin E-mediated anaphylactic food allergy. J Interferon Cytokine Res 2009;29(10):667–75.
55. Noh G, Jang EH. Dual specific oral tolerance induction using interferon gamma for IgE-mediated anaphylactic food allergy and the dissociation of local skin allergy and systemic oral allergy: tolerance or desensitization? J Investig Allergol Clin Immunol 2014;24(2):87–97.
56. Chu RS, Targoni OS, Krieg AM, et al. CpG oligodeoxynucleotides act as adjuvants that switch on T helper 1 (Th1) immunity. J Exp Med 1997;186(10):1623–31.
57. Moseman EA, Liang X, Dawson AJ, et al. Human plasmacytoid dendritic cells activated by CpG oligodeoxynucleotides induce the generation of CD4+CD25+ regulatory T cells. J Immunol 2004;173(7):4433–42.
58. Zhu FG, Kandimalla ER, Yu D, et al. Oral administration of a synthetic agonist of Toll-like receptor 9 potently modulates peanut-induced allergy in mice. J Allergy Clin Immunol 2007;120(3):631–7.
59. Kulis M, Gorentla B, Burks AW, et al. Type B CpG oligodeoxynucleotides induce Th1 responses to peanut antigens: modulation of sensitization and utility in a truncated immunotherapy regimen in mice. Mol Nutr Food Res 2013;57(5):906–15.
60. Srivastava KD, Siefert A, Fahmy TM, et al. Investigation of peanut oral immunotherapy with CpG/peanut nanoparticles in a murine model of peanut allergy. J Allergy Clin Immunol 2016;138(2):536–43.e4.
61. Vickery BP, Ebisawa M, Shreffler WG, et al. Current and future treatment of peanut allergy. J Allergy Clin Immunol Pract 2019;7(2):357–65.
62. Su Y, Connolly M, Marketon A, et al. CryJ-LAMP DNA vaccines for Japanese red cedar allergy induce robust Th1-type immune responses in murine model. J Immunol Res 2016;2016:4857869.

63. Su Y, Romeu-Bonilla E, Anagnostou A, et al. Safety and long-term immunological effects of CryJ2-LAMP plasmid vaccine in Japanese red cedar atopic subjects: a phase I study. Hum Vaccin Immunother 2017;13(12):2804–13.
64. Mertes PM, Tajima K, Regnier-Kimmoun MA, et al. Perioperative anaphylaxis. Med Clin North Am 2010;94(4):761–89.
65. Murphy A, Campbell DE, Baines D, et al. Allergic reactions to propofol in egg-allergic children. Anesth Analg 2011;113(1):140–4.
66. van der Kleij HPM, Warmenhoven HJM, van Ree R, et al. Chemically modified peanut extract shows increased safety while maintaining immunogenicity. Allergy 2019;74(5):986–95.
67. Bindslev-Jensen C, de Kam P-J, van Twuijver E, et al. SCIT-treatment with a chemically modified, aluminum hydroxide adsorbed peanut extract (HAL-MPE1) was generally safe and well tolerated and showed immunological changes in peanut allergic patients. J Allergy Clin Immunol 2017;139(2):AB191.
68. Oh HE, Chetty R. Eosinophilic gastroenteritis: a review. J Gastroenterol 2008;43(10):741–50.
69. Zuidmeer-Jongejan L, Huber H, Swoboda I, et al. Development of a hypoallergenic recombinant parvalbumin for first-in-man subcutaneous immunotherapy of fish allergy. Int Arch Allergy Immunol 2015;166(1):41–51.
70. Masterson JC, Furuta GT, Lee JJ. Update on clinical and immunological features of eosinophilic gastrointestinal diseases. Curr Opin Gastroenterol 2011;27(6):515–22.
71. Prickett SR, Voskamp AL, Phan T, et al. Ara h 1 CD4+ T cell epitope-based peptides: candidates for a peanut allergy therapeutic. Clin Exp Allergy 2013;43(6):684–97.
72. Prickett SR, Hickey PLC, Bingham J, et al. Safety and tolerability of a novel peptide-based immunotherapy for peanut allergy. J Allergy Clin Immunol 2019;143(2).
73. Pali-Scholl I, Szollosi H, Starkl P, et al. Protamine nanoparticles with CpG-oligodeoxynucleotide prevent an allergen-induced Th2-response in BALB/c mice. Eur J Pharm Biopharm 2013;85(3 Pt A):656–64.
74. Li X-M, Srivastava K, Grishin A, et al. Persistent protective effect of heat-killed *Escherichia coli* producing "engineered," recombinant peanut proteins in a murine model of peanut allergy. J Allergy Clin Immunol 2003;112(1):159–67.
75. Wood RA, Sicherer SH, Burks AW, et al. A phase 1 study of heat/phenol-killed, *E. coli*-encapsulated, recombinant modified peanut proteins Ara h 1, Ara h 2, and Ara h 3 (EMP-123) for the treatment of peanut allergy. Allergy 2013;68(6):803–8.
76. Regan JA, Cao Y, Dispenza MC, et al. Ibrutinib, a Bruton's tyrosine kinase inhibitor used for treatment of lymphoproliferative disorders, eliminates both aeroallergen skin test and basophil activation test reactivity. J Allergy Clin Immunol 2017;140(3):875–9.e1.
77. Dispenza MC, Pongracic JA, Singh AM, et al. Short-term ibrutinib therapy suppresses skin test responses and eliminates IgE-mediated basophil activation in adults with peanut or tree nut allergy. J Allergy Clin Immunol 2018;141(5):1914–6.e7.
78. Andorf S, Purington N, Block WM, et al. Anti-IgE treatment with oral immunotherapy in multifood allergic participants: a double-blind, randomised, controlled trial. Lancet Gastroenterol Hepatol 2018;3(2):85–94.
79. Hsiao KC, Ponsonby AL, Axelrad C, et al. Long-term clinical and immunological effects of probiotic and peanut oral immunotherapy after treatment cessation: 4-year follow-up of a randomised, double-blind, placebo-controlled trial. Lancet Child Adolesc Health 2017;1(2):97–105.

Novel Therapies for Treatment of Food Allergy

Sultan Albuhairi, MD[a], Rima Rachid, MD[b],*

KEYWORDS

- Food allergy • Novel therapies • Biologics • Microbiome
- Fecal microbiota transplantation • Omalizumab • Dupilumab

KEY POINTS

- There is an unmet need to evaluate new therapeutic modalities that may decrease the risk of food-induced anaphylaxis and improve patients' quality of life.
- Oral, epicutaneous, and sublingual food immunotherapies have different safety and efficacy profiles, and their long-term outcome and applicability are unclear.
- Food allergy trials are currently evaluating different biologics (given as monotherapy or adjunct to immunotherapy), modified food proteins, DNA vaccines, and fecal microbiota transplantation.

INTRODUCTION

The prevalence of food allergy has significantly increased over time. The Centers of Disease Control and Prevention in the United States reported an increase in food allergy among children from 3.4% in 1997 to 2007 to 5.1% in 2009 to 2011.[1] Large surveys in the United States estimated that at least 4% to 10% of adults (26 million) and 8% of children have food allergy.[2,3] Standard of care currently consists of food allergen avoidance and keeping rescue medications including epinephrine and antihistamines for emergency use.[4] Unfortunately, food allergy can affect quality of life of affected patients and their families significantly, and can lead to significant social impact, anxiety, and dietary limitations.[5]

Although there are currently no treatments approved by the Food and Drug Administration (FDA) for food allergy, food immunotherapy via the oral (OIT), epicutaneous (EPIT), and sublingual routes (SLIT) has been evaluated in numerous trials over the

Disclosure Statement: The authors have nothing to disclose.
[a] Department of Pediatrics, College of Medicine, Majmaah University, PO Box 66, Majmaah 11952, Saudi Arabia; [b] Division of Immunology, Department of Pediatrics, Boston Children's Hospital, Harvard Medical School, 300 Longwood Avenue, Boston, MA 02115, USA
* Corresponding author.
E-mail address: rima.rachid@childrens.harvard.edu

Immunol Allergy Clin N Am 40 (2020) 175–186
https://doi.org/10.1016/j.iac.2019.09.007
0889-8561/20/© 2019 Elsevier Inc. All rights reserved.
immunology.theclinics.com

past decade.[6] The success and side effects of these techniques is variable depending on the route, build-up protocol, maintenance dose, or food used. Recently a large study on 496 children who reacted to ≤100 mg peanut protein during entry food challenge showed that 67% of participants on AR101 pharmaceutical peanut product tolerated at least 600 mg of peanut protein during exit food challenge compared with 4% on placebo. However, 4.3% of subjects on study drug developed severe allergic reactions compared with 0.8% of placebo.[7] EPIT on the other side, using Viaskin Peanut, had less efficacy in peanut-allergic children aged 4 to 11 years, as the percentage difference in responders at 12 months with the 250-μg peanut-patch therapy versus placebo was 21.7%. Systemic side effects were much less frequent compared with peanut OIT and there was no severe anaphylaxis reported.[8] None of these food immunotherapy approaches are known to lead to a permanent oral tolerance (cure). In clinical trials, the surrogate term for permanent tolerance, sustained unresponsiveness (SU) is used. SU, which is evaluated by successfully passing a food challenge after withholding immunotherapy for a defined period, was observed in only 50% of patients who were on peanut OIT for up to 5 years and interrupted therapy for 4 weeks.[9] However, SU was reported in only 15% of patients who stopped peanut OIT for 6 months, suggesting that the longer the period of avoidance, the lower SU rate.[10] A recent meta-analysis of 12 peanut OIT trials that included 1041 subjects reported that high-certainty evidence shows that the analyzed peanut OIT regimens considerably increase allergic and anaphylactic reactions compared with avoidance or placebo, despite effectively inducing desensitization.[11]

There is therefore an unmet need to explore other therapies for food allergy, which may be administered either separately or in combination with food immunotherapy. Fortunately, there are several immunomodulatory candidates that are currently being evaluated or are candidates for investigation. In this review article, the authors discuss some of these novel potential food allergy investigational therapies (**Tables 1** and **2**).

MECHANISM OF FOOD ALLERGY

Food allergy results from the immunologic loss of tolerance to specific food allergens. The exact mechanism underlying the development of food allergy and the subsequent allergic response remains to be elucidated. The modified hygiene hypothesis stipulates that the Western life style limits the gut microbiome exposure, leading to disruption in the healthy gut microbiota or dysbiosis. Healthy commensal gut bacteria protect the intestinal mucosal barrier and target both innate and adaptive immune response to promote tolerance to food.[12] Clostridia colonization of germ-free mice protects from oral allergen sensitization by inducing interleukin (IL)-22+ innate lymphoid cell C type 3 (ILC3) at the intestinal mucosa.[13] IL-22 promotes mucosal integrity, which prevents leakage of protease-resistant food allergens through the gut mucosal barrier.[13] In addition, commensal microbiota directly acts on regulatory T (Treg) cells through their toll-like receptors (TLRs) and promotes the development of induced Treg (iTreg) cells. We recently found that commensal bacteria can upregulate the development of RoRγTreg cells in a Myd88-dependent manner and that RoRγ Treg cells are essential for the development of tolerance.[14] Hence, dysbiosis leads to increased epithelial gut permeability. This in turn results in increased production of epithelial derived cytokines, including IL-25, IL-33, and thymic stromal lymphopoietin (TSLP) with subsequent upregulation of Th2-driven inflammatory response and production of cytokines IL-4, IL-5, and IL-13. This promotes recruitment of mast cells, eosinophils, and basophils and ultimately the formation of allergen-specific immunoglobulin (Ig)E antibody.[15] On exposure, the food-specific IgE bound to

Table 1		
Investigational therapies for food allergy		
Therapeutic Agents	**Clinical Trials in Food Allergy**	**References or NCT Number**
Anti-IgE		
Omalizumab (Anti-IgE mAb)	Monotherapy for peanut allergy	Savage et al,[18] 2012 Sampson et al,[19] 2011 Fiocchi et al,[20] 2019 Leung et al,[67] 2003
	Adjunct to peanut, milk or multi-food OIT	Nadeau et al,[21] 2011 MacGinnitie et al,[22] 2017 Schneider et al,[23] 2013 Wood et al,[24] 2016 Andorf et al,[25] 2017; Andorf et al,[26] 2018
Anti-IL 4R		
Dupilumab (Anti-IL4-R mAb)	Monotherapy for peanut allergy	Phase II (NCT03793608)
	Adjunct to peanut OIT	Phase II (NCT03682770)
Th1 adjuvants		
Glucopyranosyl lipid A (GLA)	Adjunct to peanut SLIT	Phase I (NCT03463135) (Trial has been terminated prematurely)
Anti-TSLP and IL-33		
Etokimab (anti-IL-33 Ab)	Peanut allergy	Phase II (NCT02920021)
DNA vaccines		
ASP0892 (ARA-LAMP-vax)	Peanut allergy	Phase I (NCT03755713) Phase I (NCT02851277)
Modified food allergen proteins		
Encapsulated, recombinant modified peanut proteins Ara h 1, Ara h 2, and Ara h 3 (EMP-123)	Peanut allergy	Wood et al,[59] 2013
HAL-MPE1	Peanut allergy	Phase I (NCT02991885)
Anti- Sialic acid binding immunoglobulin like lectin (Siglec-8) Antibody (AK002)	Eosinophilic gastritis and/or eosinophilic gastroenteritis	Phase II (NCT03496571)
Ibrutinib (Bruton's tyrosine kinase inhibitor)	Peanut allergy	Dispenza et al,[68] 2018
Targeting the microbiome		
Probiotics	Cow's milk allergy	Berni Canani et al,[61] 2012; Berni Canani et al,[69] 2017 Hol et al,[62] 2008 Zhang et al,[63] 2016
Probiotic with peanut oral immunotherapy	Peanut allergy	Tang et al,[64] 2015
Fecal microbiota transplantation (FMT)	Peanut allergy	Phase I (NCT02960074)

Abbreviations: Ig, immunoglobulin; IL, interleukin; LAMP, lysosomal-associated membrane protein; mAB, monoclonal antibody; OIT, oral immunotherapy; SLIT, sublingual immunotherapy; TSLP, thymic stromal lymphopoietin.

Table 2
Investigational therapies for other atopic diseases

Therapeutic Agents	FDA Approval or Clinical Trial for Asthma, Chronic Urticaria and/or Atopic Dermatitis Therapy
Anti-IgE	
Ligelizumab (Anti-IgE mAb)	Phase IIIb for chronic spontaneous urticaria Phase II for asthma
Anti-IL-5 and Anti-IL-5R	
Mepolizumab (Anti-IL-5 mAb)	FDA approved for asthma treatment ($\geq$12 y)
Reslizumab (Anti-IL-5 mAb)	FDA approved for asthma treatment (adults)
Benralizumab (Anti-IL-5-R mAb)	FDA approved for asthma treatment ($\geq$12 y)
Anti-IL 13	
Lebrikizumab (Anti-IL-13 mAb)	Phase III for atopic dermatitis, asthma
Tralokinumab (Anti-IL-13 mAb)	Phase III for atopic dermatitis, asthma
Th1 adjuvants	
CpG oligodeoxynucleotides	Phase II for allergic rhinitis
Monophosphoryl Lipid A (MPL)	Phase II for allergic rhinitis
Anti-TSLP and IL-33	
Tezepelumab (anti-TSLP mAb)	Phase II for asthma and atopic dermatitis in adults
Etokimab (anti-IL-33 Ab)	Phase II for atopic dermatitis in adults

Abbreviations: FDA, Food and Drug Administration; Ig, immunoglobulin; IL, interleukin; mAB, monoclonal antibody; TSLP, thymic stromal lymphopoietin.

FcεR1 on the surface of the mast cells and basophils binds to the antigen, which induces cross linking of bound IgE.[16] This leads to the release of inflammatory mediators including histamine, leukotriene, cytokines, and prostaglandin, leading to the development of an allergic reaction.[15]

ANTI–IMMUNOGLOBULIN E ANTIBODY

Omalizumab is a monoclonal antibody that targets the constant domain of the IgE molecule. Omalizumab binds free IgE, decreases its level in circulation, and prevents its binding to the surface of basophil and mast cell, hence suppressing them from degranulation on allergen exposure.[17] Omalizumab is the most evaluated biologic in food allergy.

As a monotherapy, omalizumab was administered for 6 months in 14 patients with peanut allergy. A significant increase in the threshold of reactivity to peanut was observed during food challenges after 3 to 11 weeks of omalizumab, from a median of 80 mg to 6500 peanut protein. However, no additional changes in the peanut-eliciting dose were observed after 6 months of therapy.[18] Another small trial demonstrated increase in tolerability to peanut after 24 weeks of omalizumab therapy compared with placebo.[19] A more recent study demonstrated a significant increase in food allergen threshold (milk, egg, hazelnut, and wheat) after 4 months of omalizumab administered for treatment of asthma.[20] Interestingly, tolerated food was reintroduced in the patients' diet without the need of oral immunotherapy in these severely asthmatic patients.

On the other hand, omalizumab had been successfully used to facilitate desensitization of OIT in several clinical trials.[21–26] We reported on the first trial using omalizumab as an adjunct therapy to peanut OIT in patients with very high peanut IgE (median

229 kU/L) who reacted to 50 mg peanut protein during entry food challenge. After receiving omalizumab only for 12 weeks, patients were rapidly desensitized to 2000 mg peanut protein over a median period of 8 weeks during which they received OIT combined with omalizumab.[23] A double-blind placebo-controlled milk OIT trial with omalizumab showed that although there was a significant reduction in adverse events in the omalizumab-treated arm, there was no difference in SU.[24] Omalizumab was also successfully used as an adjunct therapy in multi-food OIT, enabling safe and rapid desensitization.[26]

One anticipated multisite double-blind placebo-controlled randomized trial will aim at evaluating omalizumab as a monotherapy and in combination with multi-food OIT (NCT03881696).

Ligelizumab (QGE031) is another promising monoclonal antibody that binds free serum IgE with much higher affinity than omalizumab.[27] To date, no clinical trial has evaluated ligelizumab for treatment of food allergy. However, Phase II trials in asthma (NCT01716754) and atopic dermatitis (NCT01552629) were completed, and Phase III chronic spontaneous urticarial (NCT02851277) is still ongoing.

ANTI-TH2 CYTOKINE ANTIBODIES

As noted previously, although omalizumab allowed for faster and safer food desensitization, it was not shown to improve the SU rate.[22–24] Targeting other pathways that are involved in the allergic response has gained significant interest recently. Allergen-induced IL-4 expression in peripheral mononuclear cells was found to be associated with clinical allergy to milk and IgE-sensitization to milk and peanut.[28] Patients with mutations in IL-4 receptor alpha (IL-4Rα) and IL13 were found to have an increased risk of food allergy.[29] Dupilumab is a human monoclonal IgG4 antibody that binds to the alpha subunit of IL-4Rα and blocks IL-4 and IL-13 signaling. Dupilumab was approved by the FDA for treatment of adults with moderate to severe atopic dermatitis,[30] as an add-on maintenance therapy for moderate to severe asthma (with an eosinophilic phenotype or corticosteroid dependent) in patients age 12 years and older,[31] and recently for treatment of chronic rhinosinusitis with nasal polyposis.[32]

In patients who underwent peanut OIT initially facilitated by omalizumab,[23] we have shown that the suppressive function of peanut reactive Treg cells was recovered after blockade of IL-4 signaling.[33] Recently a 30-year-old patient with a history of allergic reaction to pistachio during food challenge and anaphylaxis to corn, received dupilumab for severe atopic dermatitis. Both pistachio and corn were subsequently tolerated during an open food challenge after 3 months of therapy.[34] There are currently 2 ongoing randomized placebo-controlled Phase II clinical trials evaluating dupilumab in food allergy. One of these studies is evaluating dupilumab as a monotherapy (NCT03793608) while the other as an adjunct therapy to peanut OIT (NCT03682770). Another single-site randomized Phase II trial is anticipated in patients with at least 3 food allergies, which aims at comparing safety and efficacy of dupilumab, omalizumab, or both as adjunct therapy to multi-food OIT (NCT03679676).

Blockage of IL-13 signaling alone has not been investigated yet in food allergy. Anti-IL-13 antibody (QAX576) was evaluated for treatment of eosinophilic esophagitis. Although it showed a decrease in esophageal eosinophilia, it did not lead to significant improvement in clinical symptoms.[35] Lebrikizumab is another IL-13 monoclonal antibody that has been investigated for treatment of asthma. In a Phase III trial in adults with mild to moderate asthma not receiving corticosteroids, therapy did not improve lung function.[36] However, a recent meta-analysis of 5 randomized controlled trials concluded that lebrikizumab decreased the rate of asthma exacerbation and improved lung function in patients with uncontrolled asthma, especially those with elevated periostin level.[37]

IL-5 is the main cytokine involved in activation of eosinophils. A Cochrane analysis supported the use of anti-IL-5 treatments as an adjunct to standard of care in people with severe eosinophilic asthma and poor control.[38] Mepolizumab and reslizumab, which are monoclonal antibodies against IL-5 and benralizumab, a monoclonal antibody against IL-5Rα, are all FDA approved for treatment of eosinophilic asthma.[39] The value of targeting eosinophils in the treatment of IgE-mediated food allergy remains, however, unclear. To date, there are no reported trials evaluating these biologics in food allergy.

TH1 ADJUVANTS

TH1 adjuvants, such as TLRs, combined with an allergen may be used to skew the TH1:TH2 balance toward TH1polarization.[40] Murine studies have shown that anaphylactic reactions were reduced when CpG oligodeoxynucleotide, a TLR agonist was combined with ovalbumin and peanut allergens.[41–44] There are currently no trials evaluating CpG in food allergy. However, clinical improvement was reported in patients with allergic rhinitis given CpG coupled to ragweed allergen.[45,46]

Monophosphoryl lipid A (MPL) is a TRL4 agonist that was also shown to be effective as an adjuvant therapy to immunotherapy for allergic rhinitis.[47–49] Glucopyranosyl lipid A, a synthetic form of MPL, has shown promising results in a peanut-allergic mouse model.[50] It is currently is being investigated in a Phase I trial as adjunctive therapy to peanut SLIT (NCT03463135).

Chitosan is a biodegradable polymer that was shown in a mouse model to be prevent peanut-induced anaphylaxis and suppress peanut-specific IgE and TH2 cytokines.[51] It has not been evaluated yet for food allergy.

EPITHELIAL CELL–DERIVED CYTOKINES (INTERLEUKIN-33 AND THYMIC STROMAL LYMPHOPOIETIN) ANTIBODIES

As noted previously, antigen sensitization is associated with increased epithelial cell permeability.[52] Epithelial cytokines thymic stromal lymphopoietin (TSLP) and IL-33 promote TH2 response.[53,54] Targeting these cytokines could be a potential approach in treating food allergy.

Etokimab, also known as ANB020, is an anti-IL-33 antibody that has been evaluated in a Phase 2 trial in adults with peanut allergy. The results of this study have not been published yet (NCT02920021). Another trial is ongoing to evaluate its use in atopic dermatitis (NCT03533751).

Tezepelumab is a humanized monoclonal antibody against TSLP that was investigated in a Phase 2 clinical trial in adults with uncontrolled asthma. Patients who received tezepelumab had lower rates of asthma exacerbation compared with placebo.[55] In adults with moderate to severe atopic dermatitis treated with a combination of topical corticosteroids combined with tezepelumab or placebo, there was improvement in the eczema area and severity index in tezepelumab-treated patients, although it did not reach statistical significance.[56] Treatment-emergent adverse effects were similar in the 2 groups. Anti-TSLP therapy has not been evaluated yet in food allergy.

DNA VACCINES

DNA vaccines stimulate an immune response to a specific DNA-encoded protein inserted to a bacterial plasmid.[57] The immunogenicity of DNA vaccines was shown to be enhanced by inclusion of lysosomal-associated membrane protein-1 (LAMP-1).[58] After intradermal or intramuscular administration, uptake of the plasmid by antigen-presenting cells results in the synthesis of an allergen-LAMP fusion protein. The LAMP component directs the fusion protein toward cellular lysosomes where the allergen is subsequently processed and added to major histocompatibility complex-II antigens, which induces a CD4+ helper T-cell response.[57,58] ASP0892 (ARA-LAMP-vax) is a recently developed single multivalent peanut (Ara h1, h2, h3) LAMP DNA Plasmid Vaccine. A Phase I trial is currently ongoing to evaluate its safety, tolerability, and subsequent immune responses in peanut-allergic adolescents when administered via the intradermal route (NCT03755713) after it was evaluated in adults (NCT02851277).

MODIFIED FOOD ALLERGEN PROTEINS

Using modified food allergen proteins is another approach that stipulates that desensitization may be achieved with lesser risk of allergic reactions compared with the natural protein. In a Phase I study by Wood and colleagues,[59] heat/phenol killed, *Escherichia coli* encapsulated, recombinant modified peanut proteins Ara h 1, Ara h 2, and Ara h 3 (EMP-123) was used for treatment of peanut allergy. A rectal administration of EMP-123 in 10 peanut-allergic patients resulted in frequent adverse events, including anaphylaxis in 20% of peanut-allergic patients, whereas no significant adverse events occurred in 5 healthy volunteers.

HAL-MPE1 is a chemically modified, aluminum hydroxide–adsorbed peanut extract for subcutaneous use, and is currently being evaluated in a Phase I trial that aims at assessing its safety in peanut-allergic adolescents and children (NCT02991885).

TARGETING THE MICROBIOME FOR THE TREATMENT OF FOOD ALLERGY

Manipulation of the microbiome may be considered for both preventive and therapeutic interventions.

Several studies evaluated the role of the gut microbiota in food allergy. There has been, however, significant heterogeneity between these studies in design, sample size, age at time fecal collection, methods of bacterial analysis, and geographic location among others.[12] Most studies evaluated subjects for evidence of sensitization to food (ie, positive food-specific skin or IgE) without history of food allergy per se. The small number of patients in these studies did not allow for robust statistical analysis of the effect of potential confounding variables, such as cesarean delivery, diet, antibiotic intake, number of siblings, infections, and pets.[60] We recently reported on a large longitudinal observational study in infants with a history of IgE-mediated allergic reaction to food confirmed by positive skin prick test and/ or serum food-specific IgE. Fifty-six infants with food allergy and 98 healthy controls were enrolled. Stool samples were collected every 6 months for a total of 30 months; 16S ribosomal DNA sequencing showed no difference in ecological diversity or microbial richness. However, evolving dysbiosis was identified: compositional differences in relative abundance among 77 Operational Taxonomic Units were observed in the fecal microbiome between age-stratified food-allergic subjects and controls, some spanning several age groups, whereas others were significant only within a specific age group.[14]

The role of currently available probiotics in the prevention of treatment of food allergy is inconclusive. In a prospective randomized trial in infants with cow's milk allergy, those who received extensively hydrolyzed milk formula (EHMF) supplemented with *Lactobacillus GG* (LGG) acquired tolerance to cow's milk faster than those who were consuming EHMF without probiotic.[61] On the other hand, in a double-blind placebo-controlled trial with 119 infants with cow's milk allergy fed either EHMF alone, or EHMF supplemented with *Lactobacillus casei* and *Bifidobacterium lactis*, there was no difference in the rate of acquisition of tolerance to cow's milk between the 2 groups.[62] A systemic review and meta-analysis of 17 randomized controlled trials involving 2947 infants showed that when probiotics were given either only prenatally or postnatally, no effects of probiotics on atopy and food sensitivity (positive skin and/or specific IgE testing) were observed. When administered to pregnant mothers prenatally and to the child postnatally, the analysis suggested that probiotics could reduce the risk of atopy and food sensitivity.[63]

A double-blind randomized placebo-controlled trial evaluated the effect of administering orally *Lactobacillus rhamnosus* CGMCC combined with peanut OIT for 18 months on SU. Eighty-two percent of subjects in the peanut OIT/probiotic were noted to have possible SU after withholding OIT for 2 to 5 weeks. The study, however, did not have a peanut OIT arm without probiotic or a probiotic arm without peanut OIT.[64] It is also possible that the higher rate of SU compared with other studies was affected in part by a shorter duration of interruption of therapy in some patients.

In $Il4ra^{F709}$ mice that are genetically prone to food allergy, we found that bacteriotherapy with 6 commensal Clostridiales strains and separately with 5 Bacteroidales strains, chosen as representative of clusters impacted by the dysbiosis in infants, both prevented and treated food allergy. In addition, bacteriotherapy led to upregulation of RoR γTreg cells, and decrease in total and ova-specific serum IgE, IL-4 production, and GATA3 expression by Treg cells.[14] Protection from anaphylaxis was also noted when treating these mice with a single Clostridial species, *Subdoligranulum variabilis,* which was also impacted by the dysbiosis in food-allergic infants.[14] In a different food allergy mouse model, *Anaerostipes caccae,* another Clostridial species, also protected against allergic reaction. Developing targeted bacterial therapies for food allergy may thus be promising for treatment and prevention of food allergy.

Another approach in microbial intervention is to attempt a more general modification of the gut microbiome. Fecal microbiota transplantation (FMT) is the transfer of stool from a healthy donor into the gastrointestinal tract of a diseased individual. FMT may be performed by different routes, including colonoscopy, nasogastric tube, or oral capsules. In humans, FMT has been successfully used to treat recurrent refractory *Clostridium difficile* colitis.[65] We and others have found that FMT using stools taken from healthy human infants and transplanted into a food-allergic mouse model protects from anaphylaxis after allergen exposure, whereas anaphylaxis was not abrogated when FMT was performed with stools taken from food-allergic infants.[14,66] We are currently conducting a Phase I trial to evaluate the safety and efficacy of frozen encapsulated FMT peanut-allergic adults age 18 to 40 years (NCT02960074).

SUMMARY

There is currently no cure for food allergy. There is an unmet need to evaluate different therapeutic modalities that aims at abolishing or decreasing the risk of anaphylaxis and improving the quality of life of affected patients and their families. Trials are currently ongoing evaluating biologics, modified food proteins, DNA vaccines, and

FMT. Although these are exciting times for food allergy research, the safety, efficacy, long-term effect, and ultimately cost of these interventions will need to be carefully evaluated.

REFERENCES

1. Branum AM, Lukacs SL. Food allergy among U.S. children: trends in prevalence and hospitalizations. NCHS Data Brief 2008;(10):1–8.
2. Gupta RS, Springston EE, Warrier MR, et al. The prevalence, severity, and distribution of childhood food allergy in the United States. Pediatrics 2011;128:e9–17.
3. Gupta RS, Warren CM, Smith BM, et al. Prevalence and severity of food allergies among US adults. JAMA Netw open 2019;2:e185630.
4. Sicherer SH, Sampson HA. Food allergy: epidemiology, pathogenesis, diagnosis, and treatment. J Allergy Clin Immunol 2014;133:291–307 [quiz: 308].
5. Patel N, Herbert L, Green TD. The emotional, social, and financial burden of food allergies on children and their families. Allergy Asthma Proc 2017;38:88–91.
6. Yee CS, Rachid R. The heterogeneity of oral immunotherapy clinical trials: implications and future directions. Curr Allergy Asthma Rep 2016;16:25.
7. Vickery BP, Vereda A, Casale TB, et al. AR101 oral immunotherapy for peanut allergy. N Engl J Med 2018;379:1991–2001.
8. Fleischer DM, Greenhawt M, Sussman G, et al. Effect of epicutaneous immunotherapy vs placebo on reaction to peanut protein ingestion among children with peanut allergy: the PEPITES randomized clinical trial. JAMA 2019;321(10):946–55.
9. Vickery BP, Scurlock AM, Kulis M, et al. Sustained unresponsiveness to peanut in subjects who have completed peanut oral immunotherapy. J Allergy Clin Immunol 2014;133:468–75.
10. Syed A, Garcia MA, Lyu SC, et al. Peanut oral immunotherapy results in increased antigen-induced regulatory T-cell function and hypomethylation of forkhead box protein 3 (FOXP3). J Allergy Clin Immunol 2014;133:500–10.
11. Chu DK, Wood RA, French S, et al. Oral immunotherapy for peanut allergy (PACE): a systematic review and meta-analysis of efficacy and safety. Lancet 2019;393(10187):2222–32.
12. Rachid R, Chatila TA. The role of the gut microbiota in food allergy. Curr Opin Pediatr 2016;28:748–53.
13. Stefka AT, Feehley T, Tripathi P, et al. Commensal bacteria protect against food allergen sensitization. Proc Natl Acad Sci U S A 2014;111:13145–50.
14. Abdel-Gadir A, Stephen-Victor E, Gerber GK, et al. Microbiota therapy acts via a regulatory T cell MyD88/RORgammat pathway to suppress food allergy. Nat Med 2019;25(7):1164–74.
15. Bauer RN, Manohar M, Singh AM, et al. The future of biologics: applications for food allergy. J Allergy Clin Immunol 2015;135:312–23.
16. Sampath V, Sindher SB, Zhang W, et al. New treatment directions in food allergy. Ann Allergy Asthma Immunol 2018;120:254–62.
17. Liu J, Lester P, Builder S, et al. Characterization of complex formation by humanized anti-IgE monoclonal antibody and monoclonal human IgE. Biochemistry 1995;34:10474–82.
18. Savage JH, Courneya JP, Sterba PM, et al. Kinetics of mast cell, basophil, and oral food challenge responses in omalizumab-treated adults with peanut allergy. J Allergy Clin Immunol 2012;130:1123–9.e2.

19. Sampson HA, Leung DY, Burks AW, et al. A phase II, randomized, doubleblind, parallelgroup, placebocontrolled oral food challenge trial of Xolair (omalizumab) in peanut allergy. J Allergy Clin Immunol 2011;127:1309–10.e1.
20. Fiocchi A, Artesani MC, Riccardi C, et al. Impact of omalizumab on food allergy in patients treated for asthma: a real-life study. J Allergy Clin Immunol Pract 2019; 7(6):1901–9.e5.
21. Nadeau KC, Schneider LC, Hoyte L, et al. Rapid oral desensitization in combination with omalizumab therapy in patients with cow's milk allergy. J Allergy Clin Immunol 2011;127:1622–4.
22. MacGinnitie AJ, Rachid R, Gragg H, et al. Omalizumab facilitates rapid oral desensitization for peanut allergy. J Allergy Clin Immunol 2017;139:873–81.e8.
23. Schneider LC, Rachid R, LeBovidge J, et al. A pilot study of omalizumab to facilitate rapid oral desensitization in high-risk peanut-allergic patients. J Allergy Clin Immunol 2013;132:1368–74.
24. Wood RA, Kim JS, Lindblad R, et al. A randomized, double-blind, placebo-controlled study of omalizumab combined with oral immunotherapy for the treatment of cow's milk allergy. J Allergy Clin Immunol 2016;137:1103–10.e11.
25. Andorf S, Manohar M, Dominguez T, et al. Observational long-term follow-up study of rapid food oral immunotherapy with omalizumab. Allergy Asthma Clin Immunol 2017;13:51.
26. Andorf S, Purington N, Block WM, et al. Anti-IgE treatment with oral immunotherapy in multifood allergic participants: a double-blind, randomised, controlled trial. Lancet 2018;3:85–94.
27. Kocaturk E, Zuberbier T. New biologics in the treatment of urticaria. Curr Opin Allergy Clin Immunol 2018;18:425–31.
28. Sicherer SH, Wood RA, Stablein D, et al. Immunologic features of infants with milk or egg allergy enrolled in an observational study (Consortium of Food Allergy Research) of food allergy. J Allergy Clin Immunol 2010;125:1077–83.e8.
29. Zitnik SE, Ruschendorf F, Muller S, et al. IL13 variants are associated with total serum IgE and early sensitization to food allergens in children with atopic dermatitis. Pediatr Allergy Immunol 2009;20:551–5.
30. Beck LA, Thaci D, Hamilton JD, et al. Dupilumab treatment in adults with moderate-to-severe atopic dermatitis. N Engl J Med 2014;371:130–9.
31. Rabe KF, Nair P, Brusselle G, et al. Efficacy and safety of dupilumab in glucocorticoid-dependent severe asthma. N Engl J Med 2018;378:2475–85.
32. Han JK, Bachert C, Desrosiers M, et al. Efficacy and safety of dupilumab in patients with chronic rhinosinusitis with nasal polyps: results from the randomized phase 3 sinus-24 study. J Allergy Clin Immunol 2019;143:AB422.
33. Abdel-Gadir A, Schneider L, Casini A, et al. Oral immunotherapy with omalizumab reverses the Th2 cell-like programme of regulatory T cells and restores their function. Clin Exp Allergy 2018;48:825–36.
34. Rial MJ, Barroso B, Sastre J. Dupilumab for treatment of food allergy. J Allergy Clin Immunol Pract 2019;7(2):673–4.
35. Rothenberg ME, Wen T, Greenberg A, et al. Intravenous anti-IL-13 mAb QAX576 for the treatment of eosinophilic esophagitis. J Allergy Clin Immunol 2015;135: 500–7.
36. Hanania NA, Korenblat P, Chapman KR, et al. Efficacy and safety of lebrikizumab in patients with uncontrolled asthma (LAVOLTA I and LAVOLTA II): replicate, phase 3, randomised, double-blind, placebo-controlled trials. Lancet Respir Med 2016;4:781–96.

37. Liu Y, Zhang S, Chen R, et al. Meta-analysis of randomized controlled trials for the efficacy and safety of anti-interleukin-13 therapy with lebrikizumab in patients with uncontrolled asthma. Allergy Asthma Proc 2018;39:332–7.
38. Farne HA, Wilson A, Powell C, et al. Anti-IL5 therapies for asthma. Cochrane Database Syst Rev 2017;(9):CD010834.
39. Matera MG, Calzetta L, Rogliani P, et al. Monoclonal antibodies for severe asthma: pharmacokinetic profiles. Respir Med 2019;153:3–13.
40. Keet CA, Wood RA. Emerging therapies for food allergy. J Clin Invest 2014;124:1880–6.
41. Adel-Patient K, Ah-Leung S, Bernard H, et al. Oral sensitization to peanut is highly enhanced by application of peanut extracts to intact skin, but is prevented when CpG and cholera toxin are added. Int Arch Allergy Immunol 2007;143:10–20.
42. Kulis M, Gorentla B, Burks AW, et al. Type B CpG oligodeoxynucleotides induce Th1 responses to peanut antigens: modulation of sensitization and utility in a truncated immunotherapy regimen in mice. Mol Nutr Food Res 2013;57:906–15.
43. San Roman B, Irache JM, Gomez S, et al. Co-delivery of ovalbumin and CpG motifs into microparticles protected sensitized mice from anaphylaxis. Int Arch Allergy Immunol 2009;149:111–8.
44. Xu W, Tamura T, Takatsu K. CpG ODN mediated prevention from ovalbumin-induced anaphylaxis in mouse through B cell pathway. Int Immunopharmacol 2008;8:351–61.
45. Creticos PS, Schroeder JT, Hamilton RG, et al. Immunotherapy with a ragweed-toll-like receptor 9 agonist vaccine for allergic rhinitis. N Engl J Med 2006;355:1445–55.
46. Tulic MK, Fiset PO, Christodoulopoulos P, et al. Amb a 1-immunostimulatory oligodeoxynucleotide conjugate immunotherapy decreases the nasal inflammatory response. J Allergy Clin Immunol 2004;113:235–41.
47. Patel P, Holdich T, Fischer von Weikersthal-Drachenberg KJ, et al. Efficacy of a short course of specific immunotherapy in patients with allergic rhinoconjunctivitis to ragweed pollen. J Allergy Clin Immunol 2014;133:121–9.e1-2.
48. Pfaar O, Barth C, Jaschke C, et al. Sublingual allergen-specific immunotherapy adjuvanted with monophosphoryl lipid A: a phase I/IIa study. Int Arch Allergy Immunol 2011;154:336–44.
49. Rosewich M, Schulze J, Fischer von Weikersthal-Drachenberg KJ, et al. Ultra-short course immunotherapy in children and adolescents during a 3-yrs post-marketing surveillance study. Pediatr Allergy Immunol 2010;21:e185–9.
50. Soos TJ, Li L, Graver K, et al. Glucopyranosyl Lipid a (GLA) a Toll-like receptor 4 (TLR4) agonist for use as an adjuvant in combination with peanut allergen immunotherapy. J Allergy Clin Immunol 2016;137:AB129.
51. Bae MJ, Shin HS, Kim EK, et al. Oral administration of chitin and chitosan prevents peanut-induced anaphylaxis in a murine food allergy model. Int J Biol Macromol 2013;61:164–8.
52. Turner JR. Intestinal mucosal barrier function in health and disease. Nat Rev Immunol 2009;9:799–809.
53. Chu DK, Llop-Guevara A, Walker TD, et al. IL-33, but not thymic stromal lymphopoietin or IL-25, is central to mite and peanut allergic sensitization. J Allergy Clin Immunol 2013;131:187–200.e1-8.
54. Jang S, Morris S, Lukacs NW. TSLP promotes induction of Th2 differentiation but is not necessary during established allergen-induced pulmonary disease. PLoS One 2013;8:e56433.

55. Corren J, Parnes JR, Wang L, et al. Tezepelumab in adults with uncontrolled asthma. N Engl J Med 2017;377:936–46.
56. Simpson EL, Parnes JR, She D, et al. Tezepelumab, an anti-thymic stromal lymphopoietin monoclonal antibody, in the treatment of moderate to severe atopic dermatitis: A randomized phase 2a clinical trial. J Am Acad Dermatol 2019;80: 1013–21.
57. Liu MA. DNA vaccines: an historical perspective and view to the future. Immunol Rev 2011;239:62–84.
58. Su Y, Connolly M, Marketon A, et al. CryJ-LAMP DNA vaccines for Japanese red cedar allergy induce robust Th1-type immune responses in murine model. J Immunol Res 2016;2016:4857869.
59. Wood RA, Sicherer SH, Burks AW, et al. A phase 1 study of heat/phenol-killed, *E. coli*-encapsulated, recombinant modified peanut proteins Ara h 1, Ara h 2, and Ara h 3 (EMP-123) for the treatment of peanut allergy. Allergy 2013;68:803–8.
60. Molloy J, Allen K, Collier F, et al. The potential link between gut microbiota and IgE-mediated food allergy in early life. Int J Environ Res Public Health 2013;10: 7235–56.
61. Berni Canani R, Nocerino R, Terrin G, et al. Effect of Lactobacillus GG on tolerance acquisition in infants with cow's milk allergy: a randomized trial. J Allergy Clin Immunol 2012;129:580–2, 582.e1-5.
62. Hol J, van Leer EH, Elink Schuurman BE, et al. The acquisition of tolerance toward cow's milk through probiotic supplementation: a randomized, controlled trial. J Allergy Clin Immunol 2008;121:1448–54.
63. Zhang GQ, Hu HJ, Liu CY, et al. Probiotics for prevention of atopy and food hypersensitivity in early childhood: a PRISMA-compliant systematic review and meta-analysis of randomized controlled trials. Medicine (Baltimore) 2016;95: e2562.
64. Tang ML, Ponsonby AL, Orsini F, et al. Administration of a probiotic with peanut oral immunotherapy: a randomized trial. J Allergy Clin Immunol 2015;135: 737–44.e8.
65. van Nood E, Vrieze A, Nieuwdorp M, et al. Duodenal infusion of donor feces for recurrent *Clostridium difficile*. N Engl J Med 2013;368:407–15.
66. Feehley T, Plunkett CH, Bao R, et al. Healthy infants harbor intestinal bacteria that protect against food allergy. Nat Med 2019;25:448–53.
67. Leung DY, Sampson HA, Yunginger JW, et al. Effect of anti-IgE therapy in patients with peanut allergy. N Engl J Med 2003;348:986–93.
68. Dispenza MC, Pongracic JA, Singh AM, et al. Short-term ibrutinib therapy suppresses skin test responses and eliminates IgE-mediated basophil activation in adults with peanut or tree nut allergy. J Allergy Clin Immunol 2018;141:1914–6.e7.
69. Berni Canani R, Di Costanzo M, Bedogni G, et al. Extensively hydrolyzed casein formula containing Lactobacillus rhamnosus GG reduces the occurrence of other allergic manifestations in children with cow's milk allergy: 3-year randomized controlled trial. J Allergy Clin Immunol 2017;139:1906–13.e4.

Risk Reduction in Peanut Immunotherapy

Benjamin C. Remington, PhD[a,b,*], Joseph L. Baumert, PhD[a]

KEYWORDS

- Peanut • Peanut immunotherapy • Food allergy • Risk assessment • Risk reduction
- Relative risk reduction • Quantitative risk assessment • Quantitative risk reduction

KEY POINTS

- Immunotherapy for peanut allergy is a potential treatment option being developed with the potential to reduce the risk of accidental reactions to peanut in the community.
- This article covers the epidemiology of unexpected allergic reactions to peanut, and outlines definitions of risk and risk reduction with quantitative risk assessment examples.
- Models for estimating accidental reaction risks to peanut show significant potential relative risk reductions for the peanut-allergic population and the peanut-allergic individual being treated with immunotherapy.
- However, longer-term clinical trials or commercial data will strengthen the knowledge surrounding risk and potential options for risk reduction in patients with peanut allergy.
- It is important to clearly define the specified period of time and population when risk is being assessed to enable better communication and understanding.

INTRODUCTION

Peanut allergy is a global disease and can be life threatening.[1–3] Patients must practice strict avoidance of peanut and be prepared to use rescue medication on development of symptoms caused by unintentional peanut ingestion.[1] However, because of widespread use in packaged foods, restaurants, and catered meals, complete avoidance of peanut is difficult. As such, unexpected allergic reactions to peanut are frequent and symptoms are unpredicable.[2,4–8] Peanut-allergic individuals and their caregivers experience tremendous anxiety and stress, and report poor quality of life; thus, an important goal for patients undergoing immunotherapy is to be able to live, eat, and socially interact more freely.[9–11]

[a] Food Allergy Research and Resource Program, Department of Food Science and Technology, University of Nebraska, Lincoln, NE 68588-6207, USA; [b] Remington Consulting Group B.V., Utrecht, the Netherlands
* Corresponding author. Food Innovation Center, Room 279, 1901 North 21 Street, PO Box 886207, Lincoln, NE 68588-6207.
E-mail address: bremington2@unl.edu

Immunol Allergy Clin N Am 40 (2020) 187–200
https://doi.org/10.1016/j.iac.2019.09.012
0889-8561/20/© 2019 Elsevier Inc. All rights reserved.
immunology.theclinics.com

At present there are no US Food and Drug Administration–approved therapies for treatment of peanut allergy and no treatments under development have shown the ability to cure a food allergy. However, the drugs in development have been focused on increasing the eliciting dose (ED) or reaction threshold (ie, the amount of protein ingested at which an allergic reaction is initiated) to provide protection against accidental exposure reactions.[12] Recent studies have created models to quantitatively estimate the clinical benefits of increasing a hypothetical individual's threshold through immunotherapy (nonspecific to immunotherapy method) in modeling predicted relative risk reduction (RRR) in American and European consumers.[13,14] More recently, RRRs for a phase 3 clinical trial population were modeled based on the increase in ED during a food challenge after 12 months of treatment with epicutaneous immunotherapy (EPIT).[15]

This article covers the epidemiology of unexpected allergic reactions to peanut and outlines definitions of risk and risk reduction with relevant examples. In addition, prior efforts to model potential risk reduction for peanut-allergic individuals or peanut-allergic populations undergoing immunotherapy are discussed.

EPIDEMIOLOGY
Frequency and Causes of Allergic Reactions

Previously, it has been reported that between 3% and 55% of peanut-allergic individuals experienced at least 1 unexpected allergic reaction during a 1-year period.[4–7,16–21] When the place of reaction was identifiable, most adverse events occurred at home, or at a relative's/friend's home, in restaurants, at a party, or at school or day care.[6,16–18,22] Reactions are commonly attributed to packaged foods, meals outside the home (ie, restaurants, school, friends' or relatives' homes), fresh products, products or meals in a foreign country, and meals at home.[4,23] Accidental reactions have been caused by forgetfulness, reduced supervision, not checking a product, label reading errors, cross contamination, errors in meal preparation, and manufacturer labeling errors.[4,5,21,24] When discussing unexpected reactions to packaged foods, it is acknowledged by allergic consumers that the total avoidance of food products bearing precautionary allergen labeling (PAL) is impossible. In addition, the application of PAL is voluntary and specifics for application not officially regulated within any allergen labeling framework.[25,26] As such, decisions leading to the application of PAL (or its absence) and which form of PAL (ie, may contain…, produced in the same facility as…, made on the same equipment as…) can differ, even in situations with comparable risks for unintended allergen presence.[26,27] Because of its voluntary nature and nonuniform application, PAL is often misunderstood, which leads to increased consumption of PAL containing products and increased risk taking because of more potential allergen exposures.[4,21,24,28–31] Thus it is not surprising to find packaged foods reported as a common cause for accidental allergic reactions, especially when surveys of packaged food products with PAL for peanut found roughly 10% of products contained peanut concentrations from 0.175 to 6500 ppm (mg/kg) peanut protein.[13,30,32–42] An Australian survey further showed the disconnect between PAL and consumer adherence to labeling. The foods suspected to trigger anaphylactic reactions in 38% of the study population contained PAL.[21] Peanut was also the most commonly suspected food to cause anaphylaxis in the Australian survey.[21]

Not all allergic individuals check product labels; some ignore them, and others do not inform their waitstaff of their allergy when eating out.[4] Skipping the reading of a label or informing waitstaff were done regardless of whether there was a history of severe reactions.[4,24] However, even in cases of strict avoidance or informing restaurant staff, accidental or unexpected allergic reactions still occur.[4] In these cases in which informing waitstaff did not prevent a reaction, a mistaken ingredient, shared cooking equipment or utensils, or several other factors could have played a role in an unexpected reaction. Although mistaken ingredients can lead to high exposures of peanut protein, transfers from shared, uncleaned kitchen equipment have also been shown to reach levels of peanut protein known to cause reactions in a significant portion of the peanut-allergic population.[43] However, these exposures and subsequent reactions could be deemed accidental. In contrast, there were also a surprising number of reactions reportedly caused by purposeful exposure to the allergen, which again highlights the need for better, continued education of allergic individuals and their caregivers.[5,6,44]

Frequency of Severe Allergic Reactions to Peanut

The true proportion of food-allergic reactions that are severe is difficult to estimate because of differences in data collection methods, different definitions of severity, and study heterogeneity.[45] As such, there is a wide variance in estimates, from 0.4% to 40% of food-allergic reactions that result in a severe reaction,[46] with fatal anaphylaxis being a rare but unpredictable event.[45] More recent data confirm these previously reported values, with a prospective study in Dutch adults that found 28% of unexpected allergic reactions to food were severe[4] and a parent-reported study in the United States that found 42% of children with food allergies were considered to have a history of severe reaction and 19% of food-allergic children had at least 1 food-related emergency department visit in the past year.[2] In Australia, the Victoria State Government anaphylaxis notification system reported 1200 anaphylaxis notifications over the 6-month period of November 2018 through April 2019, with an average of 46 total anaphylaxis episodes per week of which 28 per week were attributed to food.[23] There was a fairly equal proportion of reported anaphylaxis episodes to packaged foods (18%), unpacked foods from food premises (22%), and other foods (21%).[23]

Similar severity results were found when focusing on peanut alone, with wide variations in definitions of severity and anaphylaxis leading to a range of 11% to 52% of accidental exposure reactions being deemed severe.[5,6,16,17,19,20,44] If an allergic reaction was deemed severe, medical attention was sought 14% to 75% of the time.[4,6,16,17,22] Parents in the United States reported that 59.2% of children with peanut allergy were considered to have a history of severe allergy to peanut and that 22.9% of the peanut-allergic children had at least 1 food-related emergency department visit in the past year.[2]

Prediction of a Severe Reaction

The history of prior reactions is not a predictor for the severity of future reactions. Compared with previous reactions, 10% to 32% of subsequent reactions were more severe, 40% to 64% were similar in severity, and 8% to 29% were less severe.[6,16–19,47] In addition to not being able to predict the severity of reaction, recent reviews have deemed that severity and sensitivity (individual threshold) should be treated as separate factors because of the inability to predict severity from known prior data.[47,48] Severe reactions can occur to low or high doses of allergen and the ED of an allergic reaction cannot predict the symptom severity. The notion of separating severity and sensitivity was supported by Pettersson and colleagues,[8] who could explain only 23.5% of total variance when predicting severity during double-blind, placebo-controlled food challenge (DBPCFC) in a large dataset, and the ED at food challenge only contributed 4.4% to the model for severity prediction.

Single-dose studies for peanut,[49] and milk, egg, or hazelnut,[50] provide a good demonstration that very low (milligrams) doses result mostly in mild to moderate symptoms, but a severe reaction has been observed, again indicating that ED alone does not determine severity. In addition, Taylor and colleagues[51] found no difference in DBPCFC dose distributions for individuals with a history of severe reactions or with a history of nonsevere reactions before food challenge, strengthening the argument that severity and sensitivity should be treated as separate factors. There is also a theme of undertreatment regarding severe or anaphylactic reactions. Multiple studies have confirmed that most severe reactions are insufficiently treated according to current guidelines, with low epinephrine usage rates and severe reactors not seeking medical help.[4–6,16,17,20,22,52–55] These results confirm that there are many unknown factors that contribute to the severity of an allergic reaction at DBPCFC and in everyday life. However, although the severity of an individual reaction is unpredictable, it is expected that, if the number of allergic reactions were reduced, then the number of severe reactions would at least be proportionally reduced. In light of the unpredictable severity and undertreatment of reactions being common, the desire for a buffer or margin of safety against reactions to accidental peanut exposures as expressed by caregivers of allergic children is well understood.[11]

RISK AND RISK REDUCTION

In epidemiology, absolute risk (AR) is defined as the probability of an adverse event in a defined population over a specified period of time.[56] When discussing the AR of an allergic reaction, the specified period of time is an important consideration and must be clearly communicated and understood to enable further risk assessment and discussions. Periods of time that were previously used in food allergy risk assessments for unexpected allergic reactions to an accidental exposure include risk per eating occasion, per week, per month, and per year.[13–15,33,38,57,58] In addition, risks of unexpected allergic reactions have also been expressed in different populations, which can seemingly be a great influence toward the reported risk assessment results, even though most results are readily translatable into other populations. Previous risk assessments have expressed risk in one of the following populations:

- Population A: the overall population (includes allergic and nonallergic individuals, includes consumers and nonconsumers, includes products with or without unintended allergen presence)
- Population B: the allergic population (all individuals considered allergic, includes consumers and nonconsumers, includes products with or without unintended allergen presence)
- Population C: the allergic consumer population (all individuals considered allergic and all who consume the product in question, includes products with or without unintended allergen presence)
- Population D: the allergic consumer population of products containing unintended allergen presence (all individuals considered to be allergic, all are consumers of the product, and all products contain an unintended allergen presence)

With so many different combinations, it is easy to dismiss risk results when time periods and populations are not understood or provided without clear definitions. For example, a risk of 1 in 100 million (0.000001%) *per eating occasion* of a packaged food category *in the overall population* (population A) can still predict multiple reactions per day in a population as large as the United States (estimated population of

330 million people). In contrast, a risk of 1 in 100 (1%) *per eating occasion* in *the allergic consumers of a product containing unintended allergen presence* (population D) might seem large but is not likely to predict reactions if the frequency of unintended allergen presence is extremely low and only 5 products contain allergen residue out of millions of packages produced per year. In this scenario, the prevalence of allergy, the frequency of consumption, and the frequency of unintended allergen presence would still need to be accounted for before a comparison could be made in the overall population. In the second scenario, the odds of a contaminated product being consumed by the most sensitive allergic individual and triggering a reaction are low, and much lower than 1 in 100 million.

It is with this understanding of small percentages that examples from 2 studies were selected to show different specified periods of time for the risk assessments and different populations for the expression of risk results. In a study by the French Agency for Food, Environmental and Occupational Health Safety (ANSES), simulations for the peanut-allergic pediatric age group predicted risks of 0.2% to 2.0% *per eating occasion* in *the allergic consumer population* (population C) for 6 different packaged food categories.[38] To highlight the difference by removing frequency of unintended allergen presence in the risk assessment, these same risks were also expressed as 0.9% to 6.6% *per eating occasion in allergic consumers of a product containing unintended allergen presence* (population D).[38] The results for children were also modeled on a weekly basis, and, when the full pediatric consumption pattern was included, it could be predicted that up to 3.7% of *the allergic population* (population B) would be predicted to experience at least 1 allergic reaction *per week* when consuming these 6 packaged foods.[38] Similar to the ANSES results, a recent study using threshold data from children in a phase 3 immunotherapy trial population estimated risks of 1% to 4% *per eating occasion* in *allergic consumers of a product containing unintended allergen presence* (population D) for 4 commonly eaten packaged food categories.[15] When expressed on a yearly basis, including frequency of consumption and frequency of contamination, it was predicted that up to between 11% and 30% of *the allergic population* (population B) would experience an unexpected allergic reaction *per year* to one of the 4 packaged foods,[15] comparable with estimates in prior reported literature.[2,4–7,16–21] These examples are given as a reminder that not all risks are reported in similar fashion and it is important to understand how results would change if expressed in different populations or in different time frames.

Risk Reduction

When discussing the potential results, benefits, and risks related to immunotherapy for peanut allergy, it is important to understand the potential risk reduction or risk increase achieved by the immunotherapy treatment. As previously defined, the AR is the probability of an adverse event in a defined population over a specified period of time.[56] If the AR for the treatment group ($AR_{Treatment}$) is less than the AR for the control group ($AR_{Control}$), then the risk difference is defined as the AR reduction (ARR) and calculated as shown in **Table 1**.[56] Further calculations for presenting results of randomized clinical trials can include the relative risk (RR), RRR, and the number needed to treat (NNT) (see **Table 1**). The NNT is the average number of persons who need to undergo treatment in order for 1 adverse event to be prevented compared with the control group.[56] The RR is the risk ratio of the $AR_{Treatment}$ and $AR_{Control}$ and is commonly used to present clinical trial results. RR = 1 indicates that treatment did not affect the probability of an adverse event, whereas RR<1 indicates that the probability of an adverse event is decreased by the treatment and RR>1 indicates that the probability of an adverse event is increased because of treatment. The RRR, or efficacy of the treatment, is

Table 1
Absolute risk and risk reduction definitions, with equations for calculation

Term	Definition	Equation
AR	The probability of an adverse event in a defined population over a specified period of time	—
ARR	The $AR_{Control}$ minus the $AR_{Treatment}$	$AR_{Control} - AR_{Treatment}$
RR	Risk ratio or RR is the ratio of the probability of an $AR_{Treatment}$ in relation to the probability of $AR_{Control}$	$\dfrac{AR_{Treatment}}{AR_{Control}}$
RRR	The RRR or efficacy is the relative decrease in the risk of an adverse event in the treatment group compared with a control group	$\dfrac{AR_{Control} - AR_{Treatment}}{AR_{Control}}$
NNT	The number of persons needed to be treated, on average, to prevent 1 event	$\dfrac{1}{AR_{Control} - AR_{Treatment}}$

Abbreviations: NNT, number needed to treat; RR, relative risk.
   Data from Porta M, editor. A Dictionary of Epidemiology, 6th edition. New York: Oxford University Press; 2014.

the relative decrease in the $AR_{Treatment}$ compared with the $AR_{Control}$ and can be easily understood by nonexperts, and is most helpful when used in conjunction with the AR. A fictitious dataset was created as an example (**Table 2**), in which 50% of the peanut-allergic control population was predicted to experience an allergic reaction over the course of 1 year ($AR_{Control}$ = 50%), whereas only 10% of the treatment population was predicted to experience an allergic reaction after 1 year of treatment ($AR_{Treatment}$ = 10%). These ARs would correspond with a predicted ARR of 40%, an RR of 20%, an RRR of 80%, and an NNT of 2.5 (see **Table 2**).

Table 2
Example scenario of risk reduction calculations

$AR_{Control}$	$AR_{Treatment}$
0.5 (or 50%)	0.1 or 10%
ARR	0.4 or 40%
RR	0.2 or 20%
RRR	0.8 or 80%
NNT	2.5

The data in this table are not based on clinical data and are only used as examples.

Risk Increase

In cases in which a treatment option does not reduce the probability of an adverse event but increases the probability of an adverse event, resulting in an $AR_{Treatment}$ that is greater than the $AR_{Control}$, then the risk difference is defined as the AR increase (ARI) and calculated as shown in **Table 3**.[56] In addition, in cases in which the $AR_{Treatment}$ is greater than $AR_{Control}$, the RR increase (RRI) and the number needed to harm (NNH) can also be calculated (see **Table 3**). In **Table 4**, a risk increase example was created in which the sample treatment population had a higher risk after 1 year of treatment ($AR_{Treatment}$ = 60%) than the control group ($AR_{Control}$ = 50%). These ARs would correspond with a predicted ARI of 10%, an RR of 120%, an RRI of 20%, and an NNH of 10 (see **Table 4**).

Table 3
Risk increase definitions with equations for calculation

Term	Definition	Equation
AR	The probability of an adverse event in a defined population over a specified period of time	—
ARI	The $AR_{Treatment}$ minus the $AR_{Control}$	$AR_{Treatment} - AR_{Control}$
RR	Risk ratio or RR is the ratio of the probability of an adverse event in a treatment group in relation to the probability of an adverse event in a control group	$\dfrac{AR_{Treatment}}{AR_{Control}}$
RRI	The RRI is the relative increase in the risk of an adverse event in the treatment group compared with a control group	$\dfrac{AR_{Treatment} - AR_{Control}}{AR_{Control}}$
NNH	The number of persons needed to be treated, on average, to produce 1 more adverse event	$\dfrac{1}{AR_{Treatment} - AR_{Control}}$

Abbreviations: NNH, number needed to harm; RRI, relative risk increase.
Data from Porta M, editor. A Dictionary of Epidemiology, sixth edition. New York: Oxford University Press; 2014.

Table 4
Example scenario of risk increase calculations

$AR_{Control}$	$AR_{Treatment}$
0.5 (or 50%)	0.6 or 60%
ARI	0.1 or 10%
RR	1.2 or 120%
RRI	0.2 or 20%
NNH	10

The data in this table are not based on clinical data and only used as examples.

Quantitative Risk Assessment Modeling

Recently, the measure of treatment efficacy through oral food challenges in a clinic has come under question, and there was a desire for other measures focused on risk and frequency of reactions for characterizing treatment efficacy.[59] Measurable clinical results and validation through real-world outcomes are expected in other forms of allergen immunotherapy (ie, respiratory allergens), but there is no specified or harmonized methodology for this process.[60] Quantitative risk assessment modeling in food allergy provides a tool for modeling real-world exposures, frequencies of allergic reactions, and the potential impact of immunotherapy treatments.

Quantitative risk assessments are typically conducted using Monte Carlo simulations, a long-established statistical methodology used in food safety and broadly accepted across other scientific disciplines.[61–63] In short, quantitative risk assessments simulate possible exposure amounts and compare them with either a hypothetical food-allergic individual[13,14] or to a food-allergic population[33,35,38,42,57,58,64–68] in an effort to assess the risk and frequency of predicted allergic reactions in certain scenarios.

Population-based quantitative risk assessments were conducted using Monte Carlo simulations with 3 primary inputs for the risk assessment:

- Allergen thresholds
- The concentration of peanut protein in the product
- The amount of food consumed per eating occasion of the product

Risk assessments are then conducted by simulating a large number of eating occasions to obtain a predicted AR per eating occasion. Depending on the risk assessment, the allergen thresholds can be defined to focus on a single individual to assess individual risk, or the allergen thresholds are selected from the allergic population dose-response curves for population assessments. Additional secondary inputs necessary for specific population assessments may include prevalence of (peanut) allergy, frequency of consumption, frequency of unintended allergen presence, shopping habits (label avoidance), and so forth to express risk in a different population or a different specified period of time. Once the ARs have been modeled and predicted, the RRRs can be calculated.

Quantitative population risk assessment and relative risk reduction

A model estimating the quantitative risk assessment and RRR associated with 12 months of EPIT for peanut allergy with a patch containing 250 μg of peanut protein was recently published.[15] Study population dose-response curves were fitted to baseline and 12-month DBPCFC data from a recently described EPIT phase 3 clinical trial population[69] using interval-censoring survival analysis (ICSA). ICSA was chosen because it uses the interval between the previously tolerated dose and discrete ED during DBPCFC. Because the exact dose that causes the individual reaction is not known, but is in the interval between the ED and previous dose, ICSA has been used in other studies as the appropriate, conservative method for fitting food allergen dose distributions.[70–73] Risk assessments were conducted by simulating a total of 5 million eating occasions of a contaminated packaged food product and then calculating ARs and RRRs for each study population. As detailed earlier, ARs were estimated to be 1% to 4% *per eating occasion* in *allergic consumers of a product containing unintended allergen presence* (population D) for 4 commonly eaten packaged food categories; when expressed on a yearly basis, it was predicted that between 11% and 30% of *the allergic population* (population B) would experience an unexpected allergic reaction *per year* to one of the 4 packaged foods.[15] After 12 months of EPIT with a patch containing 250 μg of peanut protein, RRRs for an allergic reaction when consuming the packaged foods were estimated from 73% to 78% (RRR). The placebo group did not change at the 12-month time point.[15]

Quantitative individual risk assessment and relative risk reduction

Two previous models with similar methodologies have been published to estimate the RRR for peanut-allergic individuals who increase their ED after immunotherapy.[13,14] These models were not tied to a specific immunotherapy method and were focused only on risk reductions when consuming packaged foods achieved through an increase in ED. Scenarios in this model investigated the RRR of a hypothetical individual with a preimmunotherapy ED of 1, 3, 10, 30, or 100 mg of peanut protein who was able to achieve a postimmunotherapy ED of 300 or 1000 mg of peanut protein. The studies estimated a greater than 95% RRR for the risk of accidental allergic reactions caused by peanut in packaged foods for the peanut-allergic individual who achieved an ED of 300 mg of peanut protein (if initial ED ≤100 mg) or 1000 mg (if initial ED ≤300 mg) after immunotherapy.[13,14]

CURRENT CONTROVERSIES

Although understanding the potential benefits and risk reductions achievable through different immunotherapy options is important, the potential benefits of treatment must be weighed against the potential risks of treatment to provide a full perspective. Recent health and economic benefit analysis from Shaker and Greenhawt[74] and the

Institute for Clinical and Economic Review (ICER) regarding oral immunotherapy or EPIT for peanut allergy,[10] as well as a systematic review and meta-analysis of efficacy and safety for oral immunotherapy for peanut allergy,[59] has raised questions regarding the potential immunotherapies in development. The peanut allergen immunotherapy, clarifying the evidence (PACE) meta-analysis of oral immunotherapy trial data found that oral immunotherapy increased the risk of anaphylaxis compared with no oral immunotherapy.[59] The PACE review also found that peanut oral immunotherapy, including the AR101 treatment[75] described earlier, induced desensitization but considerably increased the number of allergic and anaphylactic reactions compared with avoidance or placebo because of reactions to treatment.[59] It was concluded that safer peanut allergy treatment approaches than current oral immunotherapy options are needed.[59] In addition, the health and economic benefit analysis by Shaker and Greenhawt[74] found that the cost-effectiveness of oral immunotherapy with AR101 or EPIT with a patch containing 250 μg of peanut protein for treatment of peanut allergy is influenced by each therapy's "probability of sustained unresponsiveness, improvement in quality-of-life, reduction in anaphylaxis risk, and cost to the patient."[74] The ICER report states that evidence for both potential therapies was inadequate to show a superior net health benefit of either compared with strict peanut avoidance; that neither trial showed a quality-of-life improvement compared with placebo; and, contrary to the prior RRR models, that neither trial showed a reduction in accidental reactions to when exposed to peanut.[10] In addition, it was voted that there were insufficient data to show a net health benefit of AR101 compared with noncommercialized peanut oral immunotherapy. Three themes arose from this concern: the seeming need for indefinite treatment without longer-term safety or efficacy data, the need to continue vigilant avoidance diets while on therapy, and the known increase in the risk of allergic reactions and epinephrine use during treatment in the 1-year clinical trials.[10] However, both analyses concluded that AR101 and EPIT with a patch containing 250 μg of peanut protein were long-term cost-effective under certain assumptions and pricing scenarios, but longer clinical trials and commercial data are still needed to investigate long-term sustained unresponsiveness and other important patient-related outcomes.[10,74] In addition, all public comments to the ICER review were positive toward the potential of immunotherapy and most argued that the review was premature in light of additional data that will soon become available.[10]

FUTURE CONSIDERATIONS/SUMMARY

It is well known that complete avoidance of peanut is difficult and accidental reactions occur, with possibly severe symptoms. Immunotherapy for peanut allergy is a potential treatment option being developed with the potential to reduce the risk of reactions to accidental exposure to peanut in the community. Models for estimating risks for reactions to accidental exposure to peanut in packaged foods show significant potential RRRs for the peanut-allergic population and peanut-allergic individuals. However, it is important to clearly define the specified period of time and population when the risk is being assessed to enable clear communication and understanding. In addition, future areas of research still exist, especially in the area of longer-term clinical trials or commercial data, which will strengthen the knowledge surrounding risk and potential options for risk reduction in people with peanut allergy.

DISCLOSURE

Dr B.C. Remington is the Managing Director of the Remington Consulting Group B.V. and is an Adjunct Assistant Professor of Food Science & Technology at the University of Nebraska-Lincoln; Dr B.C. Remington reports grants, travel support, and consulting fees from DBV Technologies. Dr J.L. Baumert is an Associate Professor of Food Science & Technology and Co-Director of the Food Allergy Research and Resource Program (FARRP) at the University of Nebraska-Lincoln; Dr J.L. Baumert reports travel support and consulting fees from DBV Technologies.

REFERENCES

1. Sicherer SH, Sampson HA. Food allergy: a review and update on epidemiology, pathogenesis, diagnosis, prevention, and management. J Allergy Clin Immunol 2018;141(1):41–58.
2. Gupta RS, Warren CM, Smith BM, et al. The public health impact of parent-reported childhood food allergies in the United States. Pediatrics 2018;142(6): e20181235.
3. Nwaru BI, Hickstein L, Panesar SS, et al. Prevalence of common food allergies in Europe: a systematic review and meta-analysis. Allergy 2014;69(8):992–1007.
4. Michelsen-Huisman AD, van Os-Medendorp H, Blom WM, et al. Accidental allergic reactions in food allergy: causes related to products and patient's management. Allergy 2018;73(12):2377–81.
5. Fleischer DM, Perry TT, Atkins D, et al. Allergic reactions to foods in preschool-aged children in a prospective observational food allergy study. Pediatrics 2012;130(1):e25–32.
6. Yu JW, Kagan R, Verreault N, et al. Accidental ingestions in children with peanut allergy. J Allergy Clin Immunol 2006;118(2):466–72.
7. Hourihane JO, Lieberman JA, Bird JA, et al. Accidental exposures to peanut and other food allergens: results from a phase 3, randomized, double-blind, placebo-controlled trial (PALISADE). J Allergy Clin Immunol 2019;143(2):AB265.
8. Pettersson ME, Koppelman GH, Flokstra-de Blok BMJ, et al. Prediction of the severity of allergic reactions to foods. Allergy 2018;73(7):1532–40.
9. Ward CE, Greenhawt MJ. Treatment of allergic reactions and quality of life among caregivers of food-allergic children. Ann Allergy Asthma Immunol 2015;114(4): 312–8.e2.
10. Institute for Clinical and Economic Review. Oral immunotherapy and viaskin ® peanut for peanut allergy: effectiveness and value. Final evidence report. 2019. Available at: https://icer-review.org/wp-content/uploads/2018/12/ICER_PeanutAllergy_Final_Report_071019.pdf. Accessed July 17, 2019.
11. Greenhawt M, Marsh R, Gilbert H, et al. Understanding caregiver goals, benefits, and acceptable risks of peanut allergy therapies. Ann Allergy Asthma Immunol 2018;121(5):575–9.
12. Shreffler WG, Baumert JL, Remington BC, et al. The importance of reducing risk in peanut allergy: current and future therapies. Ann Allergy Asthma Immunol 2018; 120(2):124–7.
13. Baumert JL, Taylor SL, Koppelman SJ. Quantitative assessment of the safety benefits associated with increasing clinical peanut thresholds through immunotherapy. J Allergy Clin Immunol Pract 2018;6(2):457–65.e4.
14. Remington BC, Krone T, Koppelman SJ. Quantitative risk reduction through peanut immunotherapy: Safety benefits of an increased threshold in Europe. Pediatr Allergy Immunol 2018;29(7):762–72.
15. Remington BC, Krone T, Kim EH, et al. Estimated risk reduction to packaged food reactions by epicutaneous immunotherapy (EPIT) for peanut allergy. Ann Allergy Asthma Immunol 2019. https://doi.org/10.1016/j.anai.2019.08.007.

16. Cherkaoui S, Ben-Shoshan M, Alizadehfar R, et al. Accidental exposures to peanut in a large cohort of Canadian children with peanut allergy. Clin Transl Allergy 2015;5(1):16.
17. Nguyen-Luu NU, Ben-Shoshan M, Alizadehfar R, et al. Inadvertent exposures in children with peanut allergy. Pediatr Allergy Immunol 2012;23(2):134–40.
18. Clark AT, Ewan PW. Good prognosis, clinical features, and circumstances of peanut and tree nut reactions in children treated by a specialist allergy center. J Allergy Clin Immunol 2008;122(2):286–9.
19. Vander Leek TK, Liu AH, Stefanski K, et al. The natural history of peanut allergy in young children and its association with serum peanut-specific IgE. J Pediatr 2000;137(6):749–55.
20. Noimark L, Wales J, Du Toit G, et al. The use of adrenaline autoinjectors by children and teenagers. Clin Exp Allergy 2012;42(2):284–92.
21. Zurzolo GA, Allen KJ, Peters RL, et al. Self-reported anaphylaxis to packaged foods in Australia. J Allergy Clin Immunol Pract 2019;7(2):687–9.
22. Sheikh A, Dhami S, Regent L, et al. Anaphylaxis in the community: a questionnaire survey of members of the UK Anaphylaxis Campaign. JRSM Open 2015; 6(7). 205427041559344.
23. Clifford E. Victoria's anaphylaxis notification system. In: FAMS2019. Melbourne, Australia. 2019. Available at: http://allergenbureau.net/wp-content/uploads/2019/05/CLIFFORD_2019-Presentation-Anaphylaxis-Notification-System-FAMS2019.pdf. Accessed September 5, 2019.
24. Zurzolo GA, Koplin JJ, Mathai ML, et al. Perceptions of precautionary labelling among parents of children with food allergy and anaphylaxis. Med J Aust 2013;198(11):621–3.
25. Gendel SM. Comparison of international food allergen labeling regulations. Regul Toxicol Pharmacol 2012;63(2):279–85.
26. Yeung J, Robert MC. Challenges and path forward on mandatory allergen labeling and voluntary precautionary allergen labeling for a global company. J AOAC Int 2018;101(1):70–6.
27. Taylor SL, Baumert JL. Cross-contamination of foods and implications for Food Allergic Patients. Curr Allergy Asthma Rep 2010;265–70. https://doi.org/10.1007/s11882-010-0112-4.
28. DunnGalvin A, Chan CH, Crevel R, et al. Precautionary allergen labelling: perspectives from key stakeholder groups. Allergy 2015;70(9):1039–51.
29. DunnGalvin A, Roberts G, Regent L, et al. Understanding how consumers with food allergies make decisions based on precautionary labelling. Clin Exp Allergy 2019. https://doi.org/10.1111/cea.13479.
30. Hefle SL, Furlong TJ, Niemann L, et al. Consumer attitudes and risks associated with packaged foods having advisory labeling regarding the presence of peanuts. J Allergy Clin Immunol 2007;120(1):171–6.
31. Zurzolo GA, de Courten M, Koplin J, et al. Is advising food allergic patients to avoid food with precautionary allergen labelling out of date? Curr Opin Allergy Clin Immunol 2016;16(3):272–7.
32. Zurzolo GA, Koplin JJ, Mathai ML, et al. Foods with precautionary allergen labeling in Australia rarely contain detectable allergen. J Allergy Clin Immunol Pract 2013;1(4):401–3.
33. Remington BC, Baumert JL, Marx DB, et al. Quantitative risk assessment of foods containing peanut advisory labeling. Food Chem Toxicol 2013;62:179–87.

34. Blom WM, Michelsen-Huisman AD, van Os-Medendorp H, et al. Accidental food allergy reactions: products and undeclared ingredients. J Allergy Clin Immunol 2018;142(3):865–75.

35. Remington BC, Baumert JL, Blom WM, et al. Unintended allergens in precautionary labelled and unlabelled products pose significant risks to UK allergic consumers. Allergy 2015;70(7):813–9.

36. Zagon J, Dittmer J, Elegbede CF, et al. Peanut traces in packaged food products consumed by allergic individuals: results of the MIRABEL project. J Food Compost Anal 2015;44:196–204.

37. Holzhauser T, Vieths S. Indirect competitive ELISA for determination of traces of peanut (Arachis hypogaea L.) protein in complex food matrices. J Agric Food Chem 1999;47(2):603–11.

38. Rimbaud L, Heraud F, La S, et al. Quantitative risk assessment relating to the inadvertent presence of peanut allergens in various food products. Int Food Risk Anal J 2013;3:1–11.

39. Vadas P, Perelman B. Presence of undeclared peanut protein in chocolate bars imported from Europe. J Food Prot 2003;66(10):1932–4.

40. Stephan O, Vieths S. Development of a real-time PCR and a sandwich ELISA for detection of potentially allergenic trace amounts of peanut (Arachis hypogaea) in processed foods. J Agric Food Chem 2004;52(12):3754–60.

41. Pele M, Brohée M, Anklam E, et al. Peanut and hazelnut traces in cookies and chocolates: Relationship between analytical results and declaration of food allergens on product labels. Food Addit Contam 2007;24(12):1334–44.

42. Robertson ON, Hourihane JO, Remington BC, et al. Survey of peanut levels in selected Irish food products bearing peanut allergen advisory labels. Food Addit Contam Part A Chem Anal Control Expo Risk Assess 2013;30(9):1467–72.

43. Remington BC, Bassa B, Koppelman SJ. Shared cooking equipment in restaurants: a quantitative risk assessment for peanut-allergic consumers. J Allergy Clin Immunol 2019;143(2):AB239.

44. Deschildre A, Elegbédé CF, Just J, et al. Peanut-allergic patients in the MIRABEL survey: characteristics, allergists' dietary advice and lessons from real life. Clin Exp Allergy 2016;46(4):610–20.

45. Turner PJ, Baumert JL, Beyer K, et al. Can we identify patients at risk of life-threatening allergic reactions to food? Allergy 2016;72(1):9.

46. Panesar SS, Javad S, De Silva D, et al. The epidemiology of anaphylaxis in Europe: A systematic review. Allergy 2013;68(11):1353–61.

47. Turner PJ, Baumert JL, Beyer K, et al. Can we identify patients at risk of life-threatening allergic reactions to food? Allergy 2016;71(9):1241–55.

48. Dubois AEJ, Turner PJ, Hourihane J, et al. How does dose impact on the severity of food-induced allergic reactions, and can this improve risk assessment for allergenic foods? Allergy 2018;73(7):1383–92.

49. Hourihane JOB, Allen KJ, Shreffler WG, et al. Peanut Allergen Threshold Study (PATS): Novel single-dose oral food challenge study to validate eliciting doses in children with peanut allergy. J Allergy Clin Immunol 2017;139(5):1583–90.

50. Hourihane J. Validating population thresholds. In: FAMS2019. Melbourne, Australia. 2019. Available at: http://allergenbureau.net/wp-content/uploads/2019/05/Hourihane-melbourne-may-2019-pdf-for-website.pdf. Accessed September 5, 2019.

51. Taylor SL, Moneret-Vautrin DA, Crevel RWR, et al. Threshold dose for peanut: Risk characterization based upon diagnostic oral challenge of a series of 286 peanut-allergic individuals. Food Chem Toxicol 2010;48(3):814–9.

52. Jacobs TS, Greenhawt MJ, Hauswirth D, et al. A survey study of index food-related allergic reactions and anaphylaxis management. Pediatr Allergy Immunol 2012;23(6):582–9.
53. Muraro A, Werfel T, Hoffmann-Sommergruber K, et al. EAACI food allergy and anaphylaxis guidelines: diagnosis and management of food allergy. Allergy 2014;69(8):1008–25.
54. Le TM, Van Hoffen E, Pasmans SG, et al. Suboptimal management of acute food-allergic reactions by patients, emergency departments and general practitioners. Allergy 2009;64(8):1227–8.
55. Greenhawt MJ, Singer AM, Baptist AP. Food allergy and food allergy attitudes among college students. J Allergy Clin Immunol 2009;124(2):323–7.
56. Porta M, editor. A dictionary of epidemiology. 6th edition. New York: Oxford University Press; 2014. https://doi.org/10.1093/acref/9780199976720.001.0001.
57. Spanjersberg MQI, Kruizinga AG, Rennen MAJ, et al. Risk assessment and food allergy: the probabilistic model applied to allergens. Food Chem Toxicol 2007; 45(1):49–54.
58. Rimbaud L, Heraud F, La Vieille S, et al. Quantitative risk assessment relating to adventitious presence of allergens in food: a probabilistic model applied to peanut in chocolate. Risk Anal 2010;30(1):7–19.
59. Chu DK, Wood RA, French S, et al. Oral immunotherapy for peanut allergy (PACE): a systematic review and meta-analysis of efficacy and safety. Lancet 2019;6736(19):1–11.
60. Jutel M, Agache I, Bonini S, et al. International consensus on allergy immunotherapy. J Allergy Clin Immunol 2015;136(3):556–68.
61. Bier V. Applying risk and decision analysis to food and animal health and security. Proc Inst Food Technol First Annu Food Prot Def Conf. 2005. Available at: http://www.ift.org/~/media/Knowledge Center/Science Reports/Conference Papers/13Bier.pdf. Accessed September 5, 2019.
62. Seynaeve D, Verbeke T. Software for Monte Carlo simulation of a simple risk assessment. EFSA Support Publ 2017;14(11). https://doi.org/10.2903/sp.efsa.2017.EN-1316.
63. Chen Y, Dennis SB, Hartnett E, et al. FDA-iRISK—a comparative risk assessment system for evaluating and ranking food-hazard pairs: case studies on microbial hazards. J Food Prot 2013;76(3):376–85.
64. Spanjersberg MQI, Knulst AC, Kruizinga AG, et al. Concentrations of undeclared allergens in food products can reach levels that are relevant for public health. Food Addit Contam Part A Chem Anal Control Expo Risk Assess 2010;27(2): 169–74.
65. Blom WM, Kruizinga AG, Rubingh CM, et al. Assessing food allergy risks from residual peanut protein in highly refined vegetable oil. Food Chem Toxicol 2017; 106:306–13.
66. Blom WM, Remington BC, Baumert JL, et al. Sensitivity analysis to derive a food consumption point estimate for deterministic food allergy risk assessment. Food Chem Toxicol 2019;125:413–21.
67. Gibert A, Kruizinga AG, Neuhold S, et al. Might gluten traces in wheat substitutes pose a risk in patients with celiac disease? A population-based probabilistic approach to risk estimation. Am J Clin Nutr 2013;97(1):109–16.
68. Remington B, Baumert JL, Marx DB, et al. Risk assessment of soy commodity contamination in wheat flour. J Allergy Clin Immunol 2011;127(2):AB114.
69. Fleischer DM, Greenhawt M, Sussman G, et al. Effect of epicutaneous immunotherapy vs placebo on reaction to peanut protein ingestion among children

with peanut allergy: the PEPITES Randomized Clinical Trial. JAMA 2019;321(10): 946–55.

70. Ballmer-Weber BK, Fernandez-Rivas M, Beyer K, et al. How much is too much? Threshold dose distributions for 5 food allergens. J Allergy Clin Immunol 2015; 135(4):964–71.

71. Taylor SL, Baumert JL, Kruizinga AG, et al. Establishment of reference doses for residues of allergenic foods: report of the VITAL expert panel. Food Chem Toxicol 2014;63:9–17.

72. Allen KJ, Remington BC, Baumert JL, et al. Allergen reference doses for precautionary labeling (VITAL 2.0): clinical implications. J Allergy Clin Immunol 2014; 133(1):156–64.

73. Taylor SL, Crevel RWR, Sheffield D, et al. Threshold dose for peanut: risk characterization based upon published results from challenges of peanut-allergic individuals. Food Chem Toxicol 2009;47(6):1198–204.

74. Shaker M, Greenhawt M. Estimation of health and economic benefits of commercial peanut immunotherapy products: a cost-effectiveness analysis. JAMA Netw Open 2019;2(5):e193242.

75. Vickery BP, PALISADE Group of Clinical Investigators. AR101 oral immunotherapy for peanut allergy. N Engl J Med 2018;379(21):1991–2001.

Moving?

Make sure your subscription moves with you!

To notify us of your new address, find your **Clinics Account Number** (located on your mailing label above your name), and contact customer service at:

Email: journalscustomerservice-usa@elsevier.com

800-654-2452 (subscribers in the U.S. & Canada)
314-447-8871 (subscribers outside of the U.S. & Canada)

Fax number: 314-447-8029

Elsevier Health Sciences Division
Subscription Customer Service
3251 Riverport Lane
Maryland Heights, MO 63043

*To ensure uninterrupted delivery of your subscription, please notify us at least 4 weeks in advance of move.

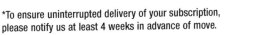

CPI Antony Rowe
Eastbourne, UK
December 31, 2019